Applied Mindfulness and Integrative Practices for Mental Well-Being

Shubhangni Jain
https://orcid.org/0009-0006-0160-9960

Amity University, India

Akanksha Singh
https://orcid.org/0000-0001-7784-1826

Chitkara School of Psychology and Counselling, Chitkara University, India

Shweta Sharma
Amity University, Gurugram, India

IGI Global Scientific Publishing
Publishing Tomorrow's Research Today

Vice President of Editorial	Melissa Wagner
Director of Acquisitions	Mikaela Felty
Director of Book Development	Jocelynn Hessler
Production Manager	Mike Brehm
Cover Design	Jose Rosado

Published in the United States of America by
IGI Global Scientific Publishing
701 East Chocolate Avenue
Hershey, PA, 17033, USA
Tel: 717-533-8845 | Fax: 717-533-7115
Website: https://www.igi-global.com E-mail: cust@igi-global.com

Library of Congress Cataloging-in-Publication Data

LCCN: (CIP Data Pending)
ISBN13: 9798260012024
Isbn13Softcover: 9798260012031
EISBN13: 9798260012048
British Cataloguing in Publication Data
A Cataloguing in Publication record for this book is available from the British Library.

Table of Contents

Detailed Table of Contents

Preface

INTRODUCTION

The contemporary world presents individuals and communities with an increasingly complex array of psychological, social, and emotional challenges. In such a context, the pursuit of mental well-being demands approaches that are not only evidence-based but also holistic, culturally grounded, and adaptable across diverse settings. Applied Mindfulness and Integrative Practices for Mental Well-Being responds to this need by offering a comprehensive exploration of mindfulness and integrative practices as transformative tools for enhancing human flourishing.

This volume brings together a wide range of perspectives that collectively emphasize the integration of contemplative traditions with modern psychological frameworks. Rooted in both global and indigenous knowledge systems—particularly those emerging from Asian contexts—the book highlights the relevance of mindfulness, yoga, and related practices in addressing mental health concerns across the lifespan and within varied socio-cultural environments. It underscores the importance of moving beyond reductionist approaches to embrace multidimensional models that consider emotional, cognitive, social, physical, and spiritual aspects of well-being.

A key strength of this collection lies in its applied orientation. The chapters demonstrate how mindfulness and integrative practices can be meaningfully embedded in community interventions, educational systems, workplaces, and clinical settings. At the same time, they critically engage with the challenges of implementation, including issues of accessibility, cultural sensitivity, stigma, and ethical responsibility. By doing so, the volume advances a nuanced understanding of both the potential and the limitations of these approaches.

CHAPTER OVERVIEWS

Chapter 1 examines the dynamics of collective trauma and healing, highlighting how contemplative practices can extend beyond individual coping to support community resilience and shared recovery within culturally grounded frameworks.

Chapter 2 explores the role of mindfulness and contemplative education in school curricula, demonstrating how culturally aligned practices can foster emotional regulation, moral development, resilience, and a sense of purpose among young learners.

Chapter 3 discusses the integration of mindfulness and yoga-based practices into language learning environments, highlighting their effectiveness in reducing anxiety, enhancing engagement, and supporting both cognitive and emotional development.

The fourth chapter presents an integrative model of workplace mental health and organizational well-being, focusing on preventive, promotive, and responsive strategies while addressing challenges such as burnout, stigma, and resource limitations.

The fifth chapter proposes an eclectic, trauma-informed clinical framework for adolescents, integrating multiple therapeutic approaches to address diverse psychological needs in a culturally sensitive and developmentally appropriate manner.

Chapter 6 addresses the unique mental health challenges faced by LGBTQIA+ individuals, exploring culturally responsive, mindfulness-based interventions that promote resilience, reduce distress, and support identity integration.

The seventh and final chapter critically examines the concept of emotional intelligence in adolescence, highlighting its complexities and proposing mindfulness-based approaches to foster ethical awareness, emotional authenticity, and balanced psychological development.

Together, these chapters reflect a shared commitment to advancing mental well-being through integrative, inclusive, and contextually sensitive approaches. This volume is intended to serve as a valuable resource for scholars, practitioners, educators, and policymakers seeking to deepen their engagement with mindfulness and its applications.

CONCLUSION

It is our hope that this work will not only contribute to academic discourse but also inspire innovative practices that promote resilience, compassion, and well-being in individuals and communities alike.

Chapter 1 Contemplating Together: An Intersection of Community Healing and Contemplative Practices in India

Ojeshavi Arya
http://orcid.org/0009-0007-6454-8373
National Forensic Sciences University, Delhi, India

Nishtha Grover
http://orcid.org/0009-0002-7609-7534
National Forensic Sciences University, Delhi, India

ABSTRACT

This chapter explores the mechanisms of collective trauma and collective healing and their manifestations in the Indian context. While mutual support, shared experiences, trauma informed approach and justice influence healing in communities, Indian texts and knowledge systems also give importance to the role of contemplative practices in healing. The chapter tries to overcome the perception that contemplative practices like yoga, meditation, mindfulness and rituals are only suited to individual bene-

DOI: 10.4018/979-8-2600-1202-4.ch001

fits and individual coping of trauma and discusses its intersection with community healing. Finally, this chapter also highlights challenges and implications of this intersection in India.

COMMUNITY: THE FOUNDATION OF WELL-BEING

Community refers to a group of people who are connected to each other, united through the thread of interpersonal connections, based on a common feature. According to the American Psychological Association (APA, 2018), human communities are characterised by commonality of interests, attitudes, and values, a general sense of belonging to a unified, socially integrated group, members' self-identification as community members, and some systems of communication, governance, education, and commerce. Communities have been viewed as a collective relationship that is bigger than the individual and lesser than social. However, this view adds ambiguity and abstractness to the definition of community and is based on territory or a common feature which may be necessary but not sufficient for a community (Fanahei, 2024). Fanahei (2024), in order to curb this ambiguity, defined community as a localized/compact and united by a common feature/problem group of people, whose sense of community is based on interpersonal connections.

Isolated environments do not present ideal conditions for holistic well-being of individuals, as humans, often referred to as social animals, have always been collective beings (Fanahei, 2024). Need for belongingness and relationships is the predominant factor in human motivation (Leary & Baumeister, 2000; Sarason, 1974; Bowlby, 1969; Maslow, 1954). In an effort to uphold collectivistic ideologies, cultures in India prioritise collective interests over individual interests resulting in attachment to groups and ensuring that groups take care of the individual. The collectivistic orientation is influenced by extended family, caste, religion and linguistic affiliations (Shah et al., 2015) and encourages individuals to value life embedded in communities and embrace the benefits of belonging. Several communities have been identified by the Government of India (n.d.) like caste based communities (SC, ST, OBC), religious communities (Hindu, Muslim, Sikh, Christians), economic communities (Business persons, workers, self employed, government employee) and rural communities etc. However it is important to note that these communities have sub sections which are more close knitted than the broader groups. While previously both theorists and practitioners have noted that primitive communities are being replaced by modern society, recently they have acknowledged that humans exist primarily in communities and not in a broad and abstract society (Fanahei, 2024). The nature of modern day communities has changed and is based on individual's own identities which are not imposed by society like LGBTQ+ community.

A positive sense of community has been shown to be correlated with identity formation (Pretty, 2002; Para, 2008), individual well-being (Farrell et al., 2003), life satisfaction (Prezza et al., 2001), mental health (Park et al., 2023; Michalski et al., 2020) and recovery from substance abuse (Jiwa et al., 2008). SM Sehgal Foundation (2021) highlighted that communities are essential in propagating economic and social development in India. Communities act like a gateway to remote areas in the country and facilitate local participation in nationwide initiatives. They are essential in growth and progress in climate change, communication, education and health and also play a role in creating awareness and sensitisation (Iyer, 2025; SM Sehgal Foundation, 2021). Iyer (2025) suggested that through the means of empowering local communities and using local resources, community development encourages participation, cooperation and sustainability and gives way to context specific solutions leading to nationwide growth and development.

While communities provide individuals with a sense of belonging, stability, and emotional support, they can also become bearers of pain and loss during times of widespread crisis. When faced with adversities, this very interconnectedness facilitates transmission of pain across the members of the community. Such shared suffering manifests as collective trauma, reflecting the deep, intertwined nature of individual and communal experiences within the social fabric.

COLLECTIVE TRAUMA: CHALLENGES AND CONSEQUENCES

Oftentimes unfortunate events like wars, death, abuse, disaster, discrimination bring people together into a community in order to cope with the trauma that comes with such events. The American Psychological Association (2018) defines trauma as any disturbing experience that results in significant fear, helplessness, dissociation, confusion, or other disruptive feelings, intense enough to have a long-lasting negative effect on a person's attitudes, behavior, and other aspects of functioning. While this definition focuses on the individual's experience of trauma and its physical, social, emotional and spiritual implications, it has been noted that implications of trauma are not limited to the individuals only but also manifest at the larger level of community or society (Mueller et al., 2021; Weisner, 2020). In fact, Fanhei (2024), noted that trauma can be a common feature or problem that unites a group of people into a community.

Community trauma is the perception of a traumatic event which may be natural, man-made and systemic in nature, by a community, resulting in severe cultural, psychological, emotional, physical, economical and ecological implications. Veerman & Ganzevoort (2001) defined community trauma, as "an aggregate of trauma experienced by community members or an event that impacts a few people but has structural and social traumatic consequences." It is also known as collective trauma. Hirschberger (2018) conceptualised collective trauma as " psychological reactions to a traumatic event that affected an entire society" e.g., holocaust, suggesting that trauma also has an intergenerational impact and is passed on from one generation to another. Eyerman et al. (2004) have focused on the cultural and psychological aspect of community trauma and defined it as "a collective feeling they have been subjected to a horrendous event that leaves indelible marks upon their group consciousness, marking their memories forever and changing their future identity in fundamental and irrevocable ways." In a compelling analogy Erikson (1991) suggests that just like physical trauma is a blow to the tissues of body, individual trauma is a "blow to the psyche through one's defenses so suddenly and with such brutal force that one cannot react to it effectively " (p. 459) and further collective trauma is a blow to " to the basic tissues of social life that damages the bonds attaching people together and impairs the prevailing sense of communality" (p. 460). Unlike individual trauma, community trauma is slow and subtle for those experiencing it; however it presents with a shock and realisation that community which was a source of support and a part of self no longer exists (Erikson, 1991).

> *"I continue to exist, though damaged and maybe even permanently changed. "You" continue to exist, though distant and hard to relate to. But "we" no longer exist as a connected pair or as linked cells in a larger communal body...." (Erikson 1976, p. 154)*

Pinderhughes et al. (2015) conceptualised the symptoms of community trauma manifested at 3 levels and suggest that interventions for community trauma should focus on these 3 areas. These symptoms occur due to isolation at economic, political and social levels as well as low investment in economic development and in maintenance and improvement of the man made environment accompanied by dwindling social capital, concentration of poverty and exposures to high levels of violence (Pinderhughes et al., 2015).

a) Social-cultural environment: It centers around the people in the community and manifests as broken social relationships and networks, dislocation of social norms and low collective, political and social efficacy.
b) Physical/built environment: It focuses on places in the community and trauma leads to deteriorated environment, dangerous public spaces and unhealthy products.
c) Economic environment: It centers around the lack of equitable opportunities due to intergenerational poverty, limited employment, long-term unemployment, relocation of businesses & jobs and disinvestment.

Figure 1. Symptoms of collective trauma

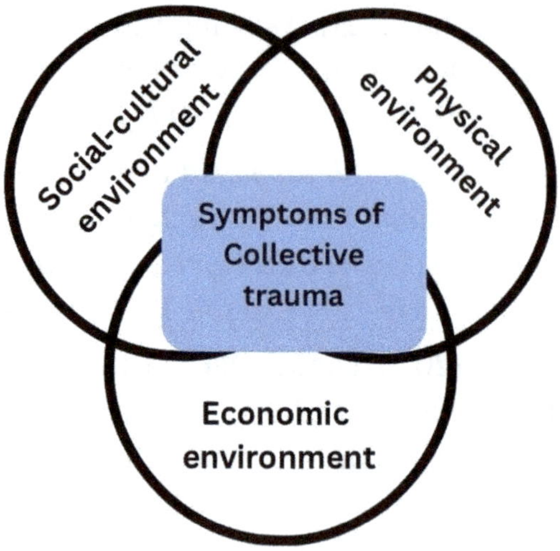

by Pinderhughes et al. (2015)

While in healthy communities these areas promote health, safety and resiliency in the community, in a traumatised community there is a distortion in these levels contributing to poor health, illness and injury of community members (Pinderhughes et al., 2015). It has been noted that trauma in communities may result in low collective efficacy and inability to come together in order to bring about positive changes and develop solutions (Pinderhughes et al., 2015). According to the Wisconsin department of health services (2020) collective trauma leads to panic attacks, nightmares, flashbacks, survivors guilt, low self-esteem, increased fear of outside threats or a hopelessness about the future. Thomson (2021) and Grover (2020) describe the experience of community trauma as dehumanisation of a person which is systemic and violent in nature leading to destruction of the sense of belonging to community and feelings of alienation and anxiety.

Many communities in India also experience collective trauma. It is multifaceted and arises from issues like intergroup conflicts, gender violence, discrimination, caste oppression, terrorism and disasters threatening individual and collective well being. Koileri (2025), highlighted the collective trauma experienced in SC/ST communities in India including intergenerational transmission of trauma along with the impact of trauma in the community and individual. Individuals in such communities internalise oppression, and inferiority feel trapped due to learned helplessness and fear based conditioning, face educational barriers resulting in low self esteem, self doubt, fear, social withdrawal, hypervigilance, lack of role models, loss of cultural identity, cultural displacement and alienation, patterns of poverty and marginalisation and mental health challenges (Koileri. V, 2025). Ahammed (2019) noted that caste based oppression of communities has led to years of humiliation, oppression and trauma as these communities faced deprivation of basic necessities, denial of access to public amenities. poverty, forced public lynching, labour including exploitation of children, forced separation from family, assaults and rapes and persecutions. Apart from caste based communities, trauma in India has also been recorded in adivasi communities. Rechsteiner (2019) noted that the Adivasi community in Pune identified several traumatic events experienced in the community like loss of a loved one, land slide and other natural calamities, work accidents, health issues, domestic violence, extreme poverty, sexual assault and animal attacks. These experiences led to the use of specific metaphors, phrases and descriptions around traumatic experiences which were common to the community like a cultural script. The devastating impact of trauma has also been seen in riot affected displaced children in Gujarat as they experience loneliness and feeling of separation from loved ones along with experiences of healing being facilitated by relationships and cultural values (Priya, 2012). Qureshi et al. (2023) viewed partition and colonisation in India through the lens of trauma and highlighted its consequences. The traumatic event of partition was characterised by religion based violence, large scale displacement, loss of life, dissolution of pre-existing community bonds, violent and forced relocation and assimilation and cultural oppression intersecting with caste, class, ethnicity, region, and religion. Partition led to intense physical and psychological violence like violence against women, divisions within community due to disruption of social networks, social stress, broken sense of collective identities, hostility, distrust and violence towards out group members. It also potentially caused trauma, poor mental health, suicidality, psychosis, substance use, family violence and poor physical health.

It can be understood through various definitions that community trauma has serious cultural, social, psychological, economic, ecological and emotional manifestations which is also expressed through 3 levels of symptoms of community trauma. It has a devastating impact on communities and social connections throughout generations along with personal implications like low self esteem, poor mental and physical health for individuals in the community. The incidences of community trauma have also been recorded in several communities in India. While the occurrence of trauma in a community is an unfortunate event with many negative implications, this trauma can also create a sense of community and can be a uniting factor among individuals (Fanahei, 2024; Erikson 1991). Trauma when experienced in community can give a shared sense of meaning, a cultural script and relatability that individuals are not alone in their sufferings. However, complexities of community trauma should be kept in mind, and the experiences of the community should not be considered from a reductionist point of view. It is therefore suggested that without diluting the negative implications of community trauma, one way to look forward is to harness the strengths of existing communities post trauma or those communities formed due to the shared experiences of trauma and work towards community healing.

COMMUNITY HEALING: RESTORING THE SOCIAL FABRIC

Healing has been defined as a personal experience of transcending suffering and transforming to a wholeness resulting in serenity, interconnectedness, and a new sense of meaning (McElligott, 2010). Community healing refers to collaborative recovery from collective trauma by a community, by harvesting personal, communal and societal resources. It is the idea of collective healing, where there is a joint process of recovery from a traumatic event that struck individuals and the community at large (Sandberg et al., 2024). It is based on the premise that members of the community have been wounded (Thomson, 2021). Community healing is a complex multidimensional process encompassing collective healing and healing of individuals (Mueller et al., 2021). It is rooted in shared experiences, social connections, collective action, justice and equity, storytelling and resistance, mutual support and trauma informed approach resulting in reduced isolation, increased resilience, improved mental health and enhanced well-being.

Community healing is impacted by the social context of the event, the community perception and conceptualization of that event, and the method of community coping (Zinner, & Williams, 1999). Healing communities are characterised by learned resourcefulness, resilience, ability to delay gratification, use of problem focused coping skills and strategies and self-regulation. It has also been suggested that a sense of coherence in the community enables them to make sense of the traumatic event and create comprehensible explanations for it (Zinner, & Williams, 1999). The effectiveness of community healing has been supported by literature in the context of black communities (Chioneso et al., 2020; Grover 2020; Gingwright, 2015), communities affected by terrorism (Boss et al., 2003), displaced populations (Theisen-Womersley, 2021; Priya, 2012), victims of violence (Harvey et al., 2007), Adivasis (Rechsteiner et al., 2019), aboriginal communities (Jiwa et al., 2008) and communities effected by genocide (Jansen et al., 2024).

Kalayjian (1995) suggested a seven stage model of community healing. It involved pre-assessment in order to investigate the nature, extent and dynamics of the community. It also involves an inquiry into the nature of the traumatic event, survivor, economic, political and sociocultural climate of the community. This is followed by on-site assessment where community leaders, intervention teams and response teams collect data which in the next stage is analysed in order to identify strengths, deficits, resources and readiness for change. The communities' response to the event is analysed next after which a comprehensive plan involving leaders and local trauma centres can be implemented. This plan should involve short-term and long-term needs of the community and achievement of goals. The last stage involves evaluation of the intervention, quality of the care, changes in community and future requirements of people. The model can potentially result in community harmony.

Figure 2. 7 stage model of community healing

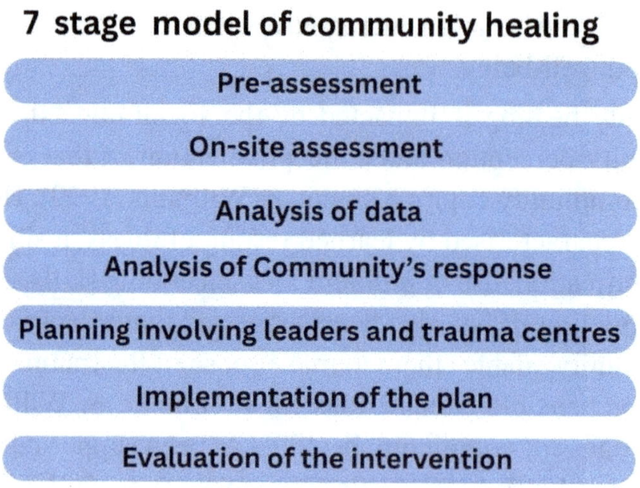

by Kalayjian (1995)

For healing the community a trauma-informed approach has also been propagated by Grover (2020) as instead of considering social inequalities as a personal characteristic, it is rather considered as a structural condition and sensitivity to historical trauma is also propagated. In order to be feasible such a framework needs to take into account the complexity, compromise, cost, culture and narratives. Ginwright (2015), suggested a healing justice framework for communities involving 3 important features of restoration, resistance, and reclamation. Restoring well being, meaning and purpose in community is essential and requires acknowledgment of collective nature of well being. Resistance acts as hope for young people as they reject the traditional notions of justice. Lastly, reclamation involves the ability to reclaim, redefine, and reimagine a possible future. This framework highlights the importance of recognition and understanding of systemic and structural issues that are faced by the community.

Figure 3. Healing justice framework

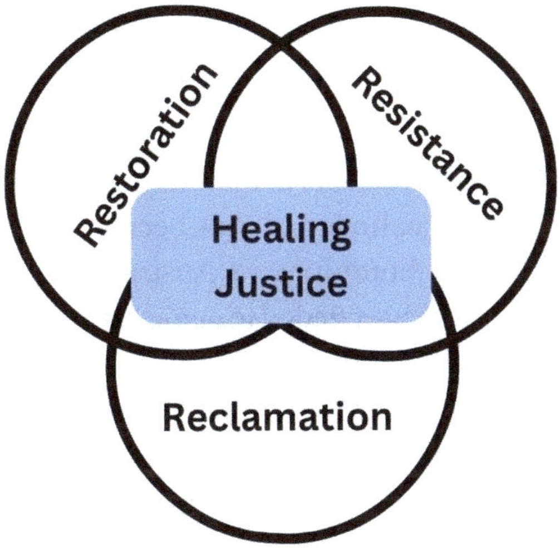

by Ginwright (2015)

With the systemic, political and economic nature of collective trauma and dehumanisation in consideration, Thomson (2021), suggested that justice is an essential aspect of community healing; however, the ways to bring about justice are neither completely political nor psychological but a collaboration between the two. It was proposed that healing can support social change and vice versa through creation of safe spaces which helps in socially recontextualising the process of healing and build a shared understanding of communities helping in overcoming oppressive structures. This would enable transcendence from local identities towards solidarity, from individual healing processes to relational healing processes. Chioneso et al. (2020), also place justice at the centre of their community healing framework called Community Healing and Resistance Through Storytelling (C-HeARTS). In this framework, processes which are responsive to culture like resistance and story telling are essential along with 3 psychological dimensions: connectedness, collective memory, and critical consciousness which are created through these processes. Mueller et al. (2021) highlighted that healing is a multidimensional process and self healing and community healing are mutual processes with interpersonal, intrapersonal and collective/structural levels. The mutual process of healing works as it cultivates hope and strengthens social ties, sense of belonging, self efficacy and collective efficacy. It is necessary to consider a person's collective experiences and ways of healing which can include prayer, family time or helping the rest of the community.

The theory of change model by Healing foundation (2019) harnesses several community related aspects in their healing model and is a practical approach to community healing. This has been applied to Aboriginal and Torres Strait Islander communities in Australia. The theory of change model highlights the elements needed to achieve real social change through collaboration between staff, funding bodies, communities and partner agencies. Understanding the impact of collective trauma and along with the preference of communities to heal collectively is a critical component in real change. Without healing at a community level, families will continue to live in a state of vulnerability as there is absence of a healthy community to assist them. On a community level healing activities include yarning circles, gatherings, healing camps, counselling, art, dance, song, weaving and cultural ceremony strengthening sense of identity and connectedness. The model is based in neuroscience as cultural practices like dance, art, song, weaving, drumming, and playing are calming trauma-informed processes which stimulate parts of the brain involved in managing emotions and memory. The model has three key domains involving quality, healing programs and initiative; healing networks, champions, and organisation and a supportive policy environment. The success of the programme is determined by local leadership, community readiness, capacity, and collaboration, understanding of impact of colonisation, intergenerational, trauma and grief in the community and building individual family and community strength (Healing foundation, 2019).

Figure 4. Theory of change model

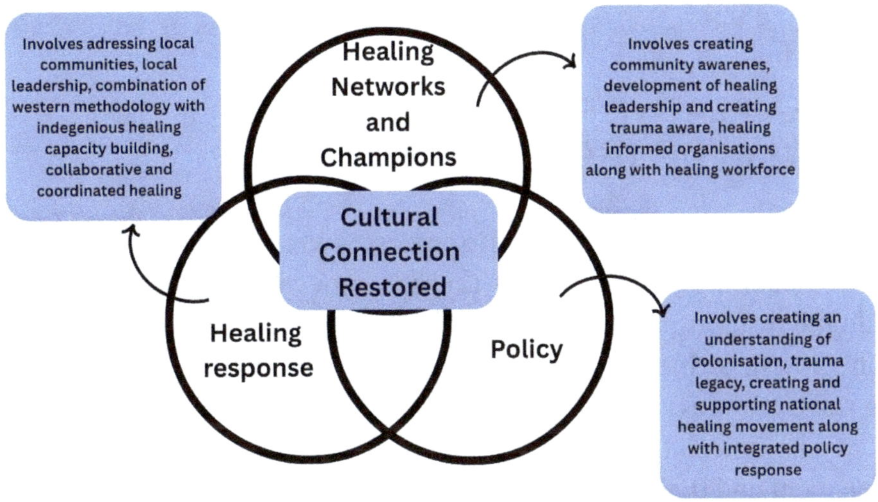

by Healing foundation (2019)

Community healing has also been demonstrated in the Indian context. Residency in the temples hold cultural power in India and are shown to result in supportive, non-threatening, and reassuring settings which are helpful in alleviating psychotic symptoms and can act as a community resource (Raguram et al., 2002). Spirituality and tribal practices are also valued as healing methods in communities. Tribals in Maharashtra, who consider themselves to be the poorest, most vulnerable and socially secluded by other communities have a unique sense of spirituality and trust within their own community and undertake individual prayer at home with their families along with engaging in communal prayer (Rowkith & Bhagwan, 2020).

Community healing has been recognised as a way of overcoming collective trauma through practices like shared narratives, social connections, justice and equity, mutual support and trauma informed approach. It has been effective in many contexts and influences healing on an individual level along with recognising structural, systemic, political injustice that the community faces. Spirituality and temple residences are some of the community healing practices prevalent in India. Parallel to these practices, several contemplative practices like yoga, meditation, mindfulness and rituals influence the Indian healing system and are rooted in ancient wisdom and scriptures.

CONTEMPLATIVE PRACTICES: A PATHWAY FOR TRAUMA RECOVERY

Contemplative practices refers to processes which enable self-realisation, self-regulation and self-control through movement, mind training and dialogue resulting in well-being of self and the community. Davidson & Dahl (2016), define contemplative practice as a form of training emphasizing self-awareness, self-regulation, and/or self-inquiry to enact a process of psychological transformation. It involves mental training, physical movement and dialogue based exercises and brings about enduring well being and inner flourishing. Qualities like equanimity and compassion, self-understanding and insight are upheld in contemplative practices. (Davidson & Dahl, 2016). An increased awareness of mental processes that is generated through contemplative practices, positively influences emotional behaviour like reducing negative affect, rumination, depression, and anxiety and increasing trait positive affect and mindfulness (Kemeny et al., 2012). Contemplative practice behaviour is also found to be positively associated with domains of well being like social connectedness, stress and resilience, experience of emotions, physical health, purpose and meaning, sense of self, financial security and satisfaction, spirituality and religiosity and exploration and creativity (Rich et al., 2022). In recent times contemplative practices have been applied to several contexts like universities where Stanford university campuses served as a case study of incorporation of contemplation and mindfulness into the daily life of student, staff, their families, alumni and retirees (Chrisinger & Rich, 2020). These practices have also been used in the workplace for reducing employee distress (Slemp, 2019) and in healthcare by building resilience to trauma in nurses (Fiske et al., 2020).

While there are several contemplative practices like prayers, pilgrimage, creative expression, the scope of the chapter will be limited to yoga, meditation, mindfulness and rituals as they are rooted in Indian tradition and therefore are more suited to this collectivistic context.

Types of Contemplative Practices

a) Yoga

Yoga is the integration of self with a higher reality or consciousness through harmony of mind, body and soul. It has originated in India and is conceptualised as union of individual self with supreme self (Moodley & West, 2005). Yoga is derived from the Sanskrit word 'Yuj', meaning 'to join' or 'to yoke' or 'to unite'.It is the process of uniting one's finite and microcosmic self with infinite macrocosmic consciousness (Moodley & West, 2005). Ancient texts like Puranas, Ramayana, Mahabharata, Bhagavad Gita and Yoga-Sutra are major contributions in the yogic tradition. In order to be more open to higher experiences in, yoga conceptualises harmony in different levels of consciousness. Patanjali highlighted 8 limbs or steps of yoga namely abstention (Yama), observances (Niyama), postures (Pranayama), breath control, sense withdrawal (Pratyahara), concentration (Dharana), meditation (Dhyana) and contemplation (Samadhi). Yoga helps the person to become more balanced and integrated. The aim of yoga is to facilitate self realisation leading to liberation (moksha) or freedom (Kaivalya) by overcoming sufferings (Moodley & West, 2005; Basavaraddi, 2015).

Yoga is very effective for holistic well being of the individual. Woodyard (2011) suggests that yoga has physical benefits like enhancing muscular strength and body flexibility, promoting and improving respiratory and cardiovascular function, along with mental health benefits like promotion of recovery and treatment of addiction, reducing stress, anxiety, depression, and chronic pain, and improving sleep patterns enhancing overall well-being and quality of life. In a review of studies (n=22) it was found that meditative movement activity practiced in yoga can meaningfully improve cardiovascular disease risk factors, physical fitness parameters, quality of life, and stress in previously inactive overweight/obese individuals (Batrakoulis, 2022). It has also been effective in smoking cessation (Bock et al., 2019), reducing perceived stress and mode of birth during pregnancy and labour (Corrigan et al., 2022) and reducing depression and anxiety in children (James-Palmer et al., 2020).

With respect to trauma, the specific modality of trauma informed yoga is found to be effective. In a review of literature (n=11) it was found that participants practicing trauma informed yoga experienced an increased sense of self-compassion, felt more centred, were able to develop coping skills and have a better mind–body relationship along with improvement in relationships with others with feelings of safety in the class being the main facilitator (English et al., 2022). Trauma sensitive yoga when applied as a complementary treatment for PTSD resulted in gratitude and compassion, relatedness, acceptance, centeredness, and empowerment in participants who were also able to change the way stress impacted their life, body and relationships (West et al., 2017). In more recent studies, Nejadghaderi et al. (2024) and Laplaud et al. (2023) also showed yoga as an effective treatment for PTSD. In the Indian context it has been found that yoga was effective in reducing sadness, and preventing an increase in anxiety in flood survivors in Bihar (Telles et al. 2010).

b) Meditation

Meditation is the practice of focusing on the mind and thoughts and achieving a state of calmness, clarity and wellbeing by eliminating distractions. The National Centre of complementary and integrative health (2022), defines "meditation" as a variety of practices that focus on mind and body integration and are used to calm the mind and enhance overall well-being. It is rooted in vedic tradition of India. It includes maintaining mental focus on a particular sensation, such as breathing, a sound, a visual image, or a mantra, which is a repeated word or phrase (National centre of complementary and integrative health, 2022).

Meditation is found to be effective in dealing with cardiovascular diseases and related factors like smoking cessation, perceived stress, myocardial ischemia, endothelial function, blood pressure (Levine et al., 2017). Mantra based meditation has profound effects on mental health as it results in reduction of anxiety, depression, stress, Post traumatic stress and improvement in mental health related quality of life (Álvarez-Pérez et al., 2022). Meditation activates vagus nerve leading relaxation and positivity along with the parasympathetic nervous system reducing the risk of heart disease and a lower heart rate and regulating blood pressure

(Sharma & Sharma, 2024). It also reduces neural activity in areas of the brain that are involved in pain mechanisms. From a psychological perspective it was shown that meditation alleviates symptoms of anxiety and depression, increases visual sensitivity, enhances focus and attention and results in improved performance in memory, intelligence and creativity (Sharma & Sharma, 2024).

Meditation is effective in reducing the impact of trauma and coping with it. Meditation appears to be effective for PTSD and depression symptoms (Hilton et al., 2017). In a review on the efficacy of meditation on the veteran population (n=15) it was found that various types of meditation like transcendental meditation, mantra meditation, breathing based meditation were effective in managing PTSD, particularly among veterans resistant to trauma-focused therapies (Haider, et al., 2021; Nidich et al., 2018). Positive impact of meditation on mental health outcomes has also been observed in female trauma survivors of interpersonal violence with co-occurring disorders. Significant changes in mental health symptoms and trauma. Symptoms were observed in the participants after six week intervention of Tibetan meditation focused on breathing, loving kindness, and compassion, meditation (Lee et al., 2015).

c) Mindfulness

Mindfulness is the non judgemental awareness of the present moment. Mindfulness, which involves maintaining attention or awareness of the present moment without making judgments (National centre of complementary and integrative health, 2022). It traces its origin in Buddhist philosophy.

Mindfulness based intervention has been found to be effective in dealing with a wide range of problems. An analysis showed that mindfulness practices among people with cancer resulted in reduced psychological distress, sleep disturbance, pain, fatigue, anxiety and depression (Cillessen et al., 2019). Mindfulness based interventions show improvement in obesity related eating behaviours in individuals who are overweight and obese and are also found to be effective in reducing weight (Carrière et al., 2018; Rogers et al., 2017). Keng et al. (2011) focused on positive effects of mindfulness on psychological markers like subjective well being, behavioral regulation and reduction in psychological symptoms and emotional reactivity. Khushid & Vythiliggam (2016) suggested that mindfulness based cognitive therapy decreases symptom severity in a current episode of depression and also reduces relapse rates.

Mindfulness is also used in navigating trauma in various sections of the population. Follette et al., (2006) suggest that behavioural treatments for trauma are integrated with mindfulness resulting in decreased avoidance towards treatment and increased efficacy. When exposure treatments are used by integrating mindfulness skills, the patient's ability to face painful memories, thoughts, and feelings without engaging in avoidance scoping increases. In veterans with PTSD, it was found that mindfulness training led to an improvement in anxiety, depression, and somatisation scores (Azadmarzabadi, 2013). High-quality structured mindfulness interventions are effective in youth facing adverse childhood exposure as it weakens the effect of stress and trauma faced due to these exposures reducing poor health outcomes, which are otherwise carried on to adulthood (Ortiz & Sibinga, 2017). In a systematic review, it was suggested that mindfulness based interventions have also been effective in reducing psychological distress, stress, depression, and burnout in nurses (Ramchandran et al., 2023). Elkayal and Metwaly (2022) also showed the effectiveness of mindful based intervention on post traumatic stress symptoms among emergency nursing students. In India after receiving mindfulness training, college students showed significant improvement in emotional regulation, psychological well-being and trade mindfulness (Antony & Neelakantam, 2025). Culturally adapted mindfulness training was effective in navigating perinatal grief among poor women in Chhattisgarh as there were changes in mental health, positive religious coping, and decrease in level of perinatal, grief, active grief, and despair along with an improved ability to cope (Roberts & Montgomery, 2016).

d) Rituals

Rituals are practices and customs which are symbolic in nature, rooted in culture, social, religious and personal traditions, undertaken to facilitate expression of values, beliefs and connections. Rituals are based in religious traditions of several cultures and is a unique contemplative practice unlike other practices it is inherently placed in community context. When performed through mindfulness, and spirituality rituals can deepen self awareness and spiritual growth. On an individual level rituals can relieve anxiety and have a beneficial effect on adjustment of individual goal or behavior and social inclusion (Zhou & Xing, 2025). They also reduce performance induced anxiety (Brooks et al., 2016). Rituals provide insight into the identities, norms, values, and goals of a community (Legare, 2022). It is important to be cautious that all rituals may not foster contemplation and some may be oppressive and discriminatory. This chapter will focus on specific rituals which enhance collaboration and growth.

Both community healing and contemplative practices are used in the Indian healing system. Contemplative practices have generated abundant research on individual benefits and navigating trauma on an individual level, their role in community settings is portrayed to be limited. The intersection between the community healing and contemplative practices is not explored sufficiently and is important to shed light on how communities can benefit and heal through an intersection of contemplative practices with community healing. This is particularly suited to the Indian context due to the collective nature of society and emphasis on contemplation in the historical texts of yoga, meditation and mindfulness.

AN INTERSECTION OF COMMUNITY HEALING AND CONTEMPLATIVE PRACTICES

Since Mueller et al. (2021) suggested that community healing and individual healing are mutually interdependent, the ability of contemplative practice in bringing improvement in physical, psychological and emotional attributes of individuals should not be undermined as it forms the basis of community healing. Contemplative practices can help in creating a safe environment in the community, create a sense of belonging, promote compassion and a shared understanding, as individuals who have experienced the same traumatic event have a better understanding of the nuances of each other's experiences which is also highlighted as essential psychological process community healing frame work by Chioneso et al. (2020). These practices are shown to cultivate a sense of purpose at a community level, nervous system regulation, prosocial qualities like humility, harmony and deep listening and community cohesion as when contemplation is done on a community level goes beyond self and other towards a sense of connection and interdependence (Draper-Clarke & Green, 2023). Contemplative practices appear to have a positive impact on not only individual health, but by extending the level of compassion and tolerance beyond self, can improve health at a public/societal level and reduce disparities (Bruce et al., 2018).

The intersection of yoga with community healing has been widely explored. Banwari (2019) suggested that Yoga along with physical healing allows social healing with yoga classes becoming separate communities. Barudin (2024), explored a unique approach to community healing called Indigenous Yoga collective (IYC) through which women engage in yoga as a reconnect to culture and spiritual reclamation. Through this collective yoga is seen as transformative, offering a holistic healing approach which aligns with indigenous knowledge system. IYC brings forth understanding of historical intergenerational and colonial trauma in order to heal from stress, grief and pain by using yoga as the core healing practice. Emotional support, creation of safe and brave spaces and community building are the pillars of IYC, which emphasise connection between healing practices and collective well-being. For bridging the gap between personal healing and systemic oppression, the collective develops a program keeping in mind a healing justice framework (Ginwright, 2015), which is based on deep trust, supportive relationship, prioritisation of Sadhana, along with reflection and collaboration.

In order to understand the impact of yoga and community healing, Mackenzie et al. (2016) explored the impact of community based yoga programs in Cancer survivors. It was found that participants experienced feelings of safety and shared understanding of the cancer experience which acted as a uniting force resulting in participants feeling comfortable and supported. The shared meaning ('everybody on the same boat') between the participants enabled them to feel safe and work together in learning yoga. When yoga was tailored, according to the needs of the participant through cancer specific instructions, it led to enhanced sense of safety and recognition of limitations. Yoga was described as a relief from symptoms of cancer, as well as acted as a means of taking back control. Other benefits reported for the ability to relax, concentrate, regulate emotions, manage symptoms of fatigue, pain, and sleep difficulties and promote physical health. Moreover, yoga resulted in participants being more confident in their ability, even when engaging in activities outside of the studio. In another group based yoga programme by Donnelly et al. (2020) community integration of people with traumatic brain injury and their caregivers was explored. The programme provided participants with an opportunity to overcome isolation through connecting with a bigger community enhancing their sense of belonging and community connection and instilled a sense of hope. On a personal level the programme offered benefits like physical health, self regulation, self efficacy and resilience. The Experience of Yoga for individuals with complex interpersonal trauma was explored also by Bennett & Starnino (2022) and it was found that the participants formed a yoga community which extended beyond classes and led to healing of trauma.

Like yoga, meditation can also facilitate community healing. Meditation when practiced in groups promotes compassion in the community, reduces collective stress and also contributes to peacebuilding in conflict-affected communities.Through meditation an individual is much less likely to blame others or experience negative emotions and is able to easily let go of minor disagreements. Sudarshan Kriya enhances oxytocin which promotes feelings of love and social bonding (Sharma &Sharma, 2024). Schneider et al. (2024) evaluated TM sidhi programme which revolves around transcendental meditation and highlighted that through these techniques individuals are trained to sustain thought and activity from the silent state of awareness and integrate experience of pure consciousness with activity resulting in amplified effects on collective and individual functioning. Condon et al. (2013) showed that meditation increased compassionate responding with higher chances of acting to relieve another person's pain. This has implications for the community and individuals inflicting oppression and discrimination obstructing justice. Engert et al. (2023) argued that meditation induced positive change can spread from practitioners to their social network. This benefits the social environment as there can be a spread of pro social action, cognitive functioning like attention, executive functioning and perspective taking and emotional functioning.

The notions of collective consciousness have been explored as well. According to Maharishi Mahesh Yogi vedic tradition in India mentions consciousness for society as a whole with its own reality and possibility of growth (Maharishi Mahesh Yogi, 1977b). Traditional meditation can potentially reduce stress at a social level and has impacted trends of collective violence. Transcendental meditation creates harmony in individual and collective life by aligning it with laws of nature (Maharishi Mahesh Yogi, 1986b). According to Maharishi 1% of the population practicing transcendental meditation could result in increased orderliness in the society known as the maharishi effect. Orme-Johnson et al. (2022) have also replicated this effect and reported that when a group reached the required threshold of meaning trend reductions in indicators of stress like homicides, aggravated assault, rape, robbery, fatalities in youth, infant mortality, drug-related deaths, motor vehicle fatalities on a societal level were observed. The potential reason brought forward was that since every individual contributes to the collective consciousness, individual effects of transcendental meditation transcend into collective consciousness, therefore, it is the duty of citizens to contribute to coherence of collective consciousness and responsibility of the government to provide means to do so. The effect of group meditation showed that when participants came together and engaged in transcendental meditation, there were improvements in measures of war and war deaths in Israel-Lebanese armed conflict showing the impact of meditation in peace building during war (Orme-Johnson et al., 1988).

The relationship between mindfulness and community healing has also been explored. Pagis & Tal (2022) argue that mindfulness is not a private practice of individual solitude but a shared practice of collective solitude. Mindfulness opposes direct social engagement and still offers a supportive social space where there is a transformation from being audience to bodily co-dwellers. Individuals experience support and togetherness without interacting with each other and relieve societal stress resulting in a sense of community. Mindfulness builds compassion which has implications for the practitioners as compassion connects the patient's suffering with healer's suffering resulting in an emotional connection which strengthens the healing relationship (Schmidt, 2004). It can help in mitigating the impact of collective trauma and is negatively associated with COVID-

19-related fear/worry, global distress, hurricane-related fear/worry, and functional impairment over time (Lorenzini et al., 2023). It is suggested that a group practice of mindfulness fosters therapeutic relatedness and generates greater group cohesiveness which enhances community healing (Tempone-Wiltshire, 2024).

Use of collective rituals in order to cope with the collective trauma is seen in several communities especially in the Indian context. Public rituals of mourning and remembrance have a profound impact in healing from collective trauma and historic trauma (Theisen-Womersley, 2021). Through collective rituals individuals are able to canalize emotional ties, temper anxiety, and prevent isolation (Veerman & Ganzevoort, 2001). Ahammed (2019) through the rituals of theyyam, a unique socio-religious tradition in Kerala, proposed that oppressed caste communities are also equipped with unique traditions and rituals for coping with trauma through catharsis, social reflection and visceral experience of being powerful. In Theyyam, the performer embodies a chosen deity creating pathways for letting out collective rage, anger and resentment faced by people of the oppressed communities over the years. Coping mechanisms were also depicted by adivasi communities in India (Rechsteiner, 2019) where the participants suggested that occupying oneself with work and seeking community support can be some ways in which trauma is processed. In order to cope with trauma self engagement and social support were perceived as a way of relaxing one's mind. Community rituals were also highlighted where in a scenario of loss of a community member, the entire community does not work until the offerings are eaten by a crow or alternatively given to a cow after 10 days (Rechsteiner, 2019). These rituals may have been useful in venting out feelings and getting support from the community in a difficult time. Rituals like songs and dance have their own special meanings and convey narratives to upcoming generations, creating communal empowerment which develops common identity and support in the community.

It has been acknowledged that social justice is an essential aspect of community healing as systematic, structural, environmental, and social barriers often cause collective trauma, impacting these communities in a negative way (Pinderhughes et al. 2015; Ginwright, 2015). India has witnessed oppression, marginalisation, and discrimination against several communities, especially caste-based communities (Ahammed, 2019;

Koileri. V,2025). Contemplative practices cultivate awareness in people, making them conscious of their experiences and turning them into an observer of experience which may provide insight into factors that may maintain or create oppression (Gordon, 2019). These practices enable the individual to reflect on social injustice and take social action. A radical healing philosophy of yoga has been propagated by Sood (2018) which is accountable for liberation of most marginalised people within a community and entails interconnectivity of relationships and struggles. In an attempt of restoration of hope and justice and spiritual balance, community-based healers are incorporating yoga into models of collective care. The framework recognizes collective trauma, suffering, and systemic oppression and encourages spiritual work (Sood, 2018). Mindfulness also brings forth social justice practice by enabling individuals to notice personal bias and making them aware of the interconnectedness in the environment inspiring them to question the structural systems they are placed in (Conway, 2022). Hick and Furlotte (2009) suggest mindfulness provides pathways observing and investigating events in everyday life that are influenced by larger social relations and structures and gives way to mindful awareness of the dynamic of social awareness. It enables the individual to address inner troubles and situate them in relation to social oppressive structures. According to number analytics (2025) rituals can also give way to social justice through creating a sense of community and solidarity, providing a platform for expression and protest, inspiring action and mobilising support.

CHALLENGES AND FUTURE IMPLICATIONS: A CRITICAL LENS

The intersection of contemplative practices and community healing is noteworthy especially in collective cultures like India. However, even though contemplative practices discussed in this chapter originated in India, the research in the Indian perspective is limited, leading to westernisation of these practices. This has led to commercialisation of these practices which can lead to superficial, inauthentic and detached interventions. There is a lack of a comprehensive framework of community healing integrated with contemplative practices in the Indian context keeping in mind the diversity, social and judicial systems that prevail in the country. This has led to a lack of interventions exploring intersection of community healing and contemplative practices in India. The socioeconomic disparities prevalent in Indian society, would limit any present intervention to urban, educated and resource rich settings exclusive of marginalised and remote communities. The uneven distribution of resources would further hamper implementation of intervention in such communities. The stigma and shame around trauma impedes collective acknowledgment of trauma restricting the transformative potential of contemplative reflection and communal dialogue. In order to facilitate healing in communities using contemplative practices, there is a need to create awareness about the use of these practices and related interventions and ensure that they are accessible and affordable to communities facing trauma. With regards to prevention of misuse of these practices, the responsibility of ensuring the presence of credible practitioners, provision of educational pathways and establishment of community centres of healing lies on regulatory bodies and other systemic structures in place. Future researches can work towards overcoming these challenges and also highlight the need to embrace and adapt contemplative practices which originated from this very context.

REFERENCES

American Psychological Association. (2018). Community. *APA Dictionary of Psychology.* APA website. https://dictionary.apa.org/community

American Psychological Association. (2018). Trauma. *APA dictionary of psychology*. APA website. https://dictionary.apa.org/trauma

Ahammed, S. (2019). Caste-based Oppression, Trauma and Collective Victimhood in Erstwhile South India: The Collective Therapeutic Potential of Theyyam. *Psychology and Developing Societies*, *31*(1), 88–105. DOI: 10.1177/0971333618825051

Álvarez-Pérez, Y., Rivero-Santana, A., Perestelo-Pérez, L., Duarte-Díaz, A., Ramos-García, V., Toledo-Chávarri, A., Torres-Castaño, A., León-Salas, B., Infante-Ventura, D., González-Hernández, N., Rodríguez-Rodríguez, L., & Serrano-Aguilar, P. (2022). Effectiveness of Mantra-Based Meditation on Mental Health: A Systematic Review and Meta-Analysis. *International Journal of Environmental Research and Public Health*, *19*(6), 3380. DOI: 10.3390/ijerph19063380

Antony, S., & Neelakantan, M. S. (2025). Exploring the effectiveness of mindfulness-based intervention among college students in India. *Current Psychology (New Brunswick, N.J.)*, *44*(10), 8232–8244. DOI: 10.1007/s12144-024-07148-1

Azadmarzabadi, E. (2013). The effectiveness of mindfulness training on psychological symptoms in veterans with post-traumatic stress disorder. *International Journal of Behavioral Sciences*, *7*(1), 67–74.

Banwari, A. (2019). Re-imaginations of Yoga in the 21st Century: A Journey of Healing and Community- Building. *University of Cape Town.* https://www.researchgate.net/publication/354076309

Barudin, J. (2024). Weaving threads of collective liberation: Intercultural wisdom among indigenous and south asian women in the indigenous yoga collective. *Race and Yoga*, *8*(1). Advance online publication. DOI: 10.5070/R38163528

Basavaraddi, I. (2015). Yoga: Its Origin, History and Development. https://doi.org/https://www.redtwigyoga.com/uploads/1/2/1/9/12195443/yoga__its_origin_history_and_development.pdf

Batrakoulis, A. (2022). Psychophysiological Adaptations to Yoga Practice in Overweight and Obese Individuals: A Topical Review. *Diseases (Basel, Switzerland)*, *10*(4), 107. DOI: 10.3390/diseases10040107

Bennett, L. M., & Starnino, V. R. (2022). The experience of yoga for persons with complex interpersonal trauma: A phenomenological approach. *Complementary Therapies in Clinical Practice*, *49*, 101674. DOI: 10.1016/j.ctcp.2022.101674

Bock, B. C., Dunsiger, S. I., Rosen, R. K., Thind, H., Jennings, E., Fava, J. L., Becker, B. M., Carmody, J., & Marcus, B. H. (2019). Yoga as a Complementary Therapy for Smoking Cessation: Results From BreathEasy, a Randomized Clinical Trial. *Nicotine & Tobacco Research: Official Journal of the Society for Research on Nicotine and Tobacco*, *21*(11), 1517–1523. DOI: 10.1093/ntr/nty212

Boss, P., Beaulieu, L., Wieling, E., Turner, W., & LaCruz, S. (2003). Healing loss, ambiguity, and trauma: A community-based intervention with families of union workers missing after the 9/11 attack in New York City. *Journal of Marital and Family Therapy*, *29*(4), 455–467. DOI: 10.1111/j

Bowlby, J. (1969). Attachment and Loss: Vol. 1. *Attachment. Attachment and Loss*. Basic Books.

Brooks, A. W., Schroeder, J., Risen, J. L., Gino, F., Galinsky, A. D., Norton, M. I., & Schweitzer, M. E. (2016). RETRACTED: Don't stop believing: Rituals improve performance by decreasing anxiety. *Organizational Behavior and Human Decision Processes*, *137*, 71–85. DOI: 10.1016/j.obhdp.2016.07.004

Bruce, M. A., Skrine Jeffers, K., King Robinson, J., & Norris, K. C. (2018). Contemplative Practices: A Strategy to Improve Health and Reduce Disparities. *International Journal of Environmental Research and Public Health*, *15*(10), 2253. DOI: 10.3390/ijerph15102253

Carrière, K., Khoury, B., Günak, M. M., & Knäuper, B. (2018). Mindfulness-based interventions for weight loss: A systematic review and meta-analysis. *Obesity Reviews*, *19*(2), 164–177. DOI: 10.1111/obr.12623

Cillessen, L., Johannsen, M., Speckens, A. E. M., & Zachariae, R. (2019). Mindfulness-based interventions for psychological and physical health outcomes in cancer patients and survivors: A systematic review and meta-analysis of randomized controlled trials. *Psycho-Oncology*, *28*(12), 2257–2269. DOI: 10.1002/pon.5214

Chioneso, N. A., Hunter, C. D., Gobin, R. L., McNeil Smith, S., Mendenhall, R., & Neville, H. A. (2020). Community Healing and Resistance Through Storytelling: A Framework to Address Racial Trauma in Africana Communities. *The Journal of Black Psychology*, *46*(2-3), 95–121. DOI: 10.1177/0095798420929468

Chrisinger, B. W., & Rich, T. (2020). Contemplation by Design: Leveraging the "Power of the Pause" on a Large University Campus Through Built and Social Environments. *Frontiers in Public Health*, *8*, 31. DOI: 10.3389/fpubh.2020.00031

Condon, P., Desbordes, G., Miller, W. B., & DeSteno, D. (2013). Meditation Increases Compassionate Responses to Suffering. *Psychological Science*, *24*(10), 2125–2127. DOI: 10.1177/0956797613485603

Conway, S. M. (2022). The role of meditation in the fight for social justice. *Mindworks Meditation & Buddhist Path*. https://mindworks.org/blog/role-meditation-social-justice/

Corrigan, L., Moran, P., McGrath, N., Eustace-Cook, J., & Daly, D. (2022). The characteristics and effectiveness of pregnancy yoga interventions: A systematic review and meta-analysis. *BMC Pregnancy and Childbirth*, *22*(1), 250. DOI: 10.1186/s12884-022-04474-9

Draper-Clarke, J. L., & Green, C. (2023). Cultivating well-being, community cohesion and sense of purpose through African contemplative practices. *University of the Witwatersrand*. https://doi.org/DOI: 10.21203/rs.3.rs-3119401/v1

Davidson, R. J., & Dahl, C. J. (2016). Varieties of Contemplative Practice. *JAMA Psychiatry*. Advance online publication. DOI: 10.1001/jamapsychiatry.2016.3469

Donnelly, K. Z., Goldberg, S., & Fournier, D. (2020). A qualitative study of LoveYourBrain Yoga: A group-based yoga with psychoeducation intervention to facilitate community integration for people with traumatic brain injury and their caregivers. *Disability and Rehabilitation*, *42*(17), 2482–2491. DOI: 10.1080/09638288.2018.1563638

ElKayal, M. M., & Metwaly, S. M. (2022). Effectiveness of mindfulness-based intervention on post-traumatic stress symptoms among emergency nursing students. *Middle East Curr Psychiatry*, *29*, 40. DOI: 10.1186/s43045-022-00208-x

Engert, V., Klimecki, O., & Kanske, P. (2023). Spreading positive change: Societal benefits of men. *Frontiers in Psychiatry*, *14*. Advance online publication. DOI: 10.3389/fpsyt.2023.1038051

English, A., McKibben, E., Sivaramakrishnan, D., Hart, N., Richards, J., & Kelly, P. (2022). A Rapid Review Exploring the Role of Yoga in Healing Psychological Trauma. *International Journal of Environmental Research and Public Health*, *19*(23), 16180. DOI: 10.3390/ijerph192316180

Erikson, K. (1976). *Everything In its Path*. Simon and Schuster.

Erikson, K. (1991). Notes on Trauma and Community. *The American Imago*, *48*(4), 455–472. http://www.jstor.org/stable/26303923

Eyerman, R., Alexander, J. C., Giesen, B., Smelser, N. J., & Sztompka, P. (2004). *Cultural Trauma and Collective Identity*. University of California Press.

Fanahei, R. (2024). Community-based social healing, community healing, and the role of "healing leader.". *Grail of Science*, *36*, 501–510. DOI: 10.36074/grail-of-science.16.02.2024.088

Farrell, S. J., Aubry, T., & Coulombe, D. (2003). Neighborhoods and neighbors: Do they contribute to personal well-being? *Journal of Community Psychology*, *32*(1), 9–25. DOI: 10.1002/jcop.10082

Fiske E, Martin S, Luetkemeyer J. (2020). Building Nurses 'Resilience to Trauma through Contemplative Practices. *Creative Nursing*. 26(4):090-096. doi:DOI: 10.1891/CRNR-D-20-00054

Follette, V. Palm, K.M. & Pearson, A.N. (2006). Mindfulness and trauma: implications for treatment. *J Rat-Emo Cognitive-Behav Ther 24*, 45–61/. https://doi.org/DOI: 10.1007/s10942-006-0025-2

Ginwright, S. A. (2015). Radically Healing Black Lives: A Love Note to Justice. *New Directions for Student Leadership, 2015*(148), 33–44. DOI: 10.1002/yd.20151

Government of India. (n.d.). Community. *National portal of India*. Retrieved July 31, 2025, from https://www.india.gov.in/people-groups/community

Grover, L. T. (2020). Surviving hell Summer: Baton Rouge, Louisiana, racial polarization, and implications for community healing. *Community Development (Columbus, Ohio), 51*(3), 283–296. 10.1080

Gordon, T. (2019). Contemplativ practices. In *Holistic healing: Theories, practice and social change*. Canadian Scholars.

Haider, T., Dai, L., & Sharma, M. (2021). Efficacy of Meditation-Based Interventions on Post-Traumatic Stress Disorder (PTSD) Among Veterans: A Narrative Review. *Advances, 35*(1).

Harvey, M. R., Mondesir, A. V., & Aldrich, H. (2007). Fostering resilience in traumatized communities: A community empowerment model of intervention. *Journal of Aggression, Maltreatment & Trauma, 14*(1–2), 265–285. DOI: 10.1300/J146v14n01_14

Healing foundation. (2019). A theory of change for healing. https://cdn.healingfoundation.org.au/app/uploads/2019/04/18122127/HF_Theory_of_Change_A4_Mar2019_WEB.pdf

Hick, S. F., & Furlotte, C. R. (2009). Mindfulness and social justice-oriented approaches: Bridging the mind and society together in social work practice. *Canadian Association for Social Work Education, 26*(1), 5–24. https://www.researchgate.net/publication/321642093

Hilton, L., Maher, A. R., Colaiaco, B., Apaydin, E., Sorbero, M. E., Booth, M., Shanman, R. M., & Hempel, S. (2017). Meditation for posttraumatic stress: Systematic review and meta-analysis. *Psychological Trauma: Theory, Research, Practice, and Policy*, *9*(4), 453–460. DOI: 10.1037/tra0000180

Hirschberger, G. (2018). Collective Trauma and the Social Construction of Meaning. *Frontiers in Psychology*, *9*, 1441. DOI: 10.3389/fpsyg.2018.01441

Iyer, S. S. (2025). Indian Community Development – A bottom-to-top Prospective. *Global Journal of Human Social Science*, *4*(3), 23–59. https://doi.org/ https://doi.org/10.55640/gjhss/Volume04Issue03-03

James-Palmer, A., Anderson, E. Z., Zucker, L., Kofman, Y., & Daneault, J. F. (2020). Yoga as an Intervention for the Reduction of Symptoms of Anxiety and Depression in Children and Adolescents: A Systematic Review. *Frontiers in Pediatrics*, *8*, 78. DOI: 10.3389/fped.2020.00078

Jansen, S., Niyonzima, J. B., & Gerbarg, P. (2024). Evaluating effects of community-based social healing model on Ubuntu, mental health and psychosocial functioning in post-genocide Rwanda: Protocol for cluster randomized control trial. *Trials*, *25*, 773. DOI: 10.1186/s13063-024-08632-6

Jiwa, A., Kelly, L., & Pierre-Hansen, N. (2008). Healing the community to heal the individual: Literature review of aboriginal community-based alcohol and substance abuse programs. *Canadian Family Physician Médecin de Famille Canadien*, *54*(7), 1000–1000.e7.

Kalayjian, A. S. (1995). Disaster and mass trauma: Global perspectives on post disaster mental health management. Long Branch, NJ: Vista.

Kemeny, M. E., Foltz, C., Cavanagh, J. F., Cullen, M., Giese-Davis, J., Jennings, P., Rosenberg, E. L., Gillath, O., Shaver, P. R., Wallace, B. A., & Ekman, P. (2012). Contemplative/emotion training reduces negative emotional behavior and promotes prosocial responses. *Emotion (Washington, D.C.)*, *12*(2), 338–350. DOI: 10.1037/a0026118

Keng, S. L., Smoski, M. J., & Robins, C. J. (2011). Effects of mindfulness on psychological health: A review of empirical studies. *Clinical Psychology Review*, *31*(6), 1041–1056. DOI: 10.1016/j.cpr.2011.04.006

Koileri, V. (2025). Healing The Psyche from Caste Violence: Addressing the Cumulative Psychological Trauma of Generations of Oppression and Deprivation Among the SC/ST Community in India. *International Journal of Indian Psychology*, *13*(2). Advance online publication. DOI: 10.25215/1302.125

Laplaud, N., Perrochon, A., & Gallou-Guyot, M. (2023). Management of post-traumatic stress disorder symptoms by yoga: An overview. *BMC Complementary Medicine and Therapies*, *23*, 258. DOI: 10.1186/s12906-023-04074-w

Leary, M. R., & Baumeister, R. F. (2000). The nature and function of self-esteem: Sociometer theory. In Vol. 32, pp. 1–62). Advances in Experimental Social Psychology. Elsevier., DOI: 10.1016/S0065-2601(00)80003-9

Lee, M. Y., Zaharlick, A., & Akers, D. (2015). Impact of Meditation on Mental Health Outcomes of Female Trauma Survivors of Interpersonal Violence With Co-Occurring Disorders: A Randomized Controlled Trial. *Journal of Interpersonal Violence*, *32*(14), 2139–2165. DOI: 10.1177/0886260515591277

Legare, C., Burger, O., Johnson, T., Mor, N., & Saldanha, N. (2022). Leverage the power of ritual to improve community health worker efficacy and public health outcomes: Lessons from Bihar, India. *The Lancet Regional Health. Southeast Asia*, *1*, 100006. DOI: 10.1016/j.lansea.2022.04.002

Levine, G. N., Lange, R. A., Bairey-Merz, C. N., Davidson, R. J., Jamerson, K., & Mehta, S. C.Jr, & American Heart Association Council on Clinical Cardiology; P. K., Michos, E. D., Norris, K., Ray, I. B., Saban, K. L., Shah, T., Stein, R., Smith, Cardiovascular and Stroke Nursing; and Council on Hypertension. (2017). Meditation and Cardiovascular Risk Reduction: A Scientific Statement From the American Heart Association. *Journal of the American Heart Association*, *6*(10), e002218. DOI: 10.1161/JAHA.117.002218

Lorenzini, J. A., Wong-Parodi, G., & Garfin, D. R. (2023). Associations between mindfulness and mental health after collective trauma: Results from a longitudinal, representative, probability-based survey. *Anxiety, Stress, and Coping*, *37*(3), 361–378. DOI: 10.1080/10615806.2023.2267454

Mackenzie, M. J., Wurz, A. J., Yamauchi, Y., Pires, L. A., & Culos-Reed, S. N. (2016). Yoga Helps Put the Pieces Back Together: A Qualitative Exploration of a Community-Based Yoga Program for Cancer Survivors. *Evidence-Based Complementary and Alternative Medicine : eCAM, 1832515*. Advance online publication. DOI: 10.1155/2016/1832515

Maharishi Mahesh Yogi. (1977b). Foreword: The scientific age is rising to be the age of enlightenment. In Orme-Johnson, D. W., & Farrow, J. T. (Eds.), *Scientific Research on the Transcendental Meditation Program. 1*. Maharishi European Research University Press.

Maharishi Mahesh Yogi. (1986b). *Life supported by natural law: Lectures by Maharishi Mahesh Yogi*. Age of Enlightenment Press.

McElligott, D. (2010). Healing. *Journal of Holistic Nursing*, *28*(4), 251–259. DOI: 10.1177/0898010110376321

Maslow, A. H. (1954). Motivation and personality. *Harper's*.

Michalski, C. A., Diemert, L. M., Helliwell, J. F., Goel, V., & Rosella, L. C. (2020). Relationship between sense of community belonging and self-rated health across life stages. *SSM - Population Health*, *12*, 100676. DOI: 10.1016/j.ssmph.2020.100676

Moodley, R., & West, W. (2005). *Integrating traditional healing practices into counseling and psychotherapy*. SAGE Publications.

Mueller, D., Bacalso, E., Ortega-Williams, A., Pate, D. J.Jr, & Topitzes, J. (2021). A mutual process of healing self and healing the community: A qualitative study of coping with and healing from stress, adversity, and trauma among diverse residents of a midwestern city. *Journal of Community Psychology*, *49*(5), 1169–1194. DOI: 10.1002/jcop.22530

National centre of complementary and integrative health. (2022). Meditation and mindfulness: Effectiveness and safety. *NCCIH*. Retrieved August 3, 2025, from https://www.nccih.nih.gov/health/meditation-and-mindfulness-effectiveness-and-safety

Nejadghaderi, S. A., Mousavi, S. E., Fazlollahi, A., Motlagh Asghari, K., & Garfin, D. R. (2024). Efficacy of yoga for posttraumatic stress disorder: A systematic review and meta-analysis of randomized controlled trials. *Psychiatry Research, 340,* 116098. DOI: 10.1016/j.psychres.2024.116098

Nidich, S., Mills, P. J., Rainforth, M., Heppner, P., Schneider, R. H., Rosenthal, N. E., Salerno, J., Gaylord-King, C., & Rutledge, T. (2018). Non-trauma-focused meditation versus exposure therapy in veterans with post-traumatic stress disorder: A randomised controlled trial. *The Lancet. Psychiatry*, *5*(12), 975–986. DOI: 10.1016/S2215-0366(18)30384-5

Number analytics. (2025). Rituals in modern society. Retrieved August 3, 2025, from https://www.numberanalytics.com/blog/rituals-in-modern-society

Orme-Johnson, D. W., Cavanaugh, K. L., Dillbeck, M. C., & Goodman, R. S. (2022). Field-effects of consciousness: A seventeen-year study of the effects of group practice of the transcendental meditation and tm-sidhi programs on reducing national stress in the united states. *World Journal of Social Science*, *9*(2), 1. DOI: 10.5430/wjss.v9n2p1

Orme-Johnson, D., Alexander, C., Davies, J., Chander, H., & Larimore, W. (1988). International peace project: The effects of the maharishi Technology of the Unified Field. *The Journal of Conflict Resolution*, *32*, 776–12. DOI: 10.1177/0022002788032004009

Ortiz, R., & Sibinga, E. (2017). The role of mindfulness in reducing the adverse effects of childhood stress and trauma. *Children (Basel, Switzerland)*, *4*(3), 16. DOI: 10.3390/children4030016

Pagis, M., & Tal, O. (2022). Collective mindfulness: Somatic attention to group and self in meditation practice in Israel. *Anthropology Today*, *38*, 13–16. DOI: 10.1111/1467-8322.12708

Para, E. A. (2008). The Role of Social Support in Identity Formation: A Literature Review. *Graduate Journal of Counseling Psychology, 1*(1). http://epublications.marquette.edu/gjcp/vol1/iss1/9

Park, E. Y., Oliver, T. R., Peppard, P. E., & Malecki, K. C. (2023). Sense of community and mental health: A cross-sectional analysis from a household survey in Wisconsin. *Family Medicine and Community Health, 11*(2). Advance online publication. DOI: 10.1136/fmch-2022-001971

Pinderhughes, H., Davis, R. A., & Williams, M. (2015). *Adverse community experiences and resilience: A framework for addressing and preventing community trauma*. Prevention Institute.

Pretty, G. M. H. (2002). Young People's Development of the Community-Minded Self. *The Plenum Series in Social. Clinical Psychology*, •••, 183–203. DOI: 10.1007/978-1-4615-0719-2_10

Prezza, M., Amici, M., Roberti, T., & Tedeschi, G. (2001). Sense of community referred to the whole town: Its relations with neighboring, loneliness, life satisfaction, and area of residence. *Journal of Community Psychology, 29*(1), 29–52. DOI: 10.1002/1520-6629(200101)29:1<29:aid-jcop3>3.0.co;2-c

Priya, K. R. (2012). Trauma Reactions, Suffering, and Healing among Riot-Affected Internally Displaced Children of Gujarat, India: A Qualitative Inquiry. *Qualitative Research in Psychology, 9*(3), 189–209. DOI: 10.1080/14780887.2010.500353

Qureshi, F., Misra, S., & Poshni, A. (2023). The partition of India through the lens of historical trauma: Intergenerational effects on immigrant health in the South Asian diaspora. *SSM. Mental Health, 4*, 100246. DOI: 10.1016/j.ssmmh.2023.100246

Raguram, R., Venkateswaran, A., Ramakrishna, J., & Weiss, M. G. (2002). Traditional community resources for mental health: A report of temple healing from India. *BMJ (Clinical Research Ed.), 325*(7354), 38–40. DOI: 10.1136/bmj.325.7354.38

Rechsteiner, K., Tol, V., & Maercker, A. (2019). "It should not have happened": Metaphorical expressions, idioms, and narrative descriptions related to trauma in an indigenous community in India. *International Journal of Qualitative Studies on Health and Well-being, 14*(1). Advance online publication. DOI: 10.1080/17482631.2019.1667134

Rich, T., Chrisinger, B. W., Kaimal, R., Winter, S. J., Hedlin, H., Min, Y., Zhao, X., Zhu, S., You, S. L., Sun, C. A., Lin, J. T., Hsing, A. W., & Heaney, C. (2022). Contemplative Practices Behavior Is Positively Associated with Well-Being in Three Global Multi-Regional Stanford WELL for Life Cohorts. *International Journal of Environmental Research and Public Health, 19*(20), 13485. DOI: 10.3390/ijerph192013485

Roberts, L., & Montgomery, S. (2016). Mindfulness-based Intervention for Perinatal Grief Education and Reduction among Poor Women in Chhattisgarh, India: A Pilot Study. *Interdisciplinary Journal of Best Practices in Global Development*, *2*(1), 1.

Rogers, J. M., Ferrari, M., Mosely, K., Lang, C. P., & Brennan, L. (2017). Mindfulness-based interventions for adults who are overweight or obese: A meta-analysis of physical and psychological health outcomes. *Obesity Reviews*, *18*(1), 51–67. DOI: 10.1111/obr.12461

Rowkith, S., & Bhagwan, R. (2020). Honoring Tribal Spirituality in India: An Exploratory Study of Their Beliefs, Rituals and Healing Practices. *Religions*, *11*(11), 549. DOI: 10.3390/rel11110549

Sandberg, B., Hurmerinta, L., & Menzfeld, M. (2024). Volunteerism and community healing. *Community Development (Columbus, Ohio)*, *55*(6), 795–809. DOI: 10.1080/15575330.2023.2301695

Sarason, S. B. (1974). *The psychological sense of community: Prospects for community psychology*. Brookline Books.

Schneider, R. H., Dillbeck, M. C., Yeola, G., & Nader, T. (2024). Peace through health: Traditional medicine meditation in the prevention of collective stress, violence, and war. *Frontiers in Public Health, 12*. Advance online publication. DOI: 10.3389/fpubh.2024.1380626

Schmidt, S. (2004). Mindfulness and healing intention: Concepts, practice, and research evaluation. *Journal of Alternative and Complementary Medicine (New York, N.Y.)*, *10*(Suppl 1), S7–S14. DOI: 10.1089/ACM.2004.10.S-7

S M Sehgal Foundation. (2021, December 29). Community participation in sustainable rural development in india. https://www.smsfoundation.org/role-of-community-participation-and-its-impact-on-sustainability-in-rural/

Shah, R., Gao, Z., & Mittal, H. (2015). Culture. In *Innovation, Entrepreneurship, and the Economy in the US, China, and India* (pp. 55–65). Elsevier. https://doi.org/DOI: 10.1016/B978-0-12-801890-3.00004-6

Sharma, D., & Sharma, B. R. (2024). The impact of yoga and meditation on mental and physical well-being. *Journal of Ayurveda and Integrated Medical Sciences*, *9*(5), 144–153. DOI: 10.21760/jaims.9.5.23

Slemp, G. R., Jach, H. K., Chia, A., Loton, D. J., & Kern, M. L. (2019). Contemplative interventions and employee distress: A meta-analysis. *Stress and Health*, *35*(3), 227–255. DOI: 10.1002/smi.2857

Sood, S. (2018). Cultivating a yogic theology of collective healing: A yogini's journey disrupting white supremacy, hindu fundamentalism, and casteism. *Race and Yoga*, *3*(1). Advance online publication. DOI: 10.5070/R331034279

Theisen-Womersley, G. (2021). *Trauma and resilience among displaced populations*. Springer., DOI: 10.1007/978-3-030-67712-1_13

Telles, S., Singh, N., & Joshi, M. (2010). Post traumatic stress symptoms and heart rate variability in Bihar flood survivors following yoga: A randomized controlled study. *BMC Psychiatry*. Advance online publication. DOI: 10.1186/1471-244X-10-18

Tempone-Wiltshire, J. (2024). The Role of Mindfulness and Embodiment in Group-Based Trauma Treatment. *Psychotherapy and Counselling Journal of Australia*, *12*(1). Advance online publication. DOI: 10.59158/001c.94979

Thomson, G. (2021). Collective Healing: Towards a Conceptual Framework, Genocide Studies and Prevention. *International Journal (Toronto, Ont.)*, *15*(3), 33–48. DOI: 10.5038/1911-9933.15.3.1843

Veerman, A. L., & Ganzevoort, R. R. (2001). Communities Coping with Collective Trauma. *Psychiatry*, *101*, 141–148.

Weisner, L. (2020). Individual and community trauma: Individual experiences in collective environment. Illinois criminal justice information authority center for violence prevention and intervention research. https://researchhub.icjia-api.cloud/uploads/Individual%20and%20Community%20Trauma-%20Individual%20Experiences%20in%20Collective%20Environments-200715T15003405.pdf

West, J., Liang, B., & Spinazzola, J. (2017). Trauma Sensitive Yoga as a complementary treatment for posttraumatic stress disorder: A Qualitative Descriptive analysis. *International Journal of Stress Management*, *24*(2), 173–195. DOI: 10.1037/str0000040

Wisconsin department of health services. (2020). *In This Together: Understanding the Effects of Collective Trauma*. https://www.dhs.wisconsin.gov/publications/p02779.pdf

Woodyard, C. (2011). Exploring the therapeutic effects of yoga and its ability to increase quality of life. *International Journal of Yoga*, *4*(2), 49–54. DOI: 10.4103/0973-6131.85485

Zhou, L., & Xing, H. (2025). Individualization of Religious Rituals and Their Healing Functions in a Mobile Society—Empirical Evidence from China. *Religions*, *16*(4), 521. DOI: 10.3390/rel16040521

Zinner, E. S., & Williams, M. B. (Eds.). (1999). *When a community weeps: Case studies in group survivorship*. Brunner/Mazel.

KEY TERMS AND DEFINITIONS

Collective Trauma: It is the perception of a traumatic event which may be natural, man made, systemic in nature, by a community, resulting in severe cultural, psychological, emotional, physical, economical and ecological implications.

Community Healing: It refers to collaborative recovery from collective trauma by a community by harvesting personal, communal and societal resources.

Community: It refers to a group of people who are connected to each other united through the thread of interpersonal connections based on a common feature.

Contemplative Practices: It is a process which enables self realisation, self regulation and self control through movement, mind training and dialogue resulting in well being of self and the community.

Meditation: It is the practice of focusing on the mind and thoughts and achieving a state of calmness, clarity and wellbeing by eliminating distractions.

Mindfulness: It is the non judgemental awareness of the present moment.

Rituals: These are practices and customs which are symbolic in nature, rooted in culture, social, religious and personal traditions, undertaken to facilitate expression of values, beliefs and connections.

Yoga: It is the integration of self with a higher reality or consciousness through harmony of mind, body and soul.

Chapter 2
Contemplative Classrooms Empowering Youth With Mindfulness, Resilience, and Well-Being Practices:
Through the Philippine Good Manners and Right Conduct and Values Education Curriculum

Marie Grace Avelino Gomez
http://orcid.org/0000-0003-0180-9875
University of the Philippines, Philippines

Jona Kristen M. Valdez
http://orcid.org/0009-0001-2548-8271
Bureau of Curriculum Development, Philippines

Liza C. Legaspino
http://orcid.org/0009-0000-0334-2928
Bureau of Curriculum Development, Philippines

DOI: 10.4018/979-8-2600-1202-4.ch002

ABSTRACT

Filipino learners face rising emotional, psychological, and social challenges that hinder academic success and personal growth. The Good Manners and Right Conduct (GMRC) and Values Education Curriculum provides a foundation for fostering moral integrity, empathy, and social responsibility through contemplative practices that are aligned with Filipino cultural values. This chapter explores how integrating contemplative education practices such as mindfulness, reflection, and compassion into GMRC and Values Education can enhance students' emotional regulation, resilience, and sense of purpose. By examining the curriculum's big ideas, linking virtues to well-being, and proposing culturally grounded strategies, it advocates for "contemplative classrooms" that cultivate focus, empathy, and ethical action in the service of self, community, and nation.

INTRODUCTION

Filipino learners increasingly face emotional, psychological, and social challenges in the ever-evolving educational landscape (Srivastava, 2023). Depression, anxiety, and emotional dysregulation are no longer issues confined to adulthood; they have emerged as pressing concerns among children and adolescents (Puyat et al., 2021), often disrupting their ability to learn, relate, and grow (Serrano et al., 2023). Amid these concerns, the Philippine Values Education and Good Manners and Right Conduct curriculum is a cornerstone in nurturing Filipino learners' moral and emotional development.

The big ideas in the Philippine Good Manners and Right Conduct and Values Education Curriculum nurture mindfulness by encouraging students to be aware of their thoughts, actions, and relationships (Philippine Department of Education, 2023). Concepts like *dignity*, *responsible decision-making*, and *inclination toward goodness* foster self-reflection and emotional regulation, which are essential in building resilience. Through *love* for self, others, family, God, and the environment, students develop compassion and connectedness, supporting their overall well-being. Values such as *love for the nation* and *solidarity with the world* promote a mindful sense of purpose, belonging, and service to others. Altogether, these big ideas guide learners to live with intention, empathy, and strength in both their inner and outer lives.

The Good Manners and Right Conduct and Values Education Curriculum is a vital part of the Philippine basic education system created to promote moral integrity, ethical judgment, and social responsibility among students. Reintroduced as an independent subject through Republic Act No. 11476, The Good Manners and Right Conduct is taught from Kindergarten to Grade 6, while Values Education is included from Grade 7 to Grade 10, and further supported through related subjects such as Life and Career Skills and Philosophy of the Human Person in Senior High School.

At its core, the curriculum aims to develop individuals who embody respect, empathy, discipline, and patriotism. The Good Manners and Right Conduct section emphasizes daily behaviors such as courtesy, honesty, cleanliness, punctuality, and respect for others, all rooted in Filipino cultural values. Lessons are suitable for the developmental stage, allowing children to learn through modeling, role-playing, storytelling, and real-world experiences. In early grades, the focus is on family and community relationships, proper manners, and cooperation.

Values education in higher grades reinforces this foundation by engaging students in moral reasoning, ethical choices, and the exploration of universal and Filipino values. It also addresses pressing contemporary issues such as environmental responsibility, social justice, digital citizenship, and diversity, ensuring that values education stays relevant and adaptable to societal changes.

The curriculum promotes active, reflective learning. Students are not only taught what is right but also guided in understanding *why* certain behaviors and principles matter. This is accomplished through strategies such as classroom discussions, service-learning projects, and collaborative activities that enable values to be practiced in real-world situations.

More importantly, the The Good Manners and Right Conduct and Values Education Curriculum aligns with the holistic goals of the K–12 program: to produce graduates who are not only academically competent but also morally upright, compassionate, and active contributors to nation-building. Teachers are called to serve as role models, integrating values formation into all aspects of the learning environment.

In cultivating respect for human dignity (*dignidad*), a sense of community, and ethical responsibility, the curriculum affirms that education is not solely about intellectual development, but about shaping character and guiding students toward becoming better persons in service of others and society as a whole.

This chapter examines the integration of mindfulness and contemplative practices into the Values Education curriculum, equipping youth with vital tools for emotional regulation, attention, and resilience. By referencing educational theory and practical applications, it advocates for the concept of "contemplative classrooms," which combine values-based education with mindful awareness, emotional literacy, and psychological well-being.

Integrating Contemplative Education into the GMRC and Values Education Curriculum

Contemplative education offers powerful tools to deepen the impact of the Good Manners and Right Conduct and Values Education Curriculum by cultivating inner awareness, emotional intelligence, and authentic moral action. At its core, contemplative education emphasizes mindful presence, reflection, and compassion, qualities that resonate strongly with the goals of character and values formation.

In Good Manners and Right Conduct, contemplative activities like guided breathing, quiet reflection, or brief moments of stillness before and after lessons can help students focus their attention and minimize impulsive actions. These practices encourage learners to pause and consider their responses, strengthening values like patience, respect, and self-control. Through reflective journaling or storytelling, children can examine how their choices relate to values such as honesty, cooperation, and kindness.

In these subjects, contemplative education deepens self-awareness by guiding learners to examine their beliefs, emotions, and actions. Activities such as perspective-taking exercises and empathy walks foster compassion and understanding of diverse experiences, making values like *pakikipagkapwa* and *malasakit* more personal and lived. Discussions can be complemented with mindful listening practices, teaching students to give full attention and respect to others' voices.

By linking reflection to concrete actions, such as service-learning projects or community engagement, students learn that values are not abstract concepts but guiding principles for daily life. Mindfulness-based focus activities, such as observing the environment with full attention, help counteract the distractions of digital life, allowing learners to engage more deeply with lessons and relationships.

Ultimately, integrating contemplative education into GMRC and Values Education ensures that students do not simply memorize moral codes but internalize and embody them. It nurtures a generation capable of thoughtful decision-making, compassionate action, and responsible citizenship and graduates who live out values not only in the classroom but in the broader community and nation.

Purpose of the Chapter

This chapter has the following objectives:

1. Describe the current issues that warrant for mindfulness, resilience, and well-being practices among the Filipino youth.
2. Discuss how the Philippine GMRC and values education curriculum can help foster mindfulness, resilience, and well-being.
3. Identify how mindfulness, resilience, and well-being are locally operationalized in the big ideas of the Philippine GMRC and values education curriculum.
4. Identify how the virtues of the Philippine GMRC and values education curriculum foster mindfulness, resilience, and well-being.
5. Recommend strategies to integrate mindfulness, resilience, and well-being in the curriculum within Filipino cultural context.

This chapter presents a comprehensive argument for integrating well-being practices into the Filipino education system. It begins by identifying the pressing challenges faced by Filipino youth today—digital overload from social media, academic pressure, and economic uncertainty—all of which contribute to anxiety, burnout, and social disconnection. These realities underscore the need for educational interventions that nurture emotional and psychological well-being alongside academic achievement.

The chapter then positions the existing GMRC and Values Education curriculum as a natural foundation for this integration. Rather than introducing new programs, it proposes enhancing current frameworks that already emphasize moral and character formation. By expanding lessons on virtues and right conduct to include mindfulness, resilience, and emotional literacy, schools can cultivate students' inner development and holistic growth.

Next, the chapter connects modern psychological concepts with Filipino cultural values. It explains that mindfulness aligns with *malasakit* (attentive compassion) and resilience reflects *bayanihan* (collective strength). These parallels ensure cultural relevance and accessibility, fostering genuine engagement among students.

Practical applications are also detailed. Core virtues such as *paggalang* (respect), *pagpapakumbaba* (humility), and *pagmamahal sa pamilya* (love for family) are linked to well-being skills like mindful listening, acceptance, and emotional regulation.

Finally, the chapter offers actionable recommendations for educators and policymakers—suggesting reflective journaling, storytelling, and brief mindfulness activities within daily routines. By aligning psychological practices with Filipino values, the education system can promote resilience, compassion, and well-being among students in a culturally grounded way.

CONTEXTUALIZING WELL-BEING IN PHILIPPINE EDUCATION

In recent years, the Filipino youth have found themselves navigating a rapidly shifting world marred by deep and complex challenges (Ballaret, 2024). Beyond the typical demands of adolescence, they now face rising levels of anxiety and depression, often compounded by the harsher realities of poverty, disintegrating family structures, and frequent natural calamities (Edyburn & Meek, 2021). Typhoons regularly displace entire communities, while many children go to school with empty stomachs, broken homes, or are orphaned because a parent might have drowned in a flash flood. For this generation, "problems of living" are not abstract; they are lived experiences that leave emotional scars and erode hope.

The modern Filipino youth face a combination of challenges that highlight the urgent need for mental health and well-being practices (Alejandria et al., 2023). A major and increasing concern is the rise of anxiety and depression (Daly & Robinson, 2022). These issues are often driven by intense academic pressure, social comparison on digital platforms, and a widespread sense of uncertainty about the future (Qiu, 2024. For many, the constant connection through social media creates an environment where validation is sought externally, leading to feelings of inadequacy and loneliness (Cao et al., 2025).

Beyond these psychosocial stressors are the deeply entrenched problems of living, particularly poverty and the devastating impact of natural calamities. Poverty affects a young person's sense of security and self-worth, leading to chronic stress that can manifest as mental and physical health issues. The daily struggle for basic needs can overshadow personal development and emotional growth, making it difficult for youth to focus on their well-being. Furthermore, living in one of the world's most disaster-prone countries means that many Filipino youth have experienced the trauma and disruption caused by typhoons, earthquakes, and volcanic eruptions. The constant threat of these events, and the prolonged recovery periods that follow, can lead to post-traumatic stress and a persistent feeling of instability.

These compounded issues, from internal emotional struggles to external socioeconomic and environmental threats, create a compelling case for educational interventions. Incorporating mindfulness, resilience, and well-being practices into the curriculum is essential not only to help youth cope with these realities but also to equip them with the skills to navigate a complex world with greater emotional strength and a sense of purpose.

Within this context, education must serve not only as a means to academic achievement but as a sanctuary that cultivates resilience, empathy, and meaning. It must be a space that recognizes the whole child, not just the mind, but also the heart. This is where Republic Act 11476, also known as the Good Manners and Right Conduct (GMRC) and Values Education Act, enters the conversation. Passed in 2020, this legislation marked a renewed commitment to values formation as a key component of basic education in the Philippines. By mandating the daily teaching of GMRC and values education from Kindergarten to Grade 6 and continuing through Junior and Senior High School, the law seeks to instill in learners respect, responsibility, compassion, and nationalism.

While this legislative move is commendable, the implementation of the GMRC and Values Education Curriculum must be more than just a return to moralistic instruction or rote memorization of virtues. It must evolve to respond meaningfully to the lived realities of our youth. The real-life challenges they face—such as anxiety over academic pressure, depression linked to social disconnection or economic deprivation, or trauma from experiencing disasters—call for a more emotionally-attuned and holistic pedagogy.

Holistic education acknowledges that intellectual growth is deeply intertwined with emotional and moral development (Ramaila, 2025). It respects the child as a complex being whose experiences, relationships, and mental health directly impact their ability to learn Webster, 2022). An emotionally-attuned pedagogy, therefore, does not merely teach "what is right" but creates safe spaces for young people to express vulnerability, process difficult emotions, and build inner strength (Brown, 2025).

This can be done by integrating mental health awareness and emotional literacy into values education. Instead of focusing solely on obedience and politeness, lessons can also explore how to manage stress, develop empathy, resolve conflicts peacefully, and practice mindfulness. For instance, a GMRC class includes activities that help students identify their emotions, build gratitude journals, or reflect on how kindness can transform their school community. This is elaborated on thoroughly in Grade 2 and Grade 8. In addition to this, teachers can be trained not just as instructors, but as compassionate mentors who can recognize signs of distress and refer students to appropriate support systems.

Moreover, a values education curriculum reflects the Filipino cultural context, drawing from local stories of resilience, bayanihan, and *pakiki-pagkapwa*. When students see their own struggles mirrored in the lessons, values become more than abstract ideals. The lessons become real life solutions to their problems. They become tools for surviving and thriving. Through storytelling, reflection, community projects, and dialogue, learners can build a strong moral foundation grounded in both tradition and personal relevance.

Ultimately, addressing the mental and emotional well-being of Filipino youth requires an education system that sees well-being not as a side concern, but as central to learning. It is not enough to teach values; we must model them in how we teach, listen, and build community within our classrooms. Equipping the youth with problem solving skills can enable them to be more resilient to the changing tim4s.

In a nation vulnerable to disasters, both literal and metaphorical, the Philippines' young citizens need more than academic knowledge. They need guidance, connection, and hope. The GMRC and Values Education Act offers an avenue where these are actualized. Now, it is up to educators, school leaders, and policymakers to build on it with compassionate, context-sensitive, and holistic practices that empower the Filipino youth to not only cope with life's challenges, but to rise above them.

UNDERSTANDING CONTEMPLATIVE EDUCATION

In a world characterized by rapid technological progress, socio-political instability, and rising psychological stress, the purpose of education is being reimagined beyond its traditional roles. While academic success and cognitive growth remain important, educators, psychologists, and philosophers are asking deeper questions: How do we nurture the whole person? How do we help learners develop presence, purpose, and inner peace amid constant noise and pressure?

This is where contemplative education enters the landscape. Contemplative Education is a growing movement in global education that seeks to balance intellectual rigor with inner transformation (Dutta & Vimal, 2025). Contemplative education integrates practices such as mindfulness, compassion, and self-awareness into teaching and learning processes (Chaptman, 2021). Its goal is not just to improve academic outcomes but to cultivate the heart and mind in ways that foster ethical, reflective, and emotionally balanced individuals (Alam, 2022).

Contemplative education is a pedagogical approach that integrates introspection and reflective practices into learning environments (Karas, 2021). Rooted in both ancient spiritual traditions and modern psychology, it encourages learners and educators to connect deeply with their inner lives while engaging meaningfully with the outer world (Bruce Martin, 2022).

At its core, contemplative education seeks to cultivate attention, emotional stability, empathy, and insight (Van Gordon et al., 2022). These qualities are vital for both personal growth and social harmony. Instead of merely focusing on transmitting knowledge, it encourages learners to pause, breathe, reflect, and become aware of their thoughts, feelings, and actions (Bak, 2025).

This approach does not promote any particular religion (Ross & Rocha Beardall, 2022). Instead, it uses secular practices that often derived from meditation, yoga, journaling, silence, deep listening, or mindful movement to deepen awareness and cultivate a more holistic learning experience (Flanagan & Clough, 2024). Its application ranges from preschool to tertiary education and across diverse cultural and educational settings (Lau, 2024).

Core Elements of Contemplative Education

Contemplative education is underpinned by several interconnected elements. Among the most prominent are mindfulness, compassion, and self-awareness.

Mindfulness refers to paying attention in a specific way: deliberately, in the present moment, and without judgment (Čopelj, 2022). In the classroom, mindfulness can be introduced through breathing exercises, mindful listening, or brief moments of silence or reflection before or after lessons (Scherer et al., 2021). The research by Alvear et al. (2022) shows that major studies on mindfulness focus on seven themes: (1) mindfulness as attention or awareness; (2) mindfulness as a non-evaluative attitude; (3) mindfulness as a strategy; (4) mindfulness through a theoretical lens; (5) mindfulness as a psycho-affective-spiritual state; (6) mindfulness as personal development; and (7) lack of understanding about mindfulness.

From these themes, it can be inferred that the collected definitions are more aligned with the scientific-academic view of mindfulness than with the academic-Buddhist perspective (Alvear et al., 2020).

In contemplative education, mindfulness practice helps students become aware of their thoughts and feelings without being overwhelmed (Vilvens et al., 2021). It enhances concentration, emotional regulation, and even resilience (Mumtazah, 2024). Teachers, likewise, benefit from mindfulness by becoming more attuned to their students' needs and managing their own stress more effectively (Carroll et al., 2022).

Compassion, the ability to recognize others' suffering and respond with kindness, is a fundamental part of contemplative education (Gilbert & Van Gordon, 2023). Unlike abstract moral lessons, contemplative education fosters compassion through real-life experiences, such as group reflections, gratitude exercises, and community service, which help learners connect with others' perspectives (Gardner, 2021).

Compassion-based education fosters inclusive classrooms, reduces bullying, and promotes prosocial behaviors (Sowmya, 2025). It encourages students to be not just intelligent, but kind—to recognize their shared humanity and act with integrity (Iloka, 2025). The Good Manners and Right Conduct and Values Education Curriculum emphasizes on *mabuting kilos loob* (the volition to do good) in decision making and relating with people.

Self-awareness is the ability to reflect on one's thoughts, emotions, and motivations. It is a vital component of personal growth, ethical decision-making, and leadership (Andres, 2025). Contemplative education creates spaces for students to develop this inner clarity through journaling, dialogue circles, and reflective questioning (Chaptman, 2021). It allows students to recognize their learning styles, emotional triggers, and values (Bak, 2025). It empowers them to make conscious choices and to engage in learning as a process of self-discovery (Crasta & Dmello, 2024).

Research on Contemplative Practice

Research on contemplative practice in education underscores its multidimensional benefits across cognitive, emotional, and social domains. Ross and Beardall (2022) found that students exposed to contemplative practices learn to accept suffering with insight rather than resignation, fostering wisdom and emotional maturity. By integrating introspection with academic inquiry, contemplative learning cultivates empathy, purpose, and intellectual depth, producing students who are emotionally grounded and socially aware.

In a study by Vilven et al. (2021), mindfulness and contemplative activities integrated into a college personal health course yielded significant emotional benefits. While emotional satisfaction showed the most notable improvement ($p = .048$), students also reported reduced stress, enhanced calmness, focus, and mood. Even brief interventions such as guided visualization left 90% of participants feeling "peaceful" and "refreshed." These results suggest that mindfulness fosters emotional regulation, mental clarity, and academic readiness—skills vital for managing modern stressors.

Gunnlaugson et al. (2022) expanded this framework through second-person contemplative approaches, emphasizing shared awareness and relational dialogue. Such practices encourage presence, deep listening, and empathy, strengthening classroom community and ethical engagement. This relational form of mindfulness transforms learning into an embodied, interconnected process that unites intellectual rigor with compassion and authenticity.

Similarly, Gardner (2021) documented transformative learning through contemplative practices in an intergenerational service-learning project. Reflection writing, embodied activities, and mindfulness helped students connect experience with theory, developing empathy and a clearer sense of self and purpose.

Collectively, these studies highlight that contemplative education builds resilience and compassion—essential traits amid mental health crises and global uncertainty. As Toukan and Tawil (2024) assert, such education aligns with trauma-informed, well-being-centered pedagogy. In the Philippine context, where communities face poverty, disasters, and social challenges, contemplative practices cultivate focus, adaptability, and hope. They empower learners to respond to adversity with mindfulness and moral clarity, reinforcing education as both an academic and humanizing endeavor.

Sherab & Schuelka's (2023) nationwide study examines how Bhutan's philosophy Gross National Happiness (GNH) shapes student well-being and contemplative dispositions in schools. The findings suggest that embedding GNH values in curricula, school culture, and pedagogical practices nurtures mindfulness, emotional balance, and social harmony among students. Students report greater awareness of interdependence, more reflective attitudes, and enhanced resilience in the face of academic and life pressures. The research highlights both successes and paradoxes: while many schools foster well-being through the GNH framework, uneven implementation, reliance on traditional academic norms, and teacher capacity gaps limit its full impact. The chapter argues that genuine integration of GNH into education can meaningfully promote student mindfulness, holistic well-being, and character development (Sherab & Schuelka, 2023).

Ultimately, contemplative education redefines learning as a holistic, humanizing process that unites intellectual depth with emotional wisdom. It prepares students not only for academic achievement but also for purposeful, compassionate living in an increasingly complex world.

Benefits of Contemplative Practice in Addressing Mental Health and Health Issues Across the Lifespan

Mental health issues like mood and anxiety issues are prevalent. Due to high levels od stress, some chronic diseases also emerge during adult years. Contemplative practice has benefits on mental and overall health across the lifespan. Studies suggest significant improvement in mood, reduced emotional reactivity, and increased health benefits.

The pilot randomized controlled trial of Sofianopoulou et al. (2021) explored a 12-week stress-management intervention for elementary school students, combining diaphragmatic breathing and contemplative practices. The program aimed to lower stress responses and improve emotional regulation. Compared to control, participating students demonstrated significant reductions in self-reported stress markers, including fewer intrusive thoughts, diminished physiological arousal, and reduced emotional reactivity. Qualitative responses also indicated that students felt calmer, more centered, and better able to manage tension in their daily lives. The results suggest that even relatively brief contemplative training in an elementary context can foster internal regulation and resilience, offering promise for integrating mindfulness and breathing techniques into school curricula to support student mental health and well-being (Sofianopoulou et al., 2021).

Doddiah et al. (2021) evaluated a mindfulness-based intervention implemented among high school students to assess its effects on mental health outcomes. Across the intervention period, students showed significant reductions in perceived stress, anxiety, and depressive symptoms; concomitantly, levels of trait mindfulness increased. Qualitative feedback indicated enhanced emotional regulation, self-awareness, and coping skills in daily academic pressures. The findings suggest that even in adolescent populations under high academic and social stress, mindfulness training can bolster psychological resilience and reduce internal distress. The authors recommend integrating mindfulness practices into secondary school curricula as a preventive mental health strategy and call for longer-term, controlled research to confirm sustained benefits and examine underlying mechanisms (Doddiah et al., 2021).

The study of Fedewa et al. (2022) evaluates the effects of an eight-week Mindfulness-Based Stress Reduction (MBSR) program applied to elementary school teachers. Using a randomized pretest-posttest control design with seven teachers and 124 students, the authors found that teachers receiving MBSR significantly increased their in-class use of mindfulness techniques and experienced marked reductions in perceived stress (pre: 24.33 vs. post: 13.67; $p = .001$) and anxiety (pre: 99.00 vs. post: 59.33; $p = .001$). However, measured changes in student-teacher relationship quality and students' self-reported mindfulness were not statistically significant. While the intervention clearly improved teacher well-being, evidence for immediate student benefits was limited. The authors conclude that mindfulness practices in elementary contexts may deliver health benefits by alleviating educator stress and anxiety, potentially improving classroom climate over time, though more research is required to verify direct student effects (Fedewa et al., 2022).

For adults, the meta-analysis article of Fisher et al. (2023) presents a systematic review and meta-analysis investigating the effectiveness of MBSR on mental health, mindfulness, and glycemic control (HbA1c) in people with diabetes. Eleven studies ($n = 718$) were synthesized, and nine were included in the meta-analysis. The results indicate that MBSR produces large effect sizes in reducing anxiety and depressive symptoms and enhancing levels of mindfulness both at post-intervention and follow-up. However, stress reduction was significant primarily at follow-up, not immediately post-intervention, and MBSR did not show a statistically significant effect on HbA1c in either post or follow-up assessments. Thus, while MBSR may not directly influence blood glucose markers in diabetes, the practice offers substantial improvements in psychological well-being, emotional regulation, and trait mindfulness among diabetic patients. The authors recommend that future research incorporate biological measures (e.g., cortisol) to understand better mechanisms linking mindfulness, stress, and metabolic health (Fisher et al., 2023)

Challenges of Implementing GMRC and Values Education

The implementation of Values Education and GMRC in Philippine schools faces several challenges that affect its effectiveness One major challenge is the lack of adequately trained teachers. Many educators handling Values Education or GMRC are not specialists in the field and may have a limited background in moral philosophy, psychology, or character education pedagogy. Though there are government efforts to provide scholarships, there is still a big gap that needs to be filled. As a result, lessons in some schools sometimes become purely theoretical or overly reliant on rote memorization instead of reflective and experiential learning.

The school environment and societal influences also pose barriers. Even when desirable virtues and contemplative practices are taught in the classroom, these can be undermined by negative behaviors observed in society, such as corruption, bullying, drug use or online disrespect. Without consistent modeling from teachers, parents, and community members, students may struggle to internalize what they learn. Further, rural and underserved schools, locally called last mile schools, located in geographically isolated and disadvantaged areas (GIDA) have challenges when it comes to resource materials in GMRC and Values Education as there are limited internet facilities. Worse, some of these schools do not even have electricity.

Finally, there is the challenge of assessment. Measuring moral development and contemplative practice is inherently complex, as it involves attitudes, behaviors, and decision-making rather than simple factual recall. Development of rubrics is necessary, but many schools rely on written tests, which fail to capture authentic demonstrations of character and ethical reasoning. Addressing these challenges requires continuous teacher training, integration of values across subjects, strong home-school partnerships, and school-wide initiatives that model and celebrate good character. Only through collective effort can Values Education and GMRC truly shape morally upright and compassionate Filipino learners.

APPLICATIONS AND STRATEGIES FOR THE GOOD MANNERS AND RIGHT CONDUCT AND VALUES EDUCATION CURRICULUM

Contemplative education is not a one-size-fits-all model. It can be adapted to suit different age groups, cultural settings, and curricular demands. Some practical applications include:

In a GMRC and Values Education class, a teacher starts each day with a Mindful Minute. The students close their eyes, focus on their breath, and center themselves before the day's lessons begin. This simple practice sets a calm and attentive tone for the classroom, helping students transition from the hustle of the hallway to a space of quiet reflection. The teacher can also let the class reflect on a good deed that they have done during the day or the day before, and ask the different positive emotions that it evoked. Through this, the class starts on a positive note.

Throughout the week, the teacher provides journaling prompts that encourage students to explore their feelings and values. For instance, a prompt might be, "Write about a time you felt grateful for a friend's help." Or, "What was one problem in life that you were able to triumph over? What strategies helped you? Who helped you? How did you feel after you have triumphed over the problem?" This practice allows students to process emotions, understand their motivations, and clarify their personal values. The journals are not graded for content, but for the effort of self-reflection, making them a safe space for honest exploration.

To deepen their understanding of empathy and community, the class engages in Deep Listening activities during group discussions. Students are instructed to listen to a classmate speak without interrupting or responding. Listening should be done without judgment or prejudice. After the speaker is done, a few moments of silence are observed before anyone else speaks. This technique teaches students the value of active listening and helps them to hear and understand different perspectives truly.

Classes could also include a Gratitude Circle once a week. Students take turns sharing one thing they are grateful for in their Good Manners and Right Conduct or Values Education Classes. This simple act cultivates a positive classroom environment and reminds students to appreciate the good in their lives, no matter how small. They also keep an Acts of Kindness Journal, where they record kind actions they have performed or witnessed, further reinforcing the values of compassion and service. These techniques, inspired by contemplative education, move beyond theoretical discussions of values and provide students with practical tools to cultivate self-awareness, empathy, and positive social behavior, making GMRC and Values Education a truly transformative experience.

In a time when students are overwhelmed by stress and distractions, contemplative education reminds us that silence, reflection, and connection are not luxuries, they are necessities. The classroom must become a sanctuary not only for knowledge but for presence, humanity, and inner peace.

Integrating Contemplative Education into the Big Ideas of the Good Manners and Right Conduct and Values Education Curriculum

The following are the Big Ideas of the Philippine Good Manners and Right Conduct and Values Education Curriculum with suggested activities to integrate contemplative education:

1. Dignidad (Dignity)

Dignidad refers to the inherent worth and equality of every person, which is the foundation of just and respectful relationships. It emphasizes that each individual, regardless of status, ability, or background, deserves to be treated with fairness and compassion. Recognizing and upholding dignity fosters empathy, mutual respect, and a culture of human rights in both personal and social life.

Contemplative activity: *Guided Mindfulness on Equality*

Procedure: Students close their eyes and are guided to imagine a circle where all people, regardless of background, are seated together. The teacher prompts them to notice shared human needs and emotions. Afterward, students journal about how dignity shapes relationships in their lives. This reflective practice nurtures empathy and reinforces equality as a lived value.

2. Mapanagutang Pagpapasya (Responsible Decision-Making)

The Good Manners and Right Curriculum and Values Education frames Mapanagutang Pagpapasya as a deliberate and thoughtful process that extends beyond a simple choice. It emphasizes the need for students to practice discernment and critically consider potential consequences before acting, ensuring their choices align with core values. Ultimately, this approach cultivates accountability by preparing students to face the responsibilities that come with their decisions, thus building integrity and character.

Contemplative activity: *Pause and Reflect Technique*

Procedure: Before making group decisions in class (e.g., project choices), students are guided to take three deep breaths, silently recall past choices, and visualize possible outcomes. This practice strengthens discernment and helps them connect decisions with accountability for results.

3. Pagkiling sa Kabutihan (Inclination toward Goodness)

Pagkiling sa Kabutihan is the active practice of ethical behavior, not just the knowledge of it. It is shaped by self-awareness and a deep understanding of what is good and right. This concept is cultivated through reflection on life experiences and the nature of being human, making goodness a conscious and intentional choice.

Contemplative activity: *Ethics Meditation*

Students reflect on a personal situation where they had to choose between right and wrong. They use a quiet, structured journaling exercise to explore how their feelings, values, and reflections influenced their choice. This builds moral awareness and habits of ethical reflection.

4. Pagmamahal (Love)

Contemplative activity: *Loving-Kindness Meditation*

Adapted for young learners, students are guided to silently wish well for themselves, a friend, a stranger, and even someone they find difficult to get along with. This softens resentment, cultivates compassion, and strengthens the habit of altruism.

5. Pagmamahal sa Diyos (Love for God)

Contemplative activity: *Silent Gratitude Prayer*

Procedure: Students spend a few minutes in silence, recalling three blessings they experienced that day. They then express their gratitude through prayer, writing, or a symbolic gesture. This strengthens spiritual connection and integrates faith with everyday awareness.

6. Pagmamahal sa Pamilya (Love for Family)

Filipinos value their families. *Pagmamahal sa Pamilya* is a nurturing expression of interpersonal care that begins within the household and extends beyond it. It serves as the foundation of the nation and is expressed by supporting the family's needs and cultivating values among its members. This concept emphasizes the importance of preserving family stability through conscious acts of love and care. When family ties are strong, students will be able to have a strong support system to help them with life's difficulties.

Contemplative activity: *Family Appreciation Circle*

Procedure: Students create a gratitude list naming the ways their family members support them. In silence, they visualize moments of family care, then write short notes of appreciation to share at home. This fosters a deeper sense of connection and reciprocity within the family.

7. Pagmamahal sa Kapwa (Love for Others)

Pagmamahal sa Kapwa is viewed as the highest form of human relationship and moral development. It is demonstrated through altruism and a genuine concern for the well-being of others, transforming empathy into concrete acts of service. This concept emphasizes that true love is not just a feeling but is shown through actions that prioritize the needs and dignity of others.

Contemplative activity: *Service Reflection Journal*

Procedure: After participating in a community or peer-help activity, students sit quietly and reflect on how their actions affected others and themselves. They write about lessons learned and feelings experienced, deepening their sense of solidarity and shared humanity.

8. Pagmamahal sa Kalikasan (Love for Nature)

Pagmamahal sa Kalikasan fosters a sense of responsibility and stewardship toward the environment. It is expressed through being a good caretaker of the natural world. This concept emphasizes that our actions today are crucial for preserving the environment for future generations.

Contemplative activity: *Mindful Nature Walk*

Procedure: Students are taken outdoors (or shown nature videos if outdoors is not possible) and guided to notice details—the texture of leaves, the sound of birds, the scent of flowers. Afterward, they discuss how this awareness leads to care for the environment.

9. Pagmamalasakit sa Kapaligiran (Concern for the Environment)

Pagmamalasakit sa Kapaligiran is the active participation in maintaining the cleanliness and order of one's surroundings. It is a commitment to the well-being and health of all living beings, including humans, plants, and animals. This concept emphasizes that concern for the environment is not passive but requires concrete, collective action to create a healthy living space for all.

Contemplative activity: *Eco-Responsibility Visualization*

Procedure: Students visualize their community in two scenarios: one where the environment is cared for and another where it is neglected. They then write commitments for personal eco-friendly actions. This visualization links awareness to practical stewardship.

10. Pagmamahal sa Bayan (Love for the Nation)

Pagmamahal sa Bayan is the conscious effort to embody Filipino values and contribute to the nation's progress. It involves prioritizing the collective interests and common good over personal gain. This concept emphasizes that love for the nation is not merely a feeling but a commitment to uplifting Filipino culture and promoting national development through one's actions.

Contemplative activity: *Silent Tribute and Reflection on Heroes*

Procedure: Students view a short presentation on Filipino heroes, then sit quietly imagining themselves upholding similar values in modern times. They journal specific ways they can contribute to the nation's development, making patriotism a personal commitment.

11. Pakikiisa sa Daigdig (Solidarity with the World)

Pakikiisa sa Daigdig (Solidarity with the World) is both an individual and collective commitment to promoting international laws and policies for the universal good. It extends the values of love and concern beyond national borders to embrace the entire global community. This concept emphasizes that our actions have a worldwide impact, calling for unity on issues like peace, justice, and environmental protection.

Contemplative activity: *Global Connection Meditation*

Procedure: Students reflect on how their actions, like conserving water or practicing kindness, can have effects beyond their own community. They visualize themselves as part of a larger global family, reinforcing unity for peace, justice, and sustainability.

Peace education can also be integrated as a contemplative practice wherein students can identify strategies to minimize conflict and increase cooperation among themselves. Hopefully, when these students become adults, they will employ the same peace-making strategies with the people around them.

Dignity as a core value in GMRC (Good Manners and Right Conduct) and Values Education can be deeply nurtured through contemplative education, which emphasizes reflection, mindfulness, and lived experience. By engaging students in structured opportunities to pause, notice, and reflect, they can develop self-awareness by becoming aware of their own values, biases, and daily actions. Activities such as guided journaling or silent reflection after classroom scenarios allow them to examine how their choices align with the respect and dignity they want to maintain.

Contemplative practices also enhance empathy by encouraging students to practice perspective-taking. Activities like role-playing, storytelling from diverse voices, and reflective dialogues help learners imagine others' experiences, fostering compassion and reducing prejudice. Through these practices, they begin to see dignity not just as an abstract idea but as a lived reality that requires care and fairness for everyone.

Mindful breathing exercises, silent observation, or nature walks can help enhance focus and presence, counteracting the distraction-heavy environment of modern life. This attentiveness supports deeper listening and more respectful interactions, which are vital to honoring dignity.

Moral grounding develops when reflection is connected to action, and students are encouraged to turn insights into practical acts of kindness, fairness, and advocacy. Finally, incorporating contemplative strategies into daily school routines, such as sincere greetings, mindful transitions, or ending the day with gratitude for classroom experiences, helps ensure that values are not only discussed but also embodied consistently.

EFFECTS OF VALUES EDUCATION ON STUDENTS

Values Education has lasting effects on students. Guerero and Estera's (2025) qualitative study explores the influence of Values Education's contemplative practice on students' classroom behavior through insights from teachers at a Philippine high school. Teachers report that when values are taught using real-life stories, participatory learning, and reflective practices, students show improved ethical behavior and moral reasoning, greater self-control, and increased responsibility. Values lessons also enhance social competencies such as empathy, cooperation, and respectful interactions. Although some learners perceive Values Education as less important than core subjects, the teachers observed meaningful behavioral changes: reduced disruptive conduct, more conscientious decision-making, and a classroom climate marked by respect and moral awareness. The findings underscore that Values Education can meaningfully shape conduct and character when delivered thoughtfully and reinforced across contexts (Guerero and Estera, 2025).

The study of E. Gomez (2024) explores the importance of Values Education in shaping students' academic, social, and personal growth. Through in-depth interviews and focus group discussions with elementary students and teachers, the research uncovers how personal values influence learning strategies, scholastic performance, and overall character. Three major themes emerge: Personal Development (e.g. responsibility, diligence, positive outlook), Academic Development (improved study habits, motivation), and Social Development (social harmony, acceptance of diversity). Key practices include creating supportive classroom environments, promoting cultural understanding, and involving the whole school community. Positive outcomes reported span emotional, psychological, social, spiritual, and educational gains. The study concludes that Values Education is crucial not only for academic success but also for developing morally upright, socially competent, and emotionally balanced individuals (Gomez, 2024).

Values Education teachers also found benefits to teaching this subject. Villasanta (2022) examined how a Values Education teacher navigated the integration of mindfulness practice into her pedagogical identity. Over time, the teacher's mindfulness practice nurtured a more introspective voice, enabling her to slow, listen, and attend to internal as well as relational dynamics in teaching. This shift fostered greater self-awareness, emotional attunement, and reflective responsiveness in the classroom. The findings suggest that mindfulness can reorient a teacher's stance, from reacting habitually to engaging more mindfully and support the development of an authentic pedagogical presence grounded in contemplative awareness (Villasanta, 2022).

Aligning with Filipino Values: Kagandahang-Loob, Pakikipagkapwa, and Malasakit

One of the most powerful aspects of developing mindfulness and resilience through GMRC is how naturally these practices align with Filipino cultural values. At the core of mindfulness is *kagandahang-loob*, or the inner goodness of a person, a moral sense that guides one's thoughts, feelings, and actions. When learners pause in silence, reflect on their experiences, and practice being fully present, they become more in tune with their *loob* (inner self). This self-knowledge becomes the foundation for moral discernment and authentic relationships.

Pakikipagkapwa-tao, another core value of Filipino culture, is brought to life through mindfulness and empathy exercises. For instance, when students take part in "listening circles," where each child gets a chance to speak while others listen quietly, they learn to respect each other's voices. They become witnesses to one another's pain, joy, and humanity—building a fellowship that goes beyond mere tolerance and moves into compassionate understanding.

Meanwhile, *malasakit* encourages students to act on their awareness, not merely to feel compassion, but to turn that compassion into helpful action. Malasakit is a concious effort to care for another person. Values Education lessons that include acts of service, peer support, or small classroom responsibilities allow learners to embody this value. As students become more mindful of their surroundings and the needs of others, they develop a sense of agency rooted in empathy.

Assessment of Values Formation and Contemplative Practice

Assessment of values formation and contemplative practices requires comprehensive and authentic approaches that capture students' internal growth, behavior, and moral reasoning. Rubrics and observation records play a vital role in ensuring that these assessments are systematic and truly reflect real-world application. Through reflective journals, portfolios, and essays, teachers can use rubrics to evaluate the depth of reflection, empathy, and ethical awareness. Likewise, teacher observations and anecdotal records enable educators to document behavioral indicators such as kindness, cooperation, and emotional regulation during classroom interactions.

Behavioral assessments such as role-plays and service-learning projects can also be rated using rubrics focused on decision-making, responsibility, and compassion, providing tangible evidence of moral action. Self- and peer assessments further encourage students to evaluate their own and others' growth in mindfulness and interpersonal respect. In addition, standardized tools like the Mindful Attention Awareness Scale for Children (MAAS-C) or VIA Character Strengths Inventory can complement qualitative data by measuring levels of mindfulness and character development.

Ultimately, a combination of rubric-based evaluations and structured observation records ensures that assessment in values education and contemplative practices remains both measurable and meaningful, highlighting not only cognitive understanding of values, but also the lived expression of mindfulness, empathy, and moral behavior.

A Call for Compassionate, Emotionally-Attuned Education

In the face of rising mental health concerns, cultivating mindfulness and emotional regulation is not a luxury—it is a necessity. Mindfulness gives children and youth a toolkit for navigating emotions, making sense of their inner world, and responding with care and wisdom.

More than just a strategy for managing behavior, contemplative education speaks to the heart of human development. It empowers learners to become not just smarter, but wiser; not just efficient, but compassionate; not just reactive, but reflective.

As educators, parents, and policymakers embrace whole-child approaches, contemplatife education must become an integral part of educational design. The science is clear: when we teach children to be contmplative, we teach them to be resilient, regulated, and ready for school, for relationships, and for life.

CONCLUSION: CULTIVATING THE WHOLE CHILD THROUGH THE GMRC AND VALUES EDUCATION CURRICULUM

Good Manners and Right Conduct and Values Education is not just a curriculum enhancement but is a moral imperative. In nurturing the inner lives of students, educators fulfill one of their deepest roles: to guide children not only toward knowledge, but toward wisdom, character, and peace.

By aligning these life skills with Filipino values such as *kagandahang-loob*, *pakikipagkapwa*, and *malasakit*, Filipino educators can ensure that our approach is both effective and culturally authentic. Through storytelling, reflection, and silence, we give learners the tools to explore their thoughts, manage their emotions, and connect with others compassionately.

Ultimately, educators are not just teaching values but enable the student to live them in every interaction, every activity, and every quiet moment. In

CHALLENGES IN PROMOTING MINDFULNESS, RESILIENCE, AND WELL-BEING IN EDUCATION

The growing call to integrate contemplative education practice into the fabric of education is a response to rising mental health concerns, student disengagement, and the broader need to support whole-child development. Across the globe and particularly in the Philippines, educators, policymakers, and parents are beginning to see the value of helping students not just excel academically, but also grow into emotionally balanced and morally grounded individuals. However, while the benefits of this movement are clear, the path to implementation is not without its challenges.

From cultural sensitivities to issues of accessibility and inclusion, and the need for robust teacher training and capacity-building, the endeavor of promoting mindfulness and well-being in schools must be approached with critical thoughtfulness and cultural responsiveness. Acknowledging and addressing these challenges is necessary not to halt the momentum of change, but to strengthen its foundations and ensure that no child or educator is left behind.

Cultural Sensitivities Around Mindfulness, Resilience, and Well-Being

One of the most complex challenges in promoting mindfulness and well-being in education lies in navigating cultural attitudes and beliefs. Mindfulness, for example, often has roots in Buddhist meditation practices and Eastern philosophies. While this may align well with some cultural contexts, it may raise skepticism or discomfort in others, particularly in deeply religious societies such as the Philippines, where Catholic and Christian teachings are dominant.

There have been instances when mindfulness activities like silent meditation or breathing exercises, have been perceived as religious rituals, potentially conflicting with parents' or school leaders' faith-based convictions. Educators may encounter resistance from stakeholders who believe these practices infringe on their religious values or appear "foreign" or unfamiliar.

To address these concerns, it is important to frame mindfulness and well-being practices in secular, science-backed, and culturally grounded ways. For instance, instead of presenting mindfulness as meditation, it can be described as a focus strategy to calm the mind and body, similar to silent prayer or moments of quiet reflection. Or, mindful prayers in the context of the student's faith can also be explored. Further, emphasizing its health and cognitive benefits, such as improving attention, reducing anxiety, and increasing empathy, can help shift the focus away from spiritual or religious associations.

Moreover, integrating Filipino values such as *pagmumuni-muni* (deep reflection), *katahimikan* (inner silence), and *kagandahang-loob* (inner goodness) into discussions of mindfulness can help ground the practice in cultural authenticity. In this way, mindfulness and emotional regulation are not seen as foreign imports, but as aligned with long-standing Filipino virtues of inner strength and relational harmony.

Ensuring Accessibility and Inclusivity

A major challenge in integrating contemplative practices like mindfulness, resilience, and well-being into education is making sure they are accessible and inclusive. Students experience school differently; those with special needs, from marginalized communities, or culturally diverse backgrounds may face obstacles if programs are not intentionally designed for them. For example, traditional mindfulness activities that depend on abstract language or long periods of silence can be hard for learners with cognitive disabilities, ADHD, or trauma histories. Likewise, under-resourced schools might not have quiet spaces, materials, or time for regular practice due to overcrowded classrooms and administrative pressures.

To promote inclusivity, mindfulness must be tailored to diverse learner needs through flexible and culturally sensitive methods. Educators can offer multiple "paths" to calming—such as movement-based mindfulness (e.g., stretching), creative activities (e.g., art or storytelling), or sensory experiences (e.g., nature walks)—to support neurodiverse learners and different learning styles. Additionally, ensuring equity in mental health education should be a priority by using localized materials, translating into native languages, and providing teacher training that helps adapt to specific student contexts.

Ultimately, inclusivity should not be an afterthought but a core design principle, ensuring that mindfulness and well-being education empower every learner, particularly those most at risk of exclusion, to thrive emotionally, socially, and academically.

Training and Capacity-Building for Teachers

The third and possibly most important challenge is the need for strong teacher training and continuous capacity-building. Teachers are the main facilitators of classroom-based mindfulness and values education. However, many may lack the background, experience, or confidence to teach these practices effectively. Even worse, they might be struggling with their own emotional well-being and lack the support they need to model mindfulness and resilience for their students.

Without proper training, there is a risk of implementing mindfulness in superficial or even counterproductive ways, such as treating it as a disciplinary tool rather than a nurturing practice, or enforcing silence without explaining its purpose. Teachers need to understand not only the how but also the *why* behind these practices, so they can embody the values they teach and create safe, compassionate environments for all learners.

Teacher capacity-building should include:

- **Pre-service training** on psychosocial skills, trauma-informed practices, and inclusive mindfulness
- **In-service workshops** that go beyond theory and provide practical tools, lesson plans, and classroom scenarios
- **Peer support groups** or learning circles where teachers can reflect on their experiences, share challenges, and co-develop strategies
- **Mentoring systems** that pair experienced well-being educators with new implementers
- **Mental health support** for teachers themselves, including access to counseling, stress management resources, and opportunities for rest and renewal

Promoting contemplative education in GMRC and Values Education requires not only student-focused interventions but also strong teacher preparation and support. Teachers are the main facilitators of reflection, empathy, and mindfulness in the classroom, and their ability to model these qualities depends on the training, tools, and care they receive. A comprehensive approach starts in pre-service training, where aspiring educators should be equipped with psychosocial skills, trauma-informed practices, and inclusive mindfulness strategies. These foundations prepare them to address the diverse emotional needs of learners, respond sensitively to students who may have experienced adversity, and incorporate reflective activities in a way that respects cultural and individual differences. For example, pre-service programs can include microteaching sessions where future teachers practice leading guided reflections or mindful breathing exercises.

Once in the profession, teachers benefit from in-service workshops that move beyond theoretical discussions of contemplative education. These workshops should offer practical tools—ready-to-use lesson plans, classroom scripts for guided reflections, and sample scenarios for empathy-building discussions. By engaging in role-plays and simulated classroom situations, teachers can build confidence in applying contemplative strategies, ensuring that the concepts translate effectively to daily practice.

To sustain momentum, peer support groups or learning circles can provide a space for teachers to reflect on their experiences, share successes, and troubleshoot challenges together. This collegial exchange not only strengthens teaching strategies but also reinforces the values of empathy, active listening, and mutual respect, mirroring the very practices they aim to instill in students. In such groups, teachers might share variations of a mindfulness activity they tried, discuss student responses, and brainstorm improvements collaboratively.

Mentoring systems further enhance the capacity of educators by pairing experienced well-being practitioners with newer teachers. These mentors can offer tailored guidance, observe classroom implementation, and provide feedback on how to deepen student engagement with contemplative practices. Such relationships encourage professional growth while fostering a supportive culture of shared responsibility for nurturing values education.

Equally important is attending to the mental health and well-being of teachers themselves. The emotional labor of guiding students through reflection, empathy, and moral decision-making can be demanding. Schools should provide access to counseling services, stress management programs, and regular opportunities for rest and renewal. Practices like staff mindfulness sessions, quiet rooms for short breaks, or scheduled well-being days can help teachers recharge. When educators are cared for, they are better able to create a calm, focused, and compassionate learning environment.

By combining robust preparation, ongoing practical training, collaborative peer engagement, mentoring, and teacher well-being support, schools can ensure that contemplative education is not just an ideal but a daily, lived reality in GMRC and Values Education classrooms. In doing so, they cultivate not only students' dignity and moral grounding but also the resilience and compassion of the teachers who guide them.

More importantly, teacher development programs should emphasize cultural humility and student-centered pedagogy. Instead of offering rigid templates, trainings should encourage teachers to listen to their students, draw from local wisdom, and adapt practices to their unique classroom contexts.

MOVING FORWARD WITH SENSITIVITY AND STRENGTH

The integration of contemplative education in the Good Manners and Right Conduct Curriculu in the form of mindfulness, resilience, and well-being into the education system is a promising and compassionate movement, but it must be pursued with deep cultural awareness, inclusive design, and strong teacher support. Challenges are not signs of failure, but reminders of the complexity of working with human hearts and minds.

By honoring the cultural and spiritual identities of learners, making practices accessible to all, and empowering teachers through thoughtful training, we create not just successful programs, but communities of care. We recognize that resilience is not developed in isolation, but in the presence of empathy, connection, and shared humanity.

Ultimately, the goal is not to force mindfulness or resilience into rigid boxes, but to weave them organically into the living, breathing culture of the classroom. When students feel seen, supported, and empowered, they do not merely survive their school years, they thrive. And when educators are equipped, valued, and guided with clarity and compassion, they do not just teach, they transform lives.

REFERENCES

Alam, A. (2022). Contemplative pedagogy: An experiment with school students for demystifying the philosophy of contemplative education. *Resilience and Transformation in Global Restructuring*, *1*, 289–300.

Alejandria, M. C. P., Casimiro, K. M. D., Gibe, J. A. L., Fernandez, N. S. F., Tumaneng, D. C., Sandoval, E. C. A., Hernandez, P. J. S., Quan-Nalus, M. A., Alipao, F. A., & Alejandria, M. A. C. P. (2023). Attaining well-being beyond the home: A socio-cultural framing of mental health among university students in the Philippines. *Health Education Journal*, *82*(2), 143–155. DOI: 10.1177/00178969221141547

Alvear, D., Soler, J., & Cebolla, A. (2022). A. Meditators' Non-academic Definition of Mindfulness. *Mindfulness*, *13*(6), 1544–1554. DOI: 10.1007/s12671-022-01899-3 PMID: 35634214

Andres, F. (2025). The Role of Emotional Intelligence in Self-Awareness and Well-Being. In *Development of Self-Awareness and Wellbeing: Global Learning Challenges in a Shifting Society* (pp. 1-46). IGI Global Scientific Publishing. DOI: 10.4018/979-8-3373-0360-4.ch001

Bak, T. (2025). Exploring the contemplative: A meditative self-inquiry of Individual Consultations practice. *Journal of Academic Language and Learning*, *19*(1), 102–122.

Ballaret, J. R. (2024). Navigating the New Normal: An in-Depth Study of Adaptation and Change in Filipino Family Structures Postpandemic. *The Family Journal (Alexandria, Va.)*, •••, 10664807231225209. DOI: 10.1177/10664807231225209

Brown, L. A. (2025). Narrative Inquiry as Contemplative Methodology. *Journal of Contemplative and Holistic Education*, *3*(1), 6. DOI: 10.25035/jche.03.01.06

Bruce-Martin, M. (2022). *Higher education lecturers' experiences of contemplative practices and mindful learning: a self-determination theory perspective*. University of Northumbria at Newcastle.

Cao, X., Hangeldiyeva, N., Ali, A., & Pitafi, A. H. (2025). A social comparison perspective to investigating the influence of social media on employee creativity. *International Journal of Human-Computer Interaction, 41*(13), 8481–8494. DOI: 10.1080/10447318.2024.2410533

Carroll, A., Hepburn, S. J., & Bower, J. (2022, August). Mindful practice for teachers: Relieving stress and enhancing positive mindsets. [). Frontiers Media SA.]. *Frontiers in Education*, *7*, 954098. DOI: 10.3389/feduc.2022.954098

Čopelj, E. (2022). Mindfulness and attention: Towards a phenomenology of mindfulness as the feeling of being tuned in. *Asian Philosophy*, *32*(2), 126–151. DOI: 10.1080/09552367.2022.2031015

Crasta, A., & Dmello, L. (2024). Empowering Women: An Analysis of Needs and Preferences for Self-Discovery, Self-Esteem, and Positive Attitude Development Training. [PIJTRCS]. *Poornaprajna International Journal of Teaching & Research Case Studies*, *1*(1), 308–325. DOI: 10.64818/PIJTRCS.3107.8494.0012

Daly, M., & Robinson, E. (2022). Depression and anxiety during COVID-19. *Lancet*, *399*(10324), 518. DOI: 10.1016/S0140-6736(22)00187-8 PMID: 35123689

Dutta, G., & Vimal, K. (2025). Educating the Whole Child: The Power of Contemplative Practices. In *Handbook of Positive Psychology and Indian Thought Systems: Transforming Education for Well-being and Happiness* (pp. 127–149). Springer Nature Singapore. DOI: 10.1007/978-981-96-4210-6_9

Edyburn, K. L., & Meek, S. (2021). Seeking safety and humanity in the harshest immigration climate in a generation: A review of the literature on the effects of separation and detention on migrant and asylum-seeking children and families in the United States during the Trump administration. *Social Policy Report*, *34*(1), 1–46.

Fedewa, A. L., Ahn, S., & Aspiranti, K. B. (2022). Mindfulness in Elementary School Teachers: Effects on Teacher Stress, Mental Health, and Mindfulness in the Classroom. Int. J. School. *Health*, *9*(2), 73–82. DOI: 10.30476/INTJSH.2022.92252.1169

Fisher, V., Li, W. W., & Malabu, U. (2023). The effectiveness of mindfulness-based stress reduction (MBSR) on the mental health, HbA1C, and mindfulness of diabetes patients: A systematic review and meta-analysis of randomised controlled trials. *Applied Psychology. Health and Well-Being, 15*(4), 1733–1749. DOI: 10.1111/aphw.12441 PMID: 36855248

Flanagan, B., & Clough, K. (Eds.). (2024). *The Routledge handbook of research methods in spirituality and contemplative studies*. Taylor & Francis. DOI: 10.4324/9781003341598

Gardner, P. (2021). Contemplative pedagogy: Fostering transformative learning in a critical service learning course. *Journal of Experiential Education, 44*(2), 152–166. DOI: 10.1177/1053825920952086

Gilbert, P., & Van Gordon, W. (2023). Compassion as a skill: A comparison of contemplative and evolution-based approaches. *Mindfulness, 14*(10), 2395–2416. DOI: 10.1007/s12671-023-02173-w

Gomez, E. C. (2024, July 8). Impact of Values Education in Daily Lives of Students: A Qualitative Study. *Southeast Asian Journal of Multidisciplinary Studies*. https://research.cmc.edu.ph/index.php/journals/article/view/161

Gunnlaugson, O., Cueto de Souza, R., Zhao, S., Yee, A., Scott, C., & Bai, H. (2022). Revisiting the Nature of Transformative Learning Experiences in Contemplative Higher Education. *Journal of Transformative Education, 21*(1), 84-101. https://doi.org/ (Original work published 2023)DOI: 10.1177/15413446211067285

Iloka, P. C. (2025). Teaching Integrity: Strategies for Fostering Ethical Behavior in Students. *UNIZIK Journal of Educational Research and Policy Studies, 19*(1).

Karas, K. J. (2021). *Discovering the Contemplative Practices, Communication Techniques and Teaching Methods of Holistic Educators Demonstrating Presence with Students*. The University of Akron.

Lau, E. N. S. (2024). Implementing Contemplative Education for Enhancing Spirituality in Hong Kong Schools. *The Routledge International Handbook of Life and Values Education in Asia*, 441-452.

Mumtazah, L. (2024). The Role of Emotion Regulation in Increasing Resilience to Stress and Life Pressure. *Asian Journal of Multidisciplinary Research, 1*(2), 88–96. DOI: 10.59613/bs2n5f66

Philippine Department of Education. (2023). Good Manners and Right Conduct and Values Education Curriculum. https:// www. deped. gov. ph/ wp - content/ uploads/ MATATAG - GMRC - and - VE - Grades - 1 - 4 - and - 7. pdf

Puyat, J. H., Gastardo-Conaco, M. C., Natividad, J., & Banal, M. A. (2021). Depressive symptoms among young adults in the Philippines: Results from a nationwide cross-sectional survey. *Journal of Affective Disorders Reports, 3*, 100073. DOI: 10.1016/j.jadr.2020.100073

Qiu, Y. (2024). Social comparison on social media platforms: a media and communication perspective. In *SHS Web of Conferences* (Vol. 185, p. 03008). EDP Sciences. DOI: 10.1051/shsconf/202418503008

Ramaila, S. M. (2025). Fostering Holistic Development: The Integral Role of Educators in Nurturing Student Growth and Learning. In *Former Educators' Roles in Supporting Student Growth and Learning* (pp. 117-146). IGI Global Scientific Publishing.

Ross, C. B., & Rocha Beardall, T. (2022). Promoting empathy and reducing hopelessness using contemplative practices. *Teaching Sociology, 50*(3), 256–268. DOI: 10.1177/0092055X221092014

Scherer, S., Talley, C., & Hill, O. (2021). Mindfulness and Silent Sitting in the Classroom. In *A Human Values Pathway for Teachers: Developing Silent Sitting and Mindful Practices in Education* (pp. 55–78). Springer Singapore. DOI: 10.1007/978-981-16-0200-9_6

Serrano, I. M. A., Cuyugan, A. M. N., Cruz, K., Mahusay, J. M. A., & Alibudbud, R. (2023). Sociodemographic characteristics, social support, and family history as factors of depression, anxiety, and stress among young adult senior high school students in metro Manila, Philippines, during the COVID-19 pandemic. *Frontiers in Psychiatry, 14*, 1225035. DOI: 10.3389/fpsyt.2023.1225035 PMID: 37772068

Sherab, K., & Schuelka, M. J. (2023). Happy students in Bhutan. In *Routledge eBooks* (pp. 56–75). https://doi.org/DOI: 10.4324/9781003037262-4

Sofianopoulou, K., Bacopoulou, F., Vlachakis, D., Kokka, I., Alexopoulos, E., Varvogli, L., Chrousos, G. P., & Darviri, C. (2021). Stress Management in Elementary School Students: A Pilot Randomised Controlled Trial. *EMBnet.Journal, 26*(1), e976. DOI: 10.14806/ej.26.1.976 PMID: 34621631

Sowmya, D. S. (2025). Embracing Self-Compassion: A Cornerstone of Student Well-Being. In *Nurturing Student Well-Being in the Modern World* (pp. 103-140). IGI Global.

Srivastava, S. (2023). The evolution of education: Navigating 21st-century challenges. *International Journal for Multidisciplinary Research, 5*(5), 1–9.

Toukan, E., & Tawil, S. (2024). A new social contract for education: Rebuilding trust in education as a common good. *Prospects, 54*(2), 259–275. DOI: 10.1007/s11125-024-09702-y

Van Gordon, W., Sapthiang, S., & Shonin, E. (2022). Contemplative psychology: History, key assumptions, and future directions. *Perspectives on Psychological Science, 17*(1), 99–107. DOI: 10.1177/1745691620984479 PMID: 34185604

Vilvens, H. L., Frame, D. L., & Owen, P. C. (2021). Promoting the inclusion of mindfulness and contemplative practices in the college classroom. *Pedagogy in Health Promotion, 7*(2), 148–158. DOI: 10.1177/2373379920925849

Webster, E. M. (2022). The impact of adverse childhood experiences on health and development in young children. *Global pediatric health, 9*, 2333794X221078708.

Chapter 3
Enhancing Mental Well-Being and Language Learning Through Mindfulness and Yoga-Based Practices

Kenneth Leow
http://orcid.org/0000-0002-7423-2889
Department of Psychology, School of Social Sciences, Heriot-Watt University, Malaysia

Yueh Yea Lo
http://orcid.org/0000-0002-6347-9835
Department of Language and Literacy Education, Faculty of Education, Universiti Malaya, Malaysia

ABSTRACT

This chapter explores the integration of mindfulness and yoga-based practices into English as a Second Language (ESL) instruction to address both the linguistic and emotional challenges faced by English Language Learners (ELLs). Drawing on classroom-based applications, student reflections, and interdisciplinary research, it argues for a holistic pedagogical approach that supports cognitive, emotional, and physical well-

DOI: 10.4018/979-8-2600-1202-4.ch003

being. Mindfulness and yoga are presented as accessible tools to reduce anxiety, enhance self-regulation, and improve academic engagement. By embedding contemplative practices in ESL classrooms, educators can create inclusive, growth-oriented environments that foster language proficiency, psychological resilience, and intercultural competence.

INTRODUCTION

Students learning English as a Second Language (ESL) often face a complex array of academic and emotional challenges that extend well beyond the traditional boundaries of language instruction (Calafato, 2023; Tajik et al., 2024). English Language Learners (ELLs), particularly those from rural or underserved backgrounds, frequently enter higher education with limited prior exposure to English reading, writing, and communicative practices (Ruecker, 2021). This linguistic disadvantage not only impedes their academic readiness but also amplifies experiences of self-doubt, anxiety, and fear of failure (Hamid & Idrus, 2021; Soomro et al., 2023). While conventional ESL pedagogy has historically prioritized grammar instruction, vocabulary development, and fluency, the psychological well-being of learners remains a neglected yet critical dimension of academic success (Serquina & Batang, 2018).

Language acquisition is a demanding and long-term process that typically spans four to seven years. However, linguistic development alone does not adequately account for the academic trajectories of ESL students (Garnett, 2010). Beyond language barriers, ELLs often encounter psychosocial stressors such as marginalization, cultural dissonance, and identity conflict (Chenowith, 2014). These affective experiences can significantly erode students' motivation, self-confidence, and sense of belonging which are factors that are vital to sustained engagement and educational persistence (Leow et al., 2023; Razi & Rahmat, 2020). This reality underscores the need for a more holistic pedagogical approach, one that transcends linguistic instruction to address the broader emotional and sociocultural contexts in which learning takes place.

The teacher-researcher further argues that academic achievement, while important, does not fully encapsulate the developmental needs of

ELL students (Hussain et al., 2020). Equally essential is the intentional cultivation of social and emotional well-being encompassing skills such as emotional regulation, interpersonal competence, and identity formation (Leow et al., 2023). These affective domains are deeply interconnected with cognitive functioning and learning outcomes. Supporting students in these areas requires deliberate long-term strategies that prioritize psychological resilience alongside academic competence (Ijadi-Maghsoodi et al., 2025).

Recent studies have highlighted a growing mental health crisis in higher education, with rising levels of stress, anxiety, and emotional burnout reported among university students globally (Rosales-Ricardo et al., 2021; Raza et al., 2023). ESL learners are particularly vulnerable within this landscape, as they navigate the dual challenges of mastering a second language while adjusting to unfamiliar cultural and academic environments (Zasiekina & Shuravlova, 2019). These realities call for a paradigm shift in instructional design, one that integrates emotional resilience and well-being as foundational pillars of student support.

This chapter advocates for the integration of mindfulness and yoga-based practices into ESL instruction as a dual intervention strategy aimed at enhancing both linguistic proficiency and student well-being. When thoughtfully implemented, mindfulness and yoga offer powerful tools for supporting emotional regulation, improving concentration, and strengthening psychological resilience. A growing body of research supports the incorporation of contemplative practices in educational contexts, with evidence suggesting that such interventions can significantly improve students' mood, behavior, self-esteem, academic performance, and overall well-being (Chauhan & Saxena, 2024; Hagins & Rundle, 2016). For ELL students, many of whom are managing the compounded pressures of second-language acquisition and cultural adaptation, these practices hold particular promise. By fostering focused attention, mindfulness and yoga not only facilitate language learning but also contribute to the development of essential social-emotional competencies (Bazzano et al., 2023). These competencies are critical not only for academic success but for students' broader development as self-aware, resilient individuals. This chapter draws on classroom-based applications, student reflections, and teacher narratives within ESL contexts to examine how contemplative pedagogy can be localized and meaningfully implemented in ESL settings.

LANGUAGE LEARNING AND PSYCHOLOGICAL STRESSORS

The global rise of English as the dominant language for international communication, commerce, and academic scholarship has significantly amplified the pressure on learners worldwide to attain high levels of proficiency in English. For many learners of English as a second or foreign language, this pressure is compounded by a range of psychological barriers, most notably such as stress, apprehension, and communicative anxiety (Malik et al., 2021). These emotional responses often manifest as what learners describe as a "mental block," which hinders their capacity to engage confidently and effectively in the language acquisition process.

Indeed, students from non-English-speaking backgrounds, especially from Asian countries often enter Western higher education systems with limited exposure to academic English. This lack of linguistic readiness compromises not only their ability to engage in complex academic tasks such as reading, writing, and oral presentations but also undermines their efforts to establish meaningful peer relationships in predominantly English-speaking environments (Lashari et al., 2023; Mak et al., 2015). The implications of such language barriers extend far beyond academic performance. When students struggle to communicate fluently or confidently, they may withdraw from classroom discussions, group projects, and collaborative learning opportunities (Xuan Mai, 2024). Over time, this disengagement can lead to a diminished sense of belonging and academic self-efficacy (Wang & Sun, 2020), all of which threaten long-term educational success.

Moreover, language proficiency challenges are intricately linked with cultural adjustment difficulties (Peng & Patterson, 2022). Limited fluency in English may prevent students from accessing informal support networks, participating in extracurricular activities, or building rapport with instructors and classmates. ESL students frequently report language anxiety driven by fear of grammatical errors, poor pronunciation, and negative peer evaluation, especially during group activities and oral assessments (Alamer & Almulhim, 2021). These limitations restrict not only their social integration but also their opportunities to practice English in authentic, low-stakes environments (Kao, 2024). Consequently, addressing language barriers is not solely a pedagogical concern but a broader matter of student well-being, intercultural engagement, and equity in international education.

Among the myriad psychological factors influencing second language acquisition, anxiety has also consistently emerged as one of the most influential and widely researched constructs in both educational and psychological literature (Russell, 2020). While anxiety can disrupt various types of learning, it becomes particularly debilitating in the context of language learning, where it is commonly referred to as second or foreign language anxiety. This form of anxiety is typically marked by heightened tension, fear of negative evaluation, and self-consciousness, especially in communicative settings. These affective responses not only undermine learners' confidence but also hinder their ability to perform effectively in the target language (Shami et al., 2025).

Second or foreign language anxiety is recognized as a complex and multidimensional phenomenon that encompasses emotional, cognitive, and physiological components (Oteir & Al-Otaibi, 2019). This definition highlights the interplay between psychological discomfort and physiological arousal, manifesting in elevated heart rate, shallow breathing, and mental distraction during language-related tasks. Empirical studies have consistently demonstrated that this type of anxiety is most acute during oral communication tasks, particularly those involving listening and speaking (Horwitz, 2001). The immediacy, unpredictability, and perceived public nature of spoken interaction often leave learners feeling exposed and vulnerable to judgment. Consequently, many language learners develop avoidant behaviors, opting out of participation to minimize discomfort. Thus, limiting their exposure to the very communicative practice necessary for proficiency development.

From an education psychological perspective, language anxiety often stems from internal self-appraisals (Tessler & Schwartz, 1972). These beliefs function as intrinsic affective filters, shaping the learner's emotional engagement, motivation, and risk-taking behavior in the classroom. Importantly, anxiety in this context is both a cause and a consequence of limited proficiency. A lack of competence may trigger anxiety in communicative situations, while persistent anxiety may impair attention, working memory, and language processing further inhibiting language development and reinforcing a cycle of underperformance (Sultan, 2012).

Moreover, the broader emotional landscape of university students must be acknowledged. Many learners face multiple intersecting stressors, including academic pressure, familial expectations, financial concerns, and social comparison (Slimmen et al., 2022). Within this context, ESL students are especially vulnerable, as they must navigate the dual demands of language acquisition and cultural adjustment, often without adequate emotional preparation or institutional support (Can et al., 2021). Despite growing discourse around 21st-century competencies, such as emotional intelligence, resilience, and adaptability, emotional well-being remains under-prioritized in ESL curricula and instructional design. Yet, ESL instructors often serve as informal emotional anchors for their students. They are in a unique position to recognize signs of distress and to cultivate learning environments that nurture both linguistic and emotional growth. With appropriate training and institutional support, language teachers can implement simple, non-clinical mindfulness and yoga-based strategies that help reduce anxiety and foster self-regulation. Practices such as mindful breathing, grounding exercises, body scans, and brief emotional check-ins can serve as valuable tools for helping students recalibrate emotionally before engaging in cognitively demanding tasks like speaking or writing in English (Tasan et al., 2021).

THE CONNECTION BETWEEN YOGA AND MINDFULNESS

Yoga, with its origins in ancient Indian philosophy, has long been regarded as a holistic discipline aimed at achieving unity of the mind, body, and spirit. Rooted in the Sanskrit word *yuj*, meaning "to unite" or "to join," yoga was traditionally conceived as a path toward spiritual liberation, integrating physical, ethical, and meditative practices to foster internal harmony and self-realization (Bryant et al., 2016; Malhotra, 2017). Rather than providing extended philosophical detail, it is sufficient to emphasize that yoga comprises ethical principles (yamas and niyamas), physical postures (asanas), breath regulation (pranayama), meditative absorption (dhyana), and disciplined concentration (dharana), each of which contributes to psychological self-regulation and overall well-being (Cook-Cottone, 2015).

Over the past several decades, yoga has undergone a global transformation, particularly in Western contexts where it is often reinterpreted through the lens of wellness, fitness, and stress reduction (Wang & Szabo, 2020). In these settings, the physical postures of Hatha Yoga tend to be emphasized, while its spiritual and philosophical underpinnings are often de-emphasized or secularized. In contrast, Eastern interpretations, particularly those grounded in Indian spiritual traditions, continue to uphold yoga as a multidimensional practice that fosters not only physical vitality but also emotional balance, ethical awareness, and spiritual growth (Csala et al., 2021). While this cultural divergence remains an important consideration, in educational contexts the discussion benefits from greater emphasis on pragmatic applications that directly enhance student well-being, thereby avoiding overemphasis on theoretical exposition.

In higher education, particularly within diverse and linguistically complex environments, both yoga and mindfulness are gaining recognition as non-stigmatizing, accessible interventions that promote psychological resilience and enhance overall student well-being (Chauhan & Saxena, 2024; Pidgeon & Keye, 2014). These practices fall within the broader category of mind-body interventions, which emphasize the intrinsic link between psychological and physiological processes in fostering health and well-being (Thomson et al., 2024). Within classroom contexts, their integration has been operationalized through brief practices such as structured breathing exercises prior to examinations, short sequences of mindful movement to alleviate physical fatigue during extended sessions, or guided reflective exercises designed to reorient attention. These pedagogical adaptations ensure that yoga and mindfulness function as feasible, non-clinical strategies that can be embedded within academic curricula.

Yoga and mindfulness are closely aligned in both principle and practice. Their shared origins in Eastern contemplative traditions provide a foundation of intentional awareness, compassion, and self-discipline, although they are often adapted to suit secular or culturally diverse settings (Gaiswinkler & Unterrainer, 2016; Van Dam et al., 2018). While yoga incorporates physical movement and postural alignment, breath control, and meditation, mindfulness is typically defined as the non-judgmental, moment-to-moment awareness of one's present experience, characterized by curiosity, openness, and acceptance (Kabat-Zinn, 2003; Bishop et al., 2004). The interrelationship between the two traditions is particularly evident in how embodied awareness during asanas or pranayama cultivates attentional stability, thereby operationalizing mindfulness within physical practice (Gaiswinkler & Unterrainer, 2016).

Among the most widely recognized mindfulness-based programs is Mindfulness-Based Stress Reduction (MBSR), developed by Jon Kabat-Zinn (2003) in the late 1970s. MBSR integrates guided meditation, body scanning, mindful movement through Hatha Yoga, and focused breath awareness as strategies to reduce stress and promote well-being across clinical and non-clinical populations (Kabat-Zinn, 2003). Similarly, Mindfulness-Based Cognitive Therapy (MBCT) combines mindfulness with cognitive-behavioral strategies to address depressive relapse by helping individuals become more aware of maladaptive thought patterns (Francis et al., 2024). For instance, Karakurt and Durmaz (2025) conducted an experimental study examining the effects of a mindfulness-based intervention on the subjective well-being of nursing students. The findings revealed that participants who engaged in an eight-week Mindfulness-Based Stress Reduction (MBSR) program demonstrated significant improvements in their levels of subjective well-being compared to the control group. These results highlight the potential of structured mindfulness programs as both accessible and cost-effective interventions that can be integrated into higher education settings to promote student mental health.

Hatha Yoga, one of the most practiced forms in educational and wellness contexts, integrates physical postures (asanas), breathing techniques (pranayama), and mindful focus to support mental clarity and emotional regulation (Luu & Hall, 2016). Adaptations of Hatha Yoga in higher education contexts often take the form of brief embodied interventions, such as seated postural adjustments or structured breathing sequences, which can be systematically evaluated for their impact on cognitive engagement, emotional regulation, and classroom participation (Shelov et al., 2009). Unlike conventional exercise, such practices cultivate embodied awareness that strengthens attentional focus and stress management capacities essential for academic success.

When practice together, yoga and mindfulness enhance one another's benefits. Hatha Yoga provides a physical and experiential grounding for mindfulness, making abstract concepts of awareness and acceptance more tangible through movement and breath. Research has shown that this integration improves outcomes related to psychological well-being, including reductions in stress and anxiety, and enhancements in focus, self-awareness, and emotion regulation (Kabat-Zinn, 2003; Khoury et al., 2015). Importantly, these benefits can be systematically documented in higher education through mixed-method evaluation strategies, combining quantitative data (e.g., pre- and post- intervention surveys) with qualitative evidence (e.g., focus group narratives).

Together, yoga and mindfulness offer a holistic framework for advancing student well-being. In contrast to approaches that compartmentalize academic performance and emotional development, these practices provide an integrative model that simultaneously cultivates attention, resilience, and emotional balance. To further strengthen the academic contribution of this chapter, the discussion expands beyond philosophical and theoretical foundations to incorporate detailed strategies for curricular integration and systematic evaluation of outcomes, thereby enhancing scholarly rigor and ensuring greater relevance for educators and policymakers. Such applications are particularly valuable in university contexts serving linguistically and culturally diverse learners, who often face elevated stress due to language barriers.

THE ROLE OF SELF-REGULATION AND YOGA

Self-regulation is the capacity to manage one's thoughts, emotions, and behaviors in pursuit of personally meaningful and long-term goals (Baumeister & Vohs, 2004). It is a foundational element of adaptive functioning and psychological well-being (Schultz & Ryan, 2015). Self-regulation encompasses a suite of executive functions, including the ability to sustain attention amid distractions, inhibit impulsive reactions in emotionally charged situations, and engage in goal-directed behavior (Wei et al., 2012). In the context of education, self-regulation plays a pivotal role in supporting emotional resilience, social adjustment, and school readiness

(Park et al., 2025). These regulatory abilities enable young learners to navigate classroom expectations, engage in peer interactions, and persist through academic challenges.

Research has consistently shown that early development of self-regulatory skills predicts a wide array of positive outcomes across the lifespan. Students who demonstrate strong self-regulation are more likely to experience favorable academic performance and social competence (Veisiy et al., 2022). Furthermore, these skills contribute to higher self-esteem and greater success in educational settings (Ohrt et al., 2014). Thus, cultivating self-regulation from an early age is not only beneficial for immediate academic engagement but also critical for long-term well-being. For example, Bergen-Cico and colleagues (2015) carried out a pilot study to investigate both the feasibility and potential effectiveness of integrating mindful yoga practices into the school curriculum as a means to strengthen self-regulation, thereby supporting academic achievement and promoting overall health among adolescents. The intervention was embedded within a sixth-grade English Language Arts classroom, where mindful yoga activities were systematically infused into lessons, and outcomes were compared against a control group that did not receive any form of yoga-based intervention. Although no substantial differences were observed in short-term self-regulation outcomes between the two groups, the findings revealed that students who participated in mindful yoga demonstrated significant improvements in broader indicators of self-regulation as well as sustained gains over the longer term when compared to their peers in the control condition. These results suggest that mindful yoga, when thoughtfully incorporated into classroom practice, may cultivate enduring self-regulatory capacities that extend beyond immediate behavioral control to encompass long-term personal and academic development.

In prevention science, self-regulation has been identified as a key protective factor that buffers against adversity and promotes positive developmental trajectories (Buckner et al., 2009). One promising avenue for fostering self-regulation is through mindfulness-based interventions, particularly when integrated into contemplative movement practices such as yoga (Razza et al., 2015). Both mindfulness and self-regulation are conceptually linked together to emphasize individual's ability to respond adaptively to internal and external stimuli (Black & Fernando, 2014;

Schultz & Ryan, 2015). Practicing mindfulness involves cultivating non-judgmental, present-moment awareness, while self-regulation draws upon this attentiveness to shape purposeful action (Leyland et al., 2019).

Yoga, when practiced mindfully, engages individuals in embodied self-awareness by directing attention to physical sensations, breath patterns, and internal emotional states. This deliberate focus fosters sensory attunement and meta-cognitive reflection, which are crucial for effective self-regulation (Wimmer et al., 2020). As such, yoga functions not only as a physical discipline but as a cognitive-emotional training ground that nurtures regulation of affect and attention (Schultz & Ryan, 2015). The physiological basis for the connection between mindfulness, yoga, and self-regulation lies in the modulation of the body's stress-response systems, particularly the hypothalamic–pituitary–adrenal (HPA) axis. This neuroendocrine system regulates cortisol secretion, which helps the body adapt to and recover from stress. Chronic dysregulation of the HPA axis manifested in elevated or blunted cortisol rhythms which is associated to impaired executive functioning leading to anxiety and depression (Blair, 2010; Sarubin et al., 2014). Mindfulness-based practices have been shown to downregulate the HPA axis response, reducing physiological arousal and improving stress management These findings suggest that mindfulness supports self-regulation not only at a cognitive-emotional level but also by recalibrating biological mechanisms that underlie behavioral control (Bergen-Cico et al., 2014).

Contemplative practices such as yoga and mindfulness are increasingly recognized as valuable tools for educational settings. When implemented systematically, they can help ESL students develop stronger attentional control, increase emotional self-awareness, and engage in more thoughtful and regulated behaviors (Lemay et al., 2019). School-based programs incorporating these practices have been linked to improvements in classroom behavior, academic performance, and psychological well-being (Qi et al., 2020; Wimmer & Bellingrath, 2020). For instance, Qi et al. (2020) conducted a comparative study to examine the psychological effects of two distinct modalities of yoga practice (meditation-focused yoga and breathing-focused yoga) among a sample of 86 undergraduate students. Their results indicated that, particularly for novice practitioners, engaging in a breathing-focused yoga intervention produced more substantial psychological benefits than the meditation-focused approach. Specifically, students in the breathing-focused group reported higher levels of energy and task engagement, greater mindfulness, and lower levels of perceived stress. The authors argue that breath-based practices may serve as a more accessible entry point for beginners, offering immediate and tangible benefits that support both mental health and academic functioning. From an educational perspective, these findings highlight the potential of integrating breathing-focused yoga into university curricula or co-curricular programs as a strategy for fostering resilience, enhancing focus, and mitigating stress. Such outcomes may be particularly salient for students experiencing heightened pressures whether due to demanding academic workloads or the additional challenges of navigating linguistic and cultural transitions in higher education contexts.

Yoga and mindfulness represent promising, evidence-informed strategies for enhancing self-regulation among ESL students. The bidirectional model of self-regulation (Blair & Ku, 2022) suggests that top-down processes (e.g., executive functions) and bottom-up processes (e.g., emotional and physiological responses) interact dynamically. Mindfulness-based practices address both domains, enhancing cognitive control through attention training while simultaneously downregulating emotional reactivity and arousal. As such, they hold significant potential for cultivating both short- and long-term self-regulation skills during critical developmental windows. Their integration into educational settings aligns with contemporary priorities in student well-being and holistic development.

YOGA AND MINDFULNESS PRACTICES IN EDUCATIONAL CONTEXT

Early intervention in student mental health is increasingly recognized as essential for preventing long-term psychological challenges. Left unaddressed, emotional distress in students can escalate into more serious clinical conditions, such as anxiety disorders, depression, or chronic disengagement from school and learning (Dimitropoulos et al., 2022). Despite the high prevalence of stress and mental health difficulties among students, many, particularly those from linguistically and culturally diverse backgrounds do not receive the support they need (Hunt, 2017). This treatment gap is often exacerbated by several interrelated factors, including cultural stigma, lack of familiarity with mental health services, and limited awareness of school-based resources. For English as a Second Language (ESL) students, these challenges are further compounded by language barriers, sociocultural dislocation, and the pressure to meet academic standards in a non-native language.

Against this backdrop, yoga and mindfulness practices offer a low-cost, accessible, and inclusive framework to address student well-being, particularly for ESL learners navigating complex educational transitions. Within school settings, these practices can be seamlessly integrated into the curriculum or classroom routines to support learners' emotional, cognitive, and physical development without requiring specialized clinical infrastructure. For ESL students, the benefits of these practices are especially salient. These learners often face dual pressures: the academic demands of mastering a second language and the psychological toll of adapting to unfamiliar cultural norms, educational expectations, and peer dynamics. Many ESL students experience heightened language anxiety, self-doubt, and social withdrawal, particularly in communicative classroom settings where they fear making mistakes or being misunderstood (Malik et al., 2021; Peng & Patterson, 2022). Embedding mindfulness-based can help reduce this affective overload by enhancing ESL students' capacity for emotional regulation and present-moment awareness (Bergen-Cico et al., 2014).

Beyond their psychological benefits, yoga and mindfulness also contribute to enhanced academic performance, especially when integrated thoughtfully into educational environments. Students participating in such programs frequently report better concentration, reduced classroom anxiety, and increased motivation (Hagins & Rundle, 2016). These outcomes are particularly significant for ESL learners, whose academic engagement is often hindered by internal stressors and the fear of negative evaluation. When students feel calmer and more in control of their internal states, they are more likely to participate actively, take linguistic risks, and persevere through the discomfort of language acquisition.

Importantly, yoga and mindfulness practices also promote non-judgmental self-awareness (Hunt et al., 2018), a critical mindset for learners who often compare themselves to native speakers or feel insecure about their accents and grammar. These contemplative practices encourage students to observe their thoughts and feelings without harsh self-criticism allowing them to build a more compassionate relationship with their own learning process. This is especially important in high-stakes ESL environments, where perfectionism and fear of failure can inhibit progress (Khezerlou, 2023). When learners are taught to notice their challenges with curiosity rather than shame, they are more likely to adopt a growth mindset and remain engaged.

Moreover, yoga and mindfulness can be culturally adaptive and respectful. In multicultural ESL classrooms, where students may come from various religious, ethnic, and cultural backgrounds, these practices can be presented in secular, inclusive formats that emphasize universal skills such as attention, emotional regulation, and self-reflection. Teachers can integrate brief mindful pauses, silent reflection, or gentle stretches into lessons without compromising cultural sensitivity (Hytman et al., 2025). In doing so, educators not only support students' well-being but also model inclusive pedagogies that honor diverse experiences and needs.

For students and other ESL learners from collectivist cultural backgrounds, the benefits of mindfulness may be especially salient. In such contexts, students often internalize high expectations from family or society and may equate academic performance with self-worth (Liao & Wei, 2014). This can lead to heightened anxiety, self-censorship, and disengagement in the classroom. Mindfulness offers a culturally adaptable tool to navigate these pressures. When implemented with care and cultural sensitivity, it enables learners to observe their inner experiences with kindness, detach from harsh self-evaluations, and gradually build the confidence to express themselves both linguistically and emotionally (DeLuca et al., 2018).

Resilience, in this context, is not simply an inherent trait but a developmental capacity that can be nurtured through relational and instructional support (Gey et al., 2025). When paired with mindfulness, resilience becomes a teachable and accessible skill (Harker et al., 2016). Practical applications may include integrating short breathing exercises before language tasks, incorporating reflective journaling to process learning experiences, and encouraging mindful listening during group work. These techniques not only build emotional literacy but also foster a stronger sense of student agency and belonging (Rajan & Sandhu, 2025).

The importance of early intervention is further reinforced by research from Noggle et al. (2012), which shows that many adult mental health conditions originate during adolescence. Approximately 7.5% of adolescents already meet the diagnostic criteria for at least one mental health disorder, emphasizing the urgency of embedding mental health promotion strategies into daily school routines. In this regard, mindfulness and yoga-based practices present as low-barrier, evidence-informed approaches that empower students with skills for managing emotional distress, cultivating focus, and building a sense of inner stability.

For ESL students, the transition into higher education can be particularly overwhelming. ESL students, in particular, must navigate a convergence of academic, linguistic, and social adjustments. The shift from familiar learning environments to more autonomous, performance-driven systems can heighten feelings of isolation, inadequacy, and culture shock. Introducing mindfulness and yoga-based practices during this period, especially through first-year seminars, transition workshops, or orientation modules can provide grounding tools that mitigate anxiety and build self-confidence.

EXPLORATION ON MINDFULNESS AND ESL LEARNERS IN HIGHER EDUCATION SETTINGS

The use of yoga and mindfulness as interventions in educational settings has been widely practiced and is not a novel approach. For example, Bazzano et al. (2018) conducted an experimental study to evaluate the impact of a yoga curriculum on elementary school students' quality of life. The findings indicated that the yoga-based intervention was associated with improvements in students' emotional and psychosocial well-being. Additionally, teachers and staff reported incorporating yoga more frequently in the classroom after the second of two training sessions. While these results were promising, the study had several limitations. The sample size was relatively small, with only 20 participants in the intervention group. Moreover, students' self-perceptions of their quality of life may fluctuate throughout the school year, raising concerns about the consistency of the baseline between the intervention groups. Finally, as the intervention integrated both yoga and mindfulness, the study could not determine whether the observed benefits were attributable to one component or the combined effect of both.

Previous research on mindfulness and yoga interventions has largely focused on elementary and high school settings, with comparatively fewer studies conducted at the university level (Bazzano et al., 2018; Strapp & Lambert, 2020). While these school-based studies consistently highlight the positive effects of yoga and mindfulness practices on students' well-being and classroom engagement, their applicability to higher education contexts remains less understood. This gap is particularly significant given that university students often face heightened levels of stress, academic pressure, and transitional challenges compared to younger students (Wilson & Gillies, 2005).

Consequently, greater attention should be directed toward investigating the effectiveness of mindfulness- and yoga-based interventions within university settings. An important consideration in this regard is the training and qualifications of staff implementing such programs. Evidence suggests that the success of these interventions is strongly influenced by the competence and preparedness of facilitators. For instance, Wimmer et al. (2020) emphasized that having adequately trained and qualified staff is essential for ensuring both the fidelity of program delivery and the achievement of desired student outcomes. This underscores the need not only to expand research in higher education contexts but also to invest in building institutional capacity through professional development and staff training.

In addition to exploratory and experimental studies, several investigations have been conducted in the form of systematic reviews (Breedvelt et al., 2019; Khalsa & Butzer, 2016; Sun et al., 2021). For instance, Chauhan and Saxena (2024) carried out a systematic review that synthesized existing evidence on the integration of yoga and mindfulness within educational settings, highlighting their potential benefits for enhancing student well-being and academic performance. While such reviews play an important role in consolidating current knowledge and identifying patterns across multiple studies, they are not without limitations. Systematic reviews are inherently dependent on the quality and scope of the included studies, and their conclusions may be constrained by factors such as narrow contextual focus, inconsistent study methodologies, and the exclusion of unpublished or non-English research. Additionally, despite protocols designed to ensure objectivity, reviewer judgment in study selection and interpretation may introduce subjective bias. These limitations underscore the importance of complementing systematic reviews with empirical studies such as exploratory or experimental research that can provide deeper, context-specific insights into the effectiveness of yoga and mindfulness interventions in education.

Finally, there remains a notable scarcity of research specifically examining the use of yoga and mindfulness interventions among ESL learners. Although studies in this area are still limited, there is emerging interest as reflected in recent theses and dissertations (Snyder, 2020; Trojan, 2020). These works indicate a growing recognition of the potential role that yoga and mindfulness can play in supporting ESL learners, who often face unique challenges such as language anxiety, acculturative stress, and academic pressure in addition to the demands of second language acquisition. The increasing momentum in this line of inquiry highlights the importance of directing more systematic and empirical research toward understanding how these interventions can enhance ESL students' well-being, resilience, and academic engagement. By addressing this gap, future studies can contribute valuable insights into culturally and contextually relevant approaches that integrate both language learning and psychological support.

CASE STUDY: MINDFULNESS PRACTICE IN AN ESL WRITING COURSE

The present study aimed to conduct a qualitative exploration of student experiences and perceptions following the implementation of a yoga-based intervention within an English as a Second Language (ESL) classroom in a private university located in federal territory of Malaysia. Utilizing focus group methodology, the study sought to assess the perceived physical, emotional, and cognitive benefits of participating in a six-month yoga program embedded within the academic curriculum. The intervention was offered exclusively to a cohort of Year 2 ESL students, comprising a total of 35 participants.

Although the program was formally referred to as a "Mindfulness Program," its content and structure were rooted in traditional yoga practices, integrating elements of mindfulness, movement, and breathwork. The primary objective of the intervention was to help students improve their concentration, emotional regulation, and ability to manage classroom-related challenges, particularly within the demanding context of second-language acquisition.

Each class session followed a structured format. Sessions typically began with a brief seated centering exercise, incorporating both physical and mental grounding techniques. This was followed by a teacher-led discussion focused on a central theme relevant to the day's lesson. Subsequently, students engaged in a sequence of physical postures (asanas), breathing exercises (pranayama), and a closing relaxation or meditation segment designed to calm the nervous system and enhance present-moment awareness.

Instruction was provided by teachers who held a minimum qualification of a 200-hour Registered Yoga Teacher (RYT 200) certification. To ensure fidelity and quality of delivery, teachers participated in biweekly meetings, attended three professional development workshops (each lasting two hours), and underwent at least four classroom observations accompanied by structured feedback from the research team.

Students received one to two sessions of yoga instruction per week over the course of the six-month program. The selection of participating students was cohort-based, and all data were collected from the Year 2 ESL group.

To evaluate the students' responses to the program, a focus group discussion was held at the end of the academic term during which the intervention was implemented. The primary aim of the focus group was to obtain in-depth qualitative insights regarding students' perceptions of the yoga program, including its short- and long-term mental and physical benefits, as well as any challenges they faced in maintaining a consistent yoga practice. The discussion lasted approximately 30 minutes. Due to institutional guidelines, the session was not audio-recorded. Instead, two trained research assistants took detailed handwritten notes during the session.

Following the focus group, each research assistant independently transcribed their notes and submitted them to the primary interviewer for cross-verification and review.

Data analysis followed a thematic approach, beginning with the development of preliminary codes informed by theoretical frameworks and prior research (Braun & Clarke, 2023; Saldaña, 2021). These codes were treated as provisional and were later refined through the identification of illustrative quotations from the participants. The interviewer conducted an initial round of open coding, during which key phrases and recurring ideas were documented. Using the constant comparative method (CCM), these codes were compared across participants and settings to identify commonalities and distinctions. Patterns that emerged were synthesized into broader themes, which reflected students' collective responses to the research questions. The final themes were named and categorized following the guidance of qualitative research authorities such as Denzin and Lincoln (2003), capturing the nuanced experiences of students as they engaged with the mindfulness-based yoga intervention.

FINDINGS AND RESULTS

The participants were asked to discuss both psychological and physical benefits to practice. There were four main themes that emerged: mindfulness, autonomous self-regulation, increased well-being, and increased confidence.

Mindfulness

Kabat-Zinn (2003) defines mindfulness as the practice of "paying attention in a particular way: on purpose, in the present moment, and nonjudgmentally." This intentional awareness fosters both emotional regulation and cognitive clarity, skills that many students in the yoga-based mindfulness program identified as crucial outcomes of their participation.

In addition to improved self-regulation, several students shared how the mindfulness practices helped reshape their thought patterns, making them more open-minded and receptive to diverse perspectives. They described becoming more understanding of others' personalities and behaviors, and better able to engage in thoughtful reflection rather than impulsive reaction.

For some, this cognitive shift had a direct impact on behavior and emotional stability. One student noted that the experience had helped her avoid acting irrationally in emotionally charged situations. This change in mindset was echoed by another student who provided a detailed reflection on how mindfulness enhanced her learning experience:

> *"Since participating in the mindfulness sessions as part of our English class, I've experienced a real shift in how I feel during lessons. I now feel more connected to what I'm learning. Before, I often found myself distracted or tense, either worrying about getting the answer wrong or thinking too far ahead. But yoga has helped me to actually focus on the present moment."*

She continued by highlighting how mindfulness influenced her emotional self-awareness:

> *"One of the biggest changes I've noticed is in how I manage my thoughts and emotions, especially when I'm speaking English in class. I used to feel really nervous, and there was always this fear of making mistakes in front of others. I would overthink every sentence and worry that people were judging me. It made me want to avoid participating."*

Through consistent practice, however, she learned to relate to these experiences differently:

> *"But now, thanks to the yoga and mindfulness practices we've learned, I've developed a different relationship with those feelings. I've learned to observe my thoughts without letting them take over. I don't judge myself as harshly anymore. If I make a mistake, I can let it go and keep going. I remind myself that learning is a process and it's okay to not be perfect. That mindset shift has made a huge difference."*

This testimony underscores how mindfulness can foster greater cognitive flexibility, emotional balance, and self-compassion, all of which contribute to more effective learning and interpersonal engagement. By learning to attend to the present moment without harsh self-evaluation, students were better able to navigate the challenges of language learning with confidence and resilience.

Autonomous Self-Regulation

Self-regulation encompasses both physical and mental processes, referring to the capacity of an individual or any system to maintain internal stability while simultaneously adapting to changing external conditions. In the context of personal development and learning, enhanced self-regulation is critical for managing emotions, controlling impulsive behavior, and fostering constructive interpersonal relationships. For students, especially those navigating the complexities of language learning and classroom dynamics, developing self-regulatory skills can significantly influence their academic engagement and emotional well-being.

Participants in the mindfulness-based yoga program spoke openly about how the practices helped them cultivate greater self-awareness and emotional control. Many students highlighted that the sessions enabled them to respond to stress and interpersonal challenges with greater composure and clarity, rather than reacting impulsively or internalizing negative experiences.

One student shared, *"Having a good teacher to explain the basics is definitely helpful, but real progress happens when you start taking charge of your learning. You get immediate feedback, which helps you figure out what works and what doesn't. Over time, that helps you become more independent and confident in how you use the language."* This testimony reflects a growing sense of learner autonomy and metacognitive awareness, both of which are essential components of self-regulated learning.

Another student reflected on the emotional regulation skills gained through yoga:

> *"One of the biggest things yoga has taught me is the difference between reacting and responding. Before, if something upset me or if someone said something annoying. I would immediately react. It was like my emotions just took over, and I'd either get angry or stressed without even thinking. But now, through yoga, I've learned to pause and reflect before responding."*

This shift from automatic emotional reactivity to intentional response demonstrates the influence of mindfulness on students' ability to manage interpersonal conflict and internal stress. The same student elaborated further: *"I especially remember the lessons about the 'fight-or-flight' response. It helped me understand how our bodies are wired to react to stress, but also how we can learn to regulate that. It's like I've started recognizing when that response is being triggered, and instead of letting it take over, I can breathe, step back, and choose how to respond."*

Such reflections illustrate a deepening of emotional intelligence and physiological awareness, both of which are fundamental to sustainable self-regulation. The student continued, *"Honestly, I feel a lot calmer. I don't get aggravated as quickly. If someone is rude or says something hurtful, I try not to take it personally. Yoga has helped me understand that people often act out of their own stress or struggles, and that makes it easier to be compassionate rather than reactive."*

Through consistent mindfulness and yoga practice, students not only reported feeling more in control of their emotions, but also more empathetic and less likely to engage in reactive or defensive behaviors. These developments signal the broader psychological and interpersonal benefits of integrating contemplative practices into educational environments, particularly for students learning in a second language context, where emotional resilience and self-regulation are essential for navigating academic and social challenges.

Increased Well-Being

Participants in the study consistently expressed how the incorporation of yoga into their English lessons had a meaningful impact on their overall sense of well-being, particularly in terms of stress reduction and emotional regulation. Students described feeling more relaxed and mentally settled during and after the yoga sessions, often emphasizing how these practices gave them the patience and calm needed to engage more positively with English language learning.

Many reflected on the contrast between the typically fast-paced, noisy, and often overwhelming school environment, and the sense of mental clarity and stillness they experienced during yoga. For them, the sessions provided a much-needed opportunity to slow down, breathe, and create psychological space in which they could refocus their energy and attention. This sense of calm was not confined to the classroom; students reported that the emotional balance cultivated through yoga often extended into their daily lives, improving their interactions with family members and reducing stress in work settings as well.

One student reflected on this transformation by saying:

"Since starting the yoga-based mindfulness sessions, I've noticed a significant change in how my body and mind respond to stress, especially when learning English. Before, I would often carry a lot of tension in my shoulders and chest whenever I had to speak in class or read aloud. Now, my body feels more at ease. I can pause, take a breath, and respond more calmly. It feels like I have more control over my emotional reactions without needing to control every little thing around me."

The student continued by highlighting the deeper emotional and motivational shifts they experienced:

"That sense of calm has helped me open up more in class and actually enjoy using English. I've also found myself more motivated to practice outside the classroom. I no longer feel intimidated by English books. In fact, I've started reading for fun again, which I never thought I'd do. Overall, I feel more confident, less tense, and genuinely happier about learning English. The mindfulness techniques have made a big difference, not just in my studies, but in how I carry myself as a learner."

This testimony, echoed by others in the study, illustrates how mindfulness-based yoga interventions can enhance not only students' academic engagement but also their broader emotional and psychological well-being. By equipping learners with tools to manage stress and cultivate inner calm, such practices contribute to a more positive learning experience, healthier emotional states, and stronger motivation, both within and beyond the educational setting.

Increased Self Confidence

Participation in the school-based yoga program appeared to play a significant role in enhancing students' self-confidence, both physically and academically. For many students, yoga was a completely new experience, and they initially approached it with hesitation and uncertainty. Several participants admitted they were unsure of their abilities at the start, expressing doubt about whether they could perform the postures or keep up with the class. However, as the weeks progressed, students shared how they were pleasantly surprised by their own progress, both in terms of physical capability and emotional resilience.

Through consistent practice, students began to explore their limits and gradually push beyond them. Many shared how they were able to go deeper into poses, hold their balance longer, and approach each session with increasing confidence. These small but meaningful achievements helped reshape their self-perceptions, reinforcing a sense of capability and personal growth. One student reflected on this transformation by noting that *"it builds confidence in stressful situations"*, emphasizing how the calm and control learned on the mat translated into everyday challenges.

This theme of confidence through challenge was echoed in the classroom setting as well. One student explained:

> *"The classroom isn't just a place to absorb information, it's a space where you're encouraged to try things out, to take risks, and to explore the language in ways that might feel uncomfortable at first. When you take that leap, you're not left guessing, you get feedback that helps you improve."*

They continued by drawing a parallel between yoga and language learning:

> *"When you're holding a balancing pose and you start to wobble, it doesn't mean you're failing, it means you're testing your limits and learning how to grow. Those moments of instability are essential for building strength and resilience. And it's the same with English. If I stumble while speaking or make a mistake with a new word or sentence, I don't see it as failure anymore. I see it as a step forward. That mindset*

has really boosted my confidence, not just in yoga or English, but in how I handle challenges in general."

These reflections highlight how yoga offered more than physical benefits; it provided a psychological framework for taking risks, embracing imperfection, and learning through experience. As students became more comfortable with discomfort, whether in a difficult yoga pose or a complex classroom discussion, they began to develop a stronger sense of self-assurance. Over time, yoga became not just an activity but a life skill that helped cultivate courage, resilience, and confidence in a wide range of situations.

IMPLICATIONS FOR LANGUAGE POLICY, TEACHER EDUCATION, AND RESEARCH

At the outset of this research study, we were genuinely curious about how ESL students would articulate the impact of yoga on their learning and overall well-being. We also reflected on our own experiences with yoga and questioned whether the students' perspectives would differ significantly from ours. What emerged from their reflections was deeply personal, affirming, and remarkably courageous. Their insights not only enriched our understanding of the student experience but also led us to reconsider and expand our own perceptions of the benefits of yoga. Their stories have profoundly shaped how we view the role of mindfulness and movement in education.

Mindfulness and yoga-based approaches demand a shift in language education policy. Social Emotional Learning (SEL) should be embedded within ESL curricula to complement linguistic goals. Curriculum reform must prioritize emotional development alongside cognitive skills. Teacher education programs should include contemplative pedagogy, trauma-informed methods, and culturally responsive strategies. Robust, longitudinal research is essential to validate these approaches. Mixed-methods studies can explore their impact across diverse demographics and educational contexts.

Implementing mindfulness and yoga interventions in higher education requires approaches that are flexible, inclusive, and sensitive to students' diverse backgrounds. The goal is not to replicate traditional yoga classes but to integrate short, evidence-informed practices that promote focus, well-being, and resilience in academic contexts. Some practical strategies include:

1. Brief centering practices at the start of class which helps students transition from external distraction into a state of focus and readiness for learning.
2. Mindful movement breaks which reduce physical tension from prolong sitting and enhance attention in class.
3. Mindful journal and reflection to encourage self-awareness and reflection.
4. Breathwork for stress regulation leading to calmness and reduce feeling of anxiety, especially during exam periods.
5. Initiate more faculty training on yoga and mindfulness practices to equip faculty with safe, inclusive, and secular approaches.

MENTAL HEALTH BENEFITS OF YOGA FOR STUDENTS

Many students experience anxiety as a common emotional response to everyday academic and social pressures. This form of anxiety is often marked by excessive and uncontrollable worry related to specific challenges such as taking exams, public speaking, or concerns about health and performance (Chugh-Gupta et al., 2013). Such anxiety, also known as state anxiety, can significantly impact a student's ability to focus, engage, and perform effectively in their academic and social lives. While professional interventions such as counseling and medication are commonly used, an increasing number of students are turning to yoga as a complementary strategy to manage their mental well-being (Chugh-Gupta et al., 2013).

Yoga, especially traditional practices that emphasize slow and controlled breathing, has been found to help students relax both mentally and physically. According to Sharma and Haider (2013), many symptoms of anxiety such as rapid, shallow breathing and a racing heartbeat can be alleviated through the deep steady breathing techniques taught in yoga. These practices help activate the parasympathetic nervous system, allowing students to calm their minds, lower their heart rate, and reduce blood pressure without relying solely on medication or formal therapy. For students looking for natural and empowering ways to manage stress, yoga provides an accessible tool for achieving greater self-control and emotional balance.

Research supports the positive impact of yoga on student mental health. For instance, Noggle et al. (2012) studied high school students who participated in 28 yoga sessions over a 10-week period. Compared to their peers in regular physical education classes, students who practiced yoga reported reduced levels of anxiety and tension. These findings suggest that integrating yoga into students' routines whether at school or independently can improve their overall emotional well-being and promote a more positive mindset.

In a follow-up study, Conboy et al. (2013) found that students experienced a range of additional benefits from practicing yoga regularly. These included greater motivation and focus, improved self-image, healthier eating habits, better sleep quality, and lower emotional reactivity. Many students also reported feeling more relaxed during stressful situations such as exams, and appreciated the social connection fostered through group yoga sessions. These outcomes demonstrate that yoga not only supports individual mental health but also encourages positive lifestyle changes and peer relationships.

Overall, students who engage in yoga often find it to be a practical and holistic approach to managing anxiety and improving mental health. By incorporating yoga into their daily lives, students can build greater self-awareness, strengthen emotional regulation, and develop the resilience needed to navigate academic and personal challenges.

CONCLUSION

Mindfulness and yoga should no longer be viewed as optional or extracurricular add-ons in education, rather, they are vital pedagogical tools that enable educators to address learners as whole individuals comprising intellectual, emotional, and physical elements. In the context of English as a Second Language (ESL) education, where students often experience a unique convergence of linguistic, cultural, and emotional challenges, the integration of contemplative practices offers a transformative opportunity to support both language development and personal well-being. Teachers play a crucial role in shaping not only the academic outcomes of ESL learners but also their emotional resilience and sense of belonging. When educators intentionally incorporate mindfulness and yoga into classroom routines, they model emotionally supportive behaviors and cultivate a safe space in which learners can thrive. Such practices help students manage anxiety, improve concentration, and regulate their emotions. Such core capacities are especially important for English Language Learners navigating unfamiliar environments and high expectations.

Providing students especially those with limited access to mental health resources with regular exposure to yoga and mindfulness equips them with life skills for emotional balance, cognitive clarity, and self-awareness. This transforms classrooms into spaces that are both linguistically enriching and emotionally supportive. Such practices enhance self-efficacy, encouraging students to learn with curiosity and communicate with greater confidence. By integrating health and wellness into ESL instruction, educators foster inclusivity and reposition the language classroom as a space for personal growth and intercultural understanding. In today's multicultural societies, where communication demands both linguistic skill and emotional intelligence, this approach is not just beneficial, but it is essential. A holistic approach cultivates resilient, self-aware, and socially conscious learners equipped to navigate the demands of a globalized world. By embedding mindfulness and yoga into everyday teaching practices, educators can help shape classrooms that empower students to flourish, not just as language learners, but as whole human beings.

REFERENCES

Alamer, A., & Almulhim, F. (2021). The interrelation between language anxiety and self-determined motivation; a mixed methods approach. *Frontiers in Education, 6*, 618655. DOI: 10.3389/feduc.2021.618655

Baumeister, R. F., & Vohs, K. D. (2004). Self-regulation. *Character strengths and virtues: A handbook and classification*, 499-516.

Bazzano, A. N., Anderson, C. E., Hylton, C., & Gustat, J. (2018). Effect of mindfulness and yoga on quality of life for elementary school students and teachers: Results of a randomized controlled school-based study. *Psychology Research and Behavior Management, 11*, 81–89. DOI: 10.2147/PRBM.S157503 PMID: 29695937

Bazzano, A. N., Sun, Y., Zu, Y., Fleckman, J. M., Blackson, E. A., Patel, T., Shorty-Belisle, A., Liederman, K. H., & Roi, C. (2023). Yoga and mindfulness for social-emotional development and resilience in 3–5 year-old children: Non-randomized, controlled intervention. *Psychology Research and Behavior Management, 16*, 109–118. DOI: 10.2147/PRBM.S385413 PMID: 36660255

Bergen-Cico, D., Possemato, K., & Pigeon, W. (2014). Reductions in cortisol associated with primary care brief mindfulness program for veterans with PTSD. *Medical Care, 52*(Supplement 5), S25–S31. DOI: 10.1097/MLR.0000000000000224 PMID: 25397819

Bishop, S. R., Lau, M., Shapiro, S., Carlson, L., Anderson, N. D., Carmody, J., Segal, Z. V., Abbey, S., Speca, M., Velting, D., & Devins, G. (2004). Mindfulness: A proposed operational definition. *Clinical Psychology : a Publication of the Division of Clinical Psychology of the American Psychological Association, 11*(3), 230–241. DOI: 10.1093/clipsy.bph077

Black, D. S., & Fernando, R. (2014). Mindfulness training and classroom behavior among lower-income and ethnic minority elementary school children. *Journal of Child and Family Studies, 23*(7), 1242–1246. DOI: 10.1007/s10826-013-9784-4 PMID: 25624749

Blair, C. (2010). Stress and the development of self-regulation in context. *Child Development Perspectives, 4*(3), 181–188. DOI: 10.1111/j.1750-8606.2010.00145.x PMID: 21779305

Blair, C., & Ku, S. (2022). A hierarchical integrated model of self-regulation. *Frontiers in Psychology, 13*, 725828. DOI: 10.3389/fpsyg.2022.725828 PMID: 35317011

Braun, V., & Clarke, V. (2023). Toward good practice in thematic analysis: Avoiding common problems and be (com) ing a knowing researcher. *International Journal of Transgender Health, 24*(1), 1–6. DOI: 10.1080/26895269.2022.2129597 PMID: 36713144

Breedvelt, J. J., Amanvermez, Y., Harrer, M., Karyotaki, E., Gilbody, S., Bockting, C. L., Cuijpers, P., & Ebert, D. D. (2019). The effects of meditation, yoga, and mindfulness on depression, anxiety, and stress in tertiary education students: A meta-analysis. *Frontiers in Psychiatry, 10*, 193. DOI: 10.3389/fpsyt.2019.00193 PMID: 31068842

Bryant, E. F., Khanna, M., Bronkhorst, J., Myrvold, K., Shaw, S., Samuel, G., & Holen, A. (2016). *Asian traditions of meditation.* University of Hawaii Press.

Calafato, R. (2023). Charting the motivation, self-efficacy beliefs, language learning strategies, and achievement of multilingual university students learning Arabic as a foreign language. *Asian-Pacific Journal of Second and Foreign Language Education, 8*(1), 20. DOI: 10.1186/s40862-023-00194-5

Can, A., Poyrazl, S., & Pillay, Y. (2021). Eleven Types of Adjustment Problems and Psychological Well-Being among International Students. *Eurasian Journal of Educational Research, 91*(91), 1–20. DOI: 10.14689/ejer.2021.91.1

Chauhan, V., & Saxena, M. T. (2024). Yoga and mindfulness in educational settings: Impact on student well-being and performance. *The Journal of Research Administration, 6*(1).

Chenowith, N. H. (2014). Cultural and linguistic obstacles for ELLs. *Beyond Words, 2*(2), 91-120. https://doi.org/DOI: 10.33508/bw.v2i2.594

Chugh-Gupta, N., Baldassarre, F. G., & Vrkljan, B. H. (2013). Canadian Journal of Occupational. *Canadian Journal of Occupational Therapy*, *80*(3), 150–170. DOI: 10.1177/0008417413500930 PMID: 24224228

Conboy, L. A., Noggle, J. J., Frey, J. L., Kudesia, R. S., & Khalsa, S. B. S. (2013). Qualitative evaluation of a high school yoga program: Feasibility and perceived benefits. *Explore (New York, N.Y.)*, *9*(3), 171–180. DOI: 10.1016/j.explore.2013.02.001 PMID: 23643372

Cook-Cottone, C. P. (2015). *Mindfulness and yoga for self-regulation: A primer for mental health professionals*. Springer Publishing Company. DOI: 10.1891/9780826198631

Csala, B., Springinsfeld, C. M., & Köteles, F. (2021). The relationship between yoga and spirituality: A systematic review of empirical research. *Frontiers in Psychology*, *12*, 695939. DOI: 10.3389/fpsyg.2021.695939 PMID: 34408712

DeLuca, S. M., Kelman, A. R., & Waelde, L. C. (2018). A systematic review of ethnoracial representation and cultural adaptation of mindfulness-and meditation-based interventions. *Psychological Studies*, *63*(2), 117–129. DOI: 10.1007/s12646-018-0452-z

Dimitropoulos, G., Cullen, E., Cullen, O., Pawluk, C., McLuckie, A., Patten, S., Bulloch, A., Wilcox, G., & Arnold, P. D. (2022). "Teachers often see the red flags first": Perceptions of school staff regarding their roles in supporting students with mental health concerns. *School Mental Health*, *14*(2), 402–415. DOI: 10.1007/s12310-021-09475-1

Francis, S. E., Shawyer, F., Cayoun, B. A., Grabovac, A., & Meadows, G. (2024). Differentiating mindfulness-integrated cognitive behavior therapy and mindfulness-based cognitive therapy clinically: The why, how, and what of evidence-based practice. *Frontiers in Psychology*, *15*, 1342592. DOI: 10.3389/fpsyg.2024.1342592 PMID: 38384351

Gaiswinkler, L., & Unterrainer, H. F. (2016). The relationship between yoga involvement, mindfulness and psychological well-being. *Complementary Therapies in Medicine*, *26*, 123–127. DOI: 10.1016/j.ctim.2016.03.011 PMID: 27261992

Garnett, B. (2010). Toward understanding the academic trajectories of ESL youth. *Canadian Modern Language Review*, *66*(5), 677–710. DOI: 10.3138/cmlr.66.5.677

Gey, J. W., Yap, C. K., Leow, K., & Lo, Y. Y. (2025). Resilience as a mediator between emotional intelligence (EI) and perceived stress among young adults in Malaysia. *Discover Mental Health*, *5*(1), 1–13. DOI: 10.1007/s44192-025-00166-w PMID: 40108032

Hagins, M., & Rundle, A. (2016). Yoga improves academic performance in urban high school students compared to physical education: A randomized controlled trial. *Mind, Brain and Education : the Official Journal of the International Mind, Brain, and Education Society*, *10*(2), 105–116. DOI: 10.1111/mbe.12107

Hamid, T. M. H. T. A., & Idrus, F. (2021). A correlational study of the English listening and speaking anxiety in rural areas. *English Language Teaching*, *14*(2), 9–19. DOI: 10.5539/elt.v14n2p9

Harker, R., Pidgeon, A. M., Klaassen, F., & King, S. (2016). Exploring resilience and mindfulness as preventative factors for psychological distress burnout and secondary traumatic stress among human service professionals. *Work (Reading, Mass.)*, *54*(3), 631–637. DOI: 10.3233/WOR-162311 PMID: 27286075

Horwitz, E. (2001). Language anxiety and achievement. *Annual Review of Applied Linguistics*, *21*, 112–126. DOI: 10.1017/S0267190501000071

Hunt, J. (2017). The impact of immigration on the educational attainment of natives. *The Journal of Human Resources*, *52*(4), 1060–1118. DOI: 10.3368/jhr.52.4.0115-6913R1

Hunt, M., Al-Braiki, F., Dailey, S., Russell, R., & Simon, K. (2018). Mindfulness training, yoga, or both? Dismantling the active components of a mindfulness-based stress reduction intervention. *Mindfulness*, *9*(2), 512–520. DOI: 10.1007/s12671-017-0793-z

Hussain, M. S., Salam, A., & Farid, A. (2020). Students' motivation in English language learning (ELL): An exploratory study of motivation-al factors for EFL and ESL adult learners. *International Journal of Applied Linguistics and English Literature*, *9*(4), 15–28. DOI: 10.7575/aiac.ija-lel.v.9n.4p.15

Hytman, L., Amestoy, M. E., Ueberholz, R. Y., & Fiocco, A. J. (2025). Cultural adaptations of mindfulness-based interventions for psychosocial well-being in ethno-racial minority populations: A systematic narrative review. *Mindfulness*, *16*(1), 21–41. DOI: 10.1007/s12671-024-02501-8

Ijadi-Maghsoodi, R., Koushkaki, S. R., Klomhaus, A., Aralis, H., Venegas-Murillo, A., Marlotte, L., Siddiqi, S., Lee, K., De La Cruz, S. A., & Kataoka, S. (2025). Resilience and traumatic stress among Latinx English language learners: A cross-sectional study of students from an urban school district. *BMC Public Health*, *25*(1), 2458. DOI: 10.1186/s12889-025-23105-4 PMID: 40665267

Kabat-Zinn, J. (2003). Mindfulness-based interventions in context: Past, present, and future. *Clinical Psychology : a Publication of the Division of Clinical Psychology of the American Psychological Association*, *10*(2), 144–156. DOI: 10.1093/clipsy.bpg016

Kao, P. C. (2024). Exploring the roles of academic expectation stress, adaptive coping, and academic resilience on perceived English proficiency. *BMC Psychology*, *12*(1), 158. DOI: 10.1186/s40359-024-01630-y PMID: 38493172

Karakurt, N., & Durmaz, H. (2025). The impact of mindfulness intervention on the subjective well-being of nursing students: An experimental study. *BMC Psychology*, *13*(1), 955. DOI: 10.1186/s40359-025-03334-3 PMID: 40846982

Khalsa, S. B. S., & Butzer, B. (2016). Yoga in school settings: A research review. *Annals of the New York Academy of Sciences*, *1373*(1), 45–55. DOI: 10.1111/nyas.13025 PMID: 26919395

Khezerlou, E. (2023). Iranian EFL Students' Perceptions of Foreign Language Writing Anxiety and Perfectionism in Essay Writing. *Journal of English Language Teaching and Linguistics, 8*(3), 277–295. DOI: 10.21462/jeltl.v8i3.1167

Khoury, B., Sharma, M., Rush, S. E., & Fournier, C. (2015). Mindfulness-based stress reduction for healthy individuals: A meta-analysis. *Journal of Psychosomatic Research, 78*(6), 519–528. DOI: 10.1016/j.jpsychores.2015.03.009 PMID: 25818837

Lambert, A. B., & Stapp, A. C. (2020). The Impact of Mindfulness-Based Yoga Interventions on Fifth-Grade Students Perceived Stress and Anxiety. *International Electronic Journal of Elementary Education, 12*(5), 471–480. DOI: 10.26822/iejee.2020562137

Lashari, S. A., Awang-Hashim, R., Lashari, T. A., & Kaur, A. (2023). Acculturation stress and social support for international students' adjustment in Malaysia: Does language proficiency matter? *Journal of Applied Research in Higher Education, 15*(2), 496–508. DOI: 10.1108/JARHE-07-2021-0285

Lemay, V., Hoolahan, J., & Buchanan, A. (2019). Impact of a yoga and meditation intervention on students' stress and anxiety levels. *American Journal of Pharmaceutical Education, 83*(5), 7001. DOI: 10.5688/ajpe7001 PMID: 31333265

Leow, S., Leow, K., & Ean, C. L. C. (2023). Satisfaction of basic psychological needs and eudaimonic well-being among first-year university students. *Cogent Social Sciences, 9*(2), 2275441. DOI: 10.1080/23311886.2023.2275441

Leyland, A., Rowse, G., & Emerson, L. M. (2019). Experimental effects of mindfulness inductions on self-regulation: Systematic review and meta-analysis. *Emotion (Washington, D.C.), 19*(1), 108–122. DOI: 10.1037/emo0000425 PMID: 29578742

Liao, K. Y. H., & Wei, M. (2014). Academic stress and positive affect: Asian value and self-worth contingency as moderators among Chinese international students. *Cultural Diversity & Ethnic Minority Psychology, 20*(1), 107–115. DOI: 10.1037/a0034071 PMID: 24491130

Lincoln, Y. S., & Denzin, N. K. (Eds.). (2003). *Turning points in qualitative research: Tying knots in a handkerchief* (Vol. 2). Rowman Altamira.

Luu, K., & Hall, P. A. (2016). Hatha yoga and executive function: A systematic review. *Journal of Alternative and Complementary Medicine (New York, N.Y.)*, *22*(2), 125–133. DOI: 10.1089/acm.2014.0091 PMID: 26398441

Mak, A. S., Bodycott, P., & Ramburuth, P. (2015). Beyond host language proficiency: Coping resources predicting international students' satisfaction. *Journal of Studies in International Education*, *19*(5), 460–475. DOI: 10.1177/1028315315587109

Malhotra, A. K. (2017). *An Introduction to Yoga Philosophy: an annotated translation of the Yoga Sutras*. Routledge. DOI: 10.4324/9781315262635

Malik, S., Qin, H., & Oteir, I. (2021). Perceived Psychological, Linguistic and Socio-Cultural Obstacles: An Investigation of English Communication Apprehension in EFL Learners. *International Journal of Instruction*, *14*(4), 733–752. DOI: 10.29333/iji.2021.14442a

Noggle, J. J., Steiner, N. J., Minami, T., & Khalsa, S. B. S. (2012). Benefits of yoga for psychosocial well-being in a US high school curriculum: A preliminary randomized controlled trial. *Journal of Developmental and Behavioral Pediatrics*, *33*(3), 193–201. DOI: 10.1097/DBP.0b013e31824afdc4 PMID: 22343481

Ohrt, J., Webster, L., & De La Garza, M. (2014). The effects of a success skills group on adolescents' self-regulation, self-esteem, and perceived learning competence. *Professional School Counseling*, *18*(1), 2156759X0001800113. https://doi.org/DOI: 10.1177/2156759X000180011

Oteir, I. N., & Al-Otaibi, A. N. (2019). Foreign language anxiety: A systematic review. *Arab World English Journal*, *10*(3), 309–317. DOI: 10.24093/awej/vol10no3.21

Park, S., Ueno, S., & Sugita, M. (2025). The Impact of Resilience and Self-Regulation on L2 Proficiency among ESL Learners. *International Journal of TESOL Studies*, *7*(1). Advance online publication. DOI: 10.58304/ijts.20250107

Peng, A., & Patterson, M. M. (2022). Relations among cultural identity, motivation for language learning, and perceived English language proficiency for international students in the United States. *Language, Culture and Curriculum, 35*(1), 67–82. DOI: 10.1080/07908318.2021.1938106

Pidgeon, A. M., & Keye, M. (2014). Relationship between resilience, mindfulness, and pyschological well-being in university students. *International Journal of Liberal Arts and Social Science*, *2*(5), 27–32. http://www.ijlass.org/data/frontImages/gallery/Vol._2_No._5/3.pdf

Qi, X., Tong, J., Chen, S., He, Z., & Zhu, X. (2020). Comparing the psychological effects of meditation-and breathing-focused yoga practice in undergraduate students. *Frontiers in Psychology*, *11*, 560152. DOI: 10.3389/fpsyg.2020.560152 PMID: 33281662

Rajan, G., & Sandhu, M. (2025). Investigating the Efficacy of an Integrative Positive Psychology Intervention (PPI) in Indian College Students: An Eclectic Approach Combining Mindfulness meditation, Guided Imagery, and Gratitude Journaling. *Journal of College Student Mental Health*, 1–25. DOI: 10.1080/28367138.2025.2513954

Raza, S. A., Ahmed, S., Asif, A., & Rani, A. (2023). The Impact of Burnout on the Psychological Well-being of ESL Students in Higher Education Environment. *Siazga Research Journal*, *2*(3), 147–156. DOI: 10.58341/srj.v2i3.21

Razi, N. I. M., & Rahmat, N. H. (2020). Barriers and motivation for learning English: A case study. *European Journal of English Language Teaching*, *6*(1). Advance online publication. DOI: 10.46827/ejel.v6i1.3301

Razza, R. A., Bergen-Cico, D., & Raymond, K. (2015). Enhancing preschoolers' self-regulation via mindful yoga. *Journal of Child and Family Studies*, *24*(2), 372–385. DOI: 10.1007/s10826-013-9847-6

Rosales-Ricardo, Y., Rizzo-Chunga, F., Mocha-Bonilla, J., & Ferreira, J. P. (2021). Prevalence of burnout syndrome in university students: A systematic review. *Salud Mental*, *44*(2), 91–102. DOI: 10.17711/SM.0185-3325.2021.013

Ruecker, T. (2021, March). Retention and persistence in writing programs: A survey of students repeating first-year writing. In *Composition Forum* (Vol. 46). Association of Teachers of Advanced Composition.

Russell, V. (2020). Language anxiety and the online learner. *Foreign Language Annals*, *53*(2), 338–352. DOI: 10.1111/flan.12461

Saldaña, J. (2021). Coding techniques for quantitative and mixed data. *The Routledge reviewer's guide to mixed methods analysis*, 151-160.

Sarubin, N., Nothdurfter, C., Schüle, C., Lieb, M., Uhr, M., Born, C., Zimmermannc, R., Bühner, M., Konopka, K., Rupprecht, R., & Baghai, T. C. (2014). The influence of Hatha yoga as an add-on treatment in major depression on hypothalamic–pituitary–adrenal-axis activity: A randomized trial. *Journal of Psychiatric Research*, *53*, 76–83. DOI: 10.1016/j.jpsychires.2014.02.022 PMID: 24655586

Schultz, P. P., & Ryan, R. M. (2015). The "why,""what," and "how" of healthy self-regulation: Mindfulness and well-being from a self-determination theory perspective. In *Handbook of mindfulness and self-regulation* (pp. 81–94). Springer New York. DOI: 10.1007/978-1-4939-2263-5_7

Serquina, E. A., & Batang, B. L. (2018). Demographic, Psychological Factors and English Proficiency of ESL Students. *TESOL International Journal*, *13*(4), 182–191.

Shami, S., Venu, C. D. V. P., Shanampoodi, G. B., & Rajeswari, T. S. (2025). Impact Of English Language Learning On Mental Health: Exploring The Relationships Between Language Anxiety, Self-Esteem, And Depression. *Journal of Neonatal Surgery*, *14*(9S, 9s), 328–333. DOI: 10.52783/jns.v14.2668

Sharma, M., & Haider, T. (2013). Yoga as an alternative and complementary treatment for patients with low back pain: A systematic review. *Journal of Evidence-Based Complementary & Alternative Medicine*, *18*(1), 23–28. DOI: 10.1177/2156587212458693

Shelov, D. V., Suchday, S., & Friedberg, J. P. (2009). A pilot study measuring the impact of yoga on the trait of mindfulness. *Behavioural and Cognitive Psychotherapy*, *37*(5), 595–598. DOI: 10.1017/S1352465809990361 PMID: 19751539

Slimmen, S., Timmermans, O., Mikolajczak-Degrauwe, K., & Oenema, A. (2022). How stress-related factors affect mental wellbeing of university students A cross-sectional study to explore the associations between stressors, perceived stress, and mental wellbeing. *PLoS One*, *17*(11), e0275925. DOI: 10.1371/journal.pone.0275925 PMID: 36342914

Snyder, B. (2020). *Yoga and mindfulness as a vehicle for language acquisition and social-emotional health for fifth grade ELL language arts students* (Master's thesis, William Paterson University of New Jersey). ProQuest Dissertations & Theses Global.

Soomro, M. A., Rajper, M. A., Koondhar, M. A., & Khan, I. K. (2023). The Relationship between Perceived Psychological Barriers, Anxiety, and Rural Affiliation of Pakistani College Students to Communicate in English. *VFAST Transactions on Education and Social Sciences*, *11*(1), 29–37. DOI: 10.21015/vtess.v11i1.1380

Sultan, S. (2012). Students' perceived competence affecting level of anxiety in learning English as a foreign language. *Pakistan Journal of Psychological Research*, *27*(2), 225–239.

Sun, Y., Lamoreau, R., O'Connell, S., Horlick, R., & Bazzano, A. N. (2021). Yoga and mindfulness interventions for preschool-aged children in educational settings: A systematic review. *International Journal of Environmental Research and Public Health*, *18*(11), 6091. DOI: 10.3390/ijerph18116091 PMID: 34198737

Tajik, M. A., Manan, S. A., Schamiloglu, U., & Namyssova, G. (2024). Gaps between policy aspirations and enactment: Graduate students' struggles with academic English amidst a turbulent transition to the EMI environment in Kazakhstani universities. *Current Issues in Language Planning*, *25*(2), 212–235. DOI: 10.1080/14664208.2023.2283651

Tasan, M., Mede, E., & Sadeghi, K. (2021). The effect of pranayamic breathing as a positive psychology exercise on foreign language learning anxiety and test anxiety among language learners at tertiary level. *Frontiers in Psychology*, *12*, 742060. DOI: 10.3389/fpsyg.2021.742060 PMID: 34659061

Tessler, R. C., & Schwartz, S. H. (1972). Help seeking, self-esteem, and achievement motivation: An attributional analysis. *Journal of Personality and Social Psychology*, *21*(3), 318–326. DOI: 10.1037/h0032321 PMID: 5060750

Thomson, C. J., Lesser, I. A., & Hatfield, G. L. (2024). Psychological and physiological effects of an acute bout of yoga before a simulated academic exam in university students. *Journal of American College Health*, •••, 1–11. DOI: 10.1080/07448481.2024.2308267 PMID: 38330344

Trojan, S. (2020). *Integrating mindfulness strategies and English as a second language instruction* (Capstone project No. 485). Hamline University, School of Education and Leadership. https://digitalcommons.hamline.edu/hse_cp/485

Van Dam, N. T., Van Vugt, M. K., Vago, D. R., Schmalzl, L., Saron, C. D., Olendzki, A., Meissner, T., Lazar, S. W., Kerr, C. E., Gorchov, J., Fox, K. C. R., Field, B. A., Britton, W. B., Brefczynski-Lewis, J. A., & Meyer, D. E. (2018). Mind the hype: A critical evaluation and prescriptive agenda for research on mindfulness and meditation. *Perspectives on Psychological Science*, *13*(1), 36–61. DOI: 10.1177/1745691617709589 PMID: 29016274

Veisiy, N., Arjmandnia, A. A., Vakili, S., & Gholamali Lavasani, M. (2022). The effect of training emotional self-regulation strategies on social competence, academic performance and behavioral problems of students with learning disabilities with comorbidity of attention deficit/hyperactivity disorder. *Journal of Psychological Science*, *21*(116), 1613–1629. DOI: 10.52547/JPS.21.116.1613

Wang, C., & Sun, T. (2020). Relationship between self-efficacy and language proficiency: A meta-analysis. *System*, *95*, 102366. DOI: 10.1016/j.system.2020.102366

Wang, F., & Szabo, A. (2020). Effects of yoga on stress among healthy adults: A systematic review. *Alternative Therapies in Health and Medicine*, *26*(4), 58–64. PMID: 32088671

Wei, F. Y. F., Wang, Y. K., & Klausner, M. (2012). Rethinking college students' self-regulation and sustained attention: Does text messaging during class influence cognitive learning? *Communication Education*, *61*(3), 185–204. DOI: 10.1080/03634523.2012.672755

Wilson, G., & Gillies, R. M. (2005). Stress associated with the transition from high school to university: The effect of social support and self-efficacy. *Australian Journal of Guidance & Counselling*, *15*(1), 77–92. DOI: 10.1375/ajgc.15.1.77

Wimmer, L., Bellingrath, S., & Von Stockhausen, L. (2020). Mindfulness training for improving attention regulation in university students: Is it effective? And do yoga and homework matter? *Frontiers in Psychology*, *11*, 719. DOI: 10.3389/fpsyg.2020.00719 PMID: 32411045

Xuan Mai, L., Ngoc, L. K., & Thao, L. T. (2024). Factors hindering Student participation in English-speaking classes: Student and Lecturer perceptions. *SAGE Open*, *14*(3), 21582440241266297. DOI: 10.1177/21582440241266297

Zasiekina, L., & Zhuravlova, O. (2019). Acculturating stress, language anxiety and procrastination of international students in the academic settings. *Psycholinguistics*, *26*(1), 126–140. DOI: 10.31470/2309-1797-2019-26-1-126-140

Chapter 4

Enhancing Workplace Mental Health and Organisational Wellness: An Integrative Approach

Abinash Sahoo
http://orcid.org/0009-0002-8715-6288
Centurion University of Technology and Management, Bhubaneswar, India

Ayush Benya
http://orcid.org/0009-0009-7242-2468
Centurion University of Technology and Management, Bhubaneswar, India

DattaSai Pamidimarri
http://orcid.org/0009-0007-3819-1331
School of Physiotherapy, BLDE University, India

Pradeep Kumar Sahoo
http://orcid.org/0000-0001-9420-743X
Centurion University, India

DOI: 10.4018/979-8-2600-1202-4.ch004

ABSTRACT

The increasing incidence of mental illness at work has highlighted the need for global action on workplace mental health and organizational well-being. This chapter looks at an integrative model of workplace mental health and organizational well-being, focusing on prevention, promotion, and responsive care. It emphasizes how burnout, stress, and negative organizational culture influence psychological as well as physical health, and how mindfulness and yoga practices improve resilience, concentration, and emotional stability. The biopsychosocial model and yoga leadership are offered as potent tools for building inclusive, ethical, and effective workplaces. The chapter also covers obstacles like stigma and resource deficits while providing techniques for sustainable, culturally responsive mental health promotion in diverse workplaces.

1. INTRODUCTION

Mental health concerns are becoming an increasingly urgent issue within today's global workforce, touching lives on personal, organizational, and societal levels. At any given moment, around 15% of working-age adults are living with a mental disorder (OECD, 2015; World Health Organization, 2022), with depression and anxiety being the most prevalent. The cost of these common disorders goes far beyond the individual—collectively, they are responsible for an estimated USD 1 trillion in lost productivity every year (Bloom et al., 2011). According to WHO, mental health is not just the absence of illness—it's a state of wellbeing in which people can use their abilities, manage life's normal stresses, work productively, and contribute meaningfully to their communities (Rugulies et al., 2023).

To tackle this complex issue effectively, it's important to recognize that mental health exists along a spectrum—ranging from diagnosable mental disorders to general mental health problems and overall mental wellbeing. One of the most promising and widely discussed frameworks in this area is the "integrated approach to workplace mental health" (LaMontagne et al., 2014, 2019). This model focuses on three interconnected areas: preventing harm by addressing work-related risks, promoting the positive by fostering strengths and supportive environments, and responding to existing mental health issues regardless of their origin. It's a holistic, systems-level approach that doesn't stop at short-term solutions but aims for long-term cultural shifts—targeting both the workplace as a whole and the individual worker. The need for such a comprehensive approach is grounded in years of research showing how deeply the conditions of our jobs can impact our mental health. Things like overwhelming workloads, low control over one's tasks, unfair compensation, workplace discrimination, and lack of peer or managerial support have all been shown to increase the risk of developing mental health problems.

Workers in lower occupational roles are more likely to face poor working conditions and are disproportionately affected by mental illness and even (Rugulies et al., 2023). This underscores how mental health is not just a personal issue—it's a matter of social equity. If we want to make lasting change, workplace mental health strategies must take into account these structural disparities and tailor interventions to meet the needs of the most vulnerable. One practical application of the integrated approach can be seen in health-promotion programs that go beyond individual wellness to consider the broader work environment. Macro ergonomics is one such strategy. It focuses on improving both physical and organizational aspects of work to empower employees and promote well-being. Instead of imposing top-down solutions, these programs encourage worker participation in setting goals, designing initiatives, and evaluating outcomes. This inclusive approach has been tested in sectors like healthcare, corrections, and manufacturing, with promising results, both in terms of program effectiveness and sustainability.

What's more, as the field has evolved, different disciplines—medicine, psychology, and public health—have contributed their own perspectives on workplace mental health. However, these efforts have often operated in silos, leading to fragmented interventions that miss the bigger picture (Sanderson & Andrews, 2006). There's now a growing consensus that we need to break down these barriers and integrate insights across fields. The only widely used model for this process so far is the Knowledge to Action (KTA) framework, which helps organizations convert research findings into usable strategies tailored to their specific context (BeyondBlue, 2019). Even then, much more needs to be done to ensure these interventions are culturally sensitive, adaptable, and effective across diverse workplace settings. Despite these challenges, the workplace holds enormous untapped potential for improving public mental health. It's not just about avoiding harm—it's about creating a culture that actively supports and uplifts mental wellbeing (International Labor Organization, n.d.).

Evidence shows that work environments that emphasize psychological safety, open communication, supportive leadership, and opportunities for personal growth serve as protective buffers against stress and burnout. This is where Yoga, as a holistic and integrative health discipline, can offer a unique and valuable contribution. The principles behind the integrated approach to workplace mental health align remarkably well with traditional yogic teachings. Yoga emphasizes balance, self-awareness, compassion, and resilience—all of which are essential components of mental wellness. Practices such as pranayama (breathing techniques), asanas (postures), and dhyana (meditation) have been shown to reduce stress hormones, regulate emotions, and even enhance cognitive functioning. These effects make Yoga an ideal complement to both preventive and therapeutic mental health strategies in the workplace.

Studies have demonstrated that yoga-based workplace interventions can improve mood, lower stress levels, and foster a greater sense of emotional and psychological stability. Moreover, Yoga doesn't just benefit individuals—it fits seamlessly into broader, systems-level models of mental health. In the same way, macro ergonomic strategies aim to reshape workplace environments. Yoga encourages people to develop a mindful relationship with their surroundings. Philosophical concepts such as *samatvam* (equanimity) and *karma yoga* (selfless action) can inspire attitudes of calm, compassion, and purposeful engagement—qualities that are vital for building inclusive, supportive, and mentally healthy workplaces. By incorporating Yoga into workplace wellness policies and programs, organizations have an opportunity to address mental health on all three levels outlined in the integrated model: prevention, promotion, and response. It can empower individuals while also contributing to a culture of care and collective responsibility. Ultimately, addressing mental health in the workplace requires more than good intentions. It calls for coordinated, comprehensive action rooted in evidence and aligned with human values.

2. THE MENTAL HEALTH LANDSCAPE IN MODERN WORKPLACES

The modern workplace has undergone a significant transformation due to technological advancements, globalization, remote work trends, and an increasing emphasis on productivity. Understanding the interplay between mental and physical health is essential, especially as the profession's scope increasingly intersects with occupational health, wellness, and rehabilitation. According to the World Health Organization (WHO), depression and anxiety contribute to a loss of productivity amounting to approximately USD 1 trillion annually (World Health Organization, 2022). In today's fast-paced work environments, chronic stress has become normalized, especially in high-demand sectors such as healthcare, information technology, education, and customer service. In the Indian context, the National Mental Health Survey (2016) reported that nearly 15% of working-age adults suffer from some form of mental illness, with stress and anxiety most commonly seen in corporate sectors (Murthy, 2017).

The COVID-19 pandemic further exacerbated these concerns by introducing new stressors such as job insecurity, social isolation, and blurred work-life boundaries due to remote work (Rajgopal, 2020). Several psychosocial and organizational factors within workplaces contribute to mental health challenges. High job demands and excessive workloads often lead to burnout, especially when combined with low decision-making autonomy. Karasek's Job Demand-Control model identifies such conditions as significant predictors of psychological strain (Karasek & Theorell, 1990). The erosion of work-life boundaries, particularly with the widespread adoption of remote and hybrid work, has also led to cognitive overload and emotional fatigue. Persistent connectivity, even during off-hours, can negatively impact recovery and mental restoration (Sonnentag et al., 2010). Interpersonal issues in the workplace, such as bullying and harassment, have been strongly linked to anxiety, depression, and decreased work motivation. Chronic exposure to such toxic environments can also result in somatic symptoms like musculoskeletal pain and fatigue, reinforcing the connection between mental and physical health (Einarsen et al., 2011). Additionally, a lack of recognition, job insecurity, and minimal growth opportunities can lead to disengagement and long-term emotional exhaustion, contributing to a toxic organizational culture (Sparks et al., 2001).

Mental health issues often manifest physically through symptoms commonly addressed by physiotherapists. Employees suffering from mental distress may report chronic neck and back pain, tension headaches, migraines, temporomandibular joint disorders (TMD), myofascial pain syndrome, generalized fatigue, and insomnia. These physical symptoms may initially mask underlying psychological distress. A 2021 study by Kanchibhotla et al. found that 47% of IT professionals experiencing work-related stress also reported co-existing musculoskeletal complaints, suggesting a psychosomatic link Kanchibhotla et al. (2021). Such conditions are often worsened by poor ergonomic practices, sedentary behavior, and lack of physical activity—areas where physiotherapists can provide direct intervention.

Traditionally, physiotherapy has emphasized the biomechanical model of health. However, growing awareness of the impact of psychological factors on physical recovery supports the shift toward a biopsychosocial (BPS) framework. First proposed by Engel (1977), the BPS model incorporates the complex interactions among biological, psychological, and social influences on health outcomes. This approach is especially relevant in chronic pain and rehabilitation contexts, where anxiety, depression, and stress can lower pain thresholds, reduce motivation, and hinder adherence to treatment protocols (Main et al., 2010). By integrating mental health awareness into their clinical reasoning, physiotherapists can play a more comprehensive role in health promotion.

The role of physiotherapists in workplace mental health is multi-dimensional:

- Physiotherapist are often among the first health professionals to recognize the somatic expressions of psychological distress. Early identification and appropriate referral to mental health professionals can facilitate timely, holistic care (Cott et al., 2004).
- Physiotherapists play a key role in ergonomic interventions. Inappropriate workstation design and static postures contribute significantly to both physical discomfort and psychological strain.

Through ergonomic assessments and employee education, physiotherapists can help prevent musculoskeletal problems and reduce stress-related symptoms (Robertson et al., 2009).

- Physiotherapists are well-positioned to lead workplace wellness and stress-reduction programs. Exercise improves mood, reduces symptoms of anxiety and depression, and enhances overall well-being. Supervised exercise interventions tailored to individual capabilities have shown benefits beyond musculoskeletal health (Paluska & Schwenk, 2000).

To foster mentally healthy workplaces, organizational commitment and policy reform are essential. Human resources and occupational health teams must work together to develop preventive strategies that address both mental and physical wellness. These include regular mental health screenings, access to Employee Assistance Programs (EAPs), and training for managers in mental health literacy, and clear policies against workplace harassment and discrimination. Importantly, physiotherapists should be integrated into multidisciplinary occupational health teams to provide a dual perspective—addressing both the physical and psychological demands of work. Such collaborative efforts can contribute to a healthier and more productive workforce.

Despite growing awareness of workplace mental health, several barriers persist. Stigma remains a significant challenge, often discouraging employees from seeking help due to fear of discrimination or professional repercussions. Additionally, many physiotherapists lack formal training in mental health first aid or the application of psychosocial principles in practice. Limited resources and poor access to integrated care in low- and middle-income countries further compound the problem. Overcoming these barriers requires a multipronged approach, including curriculum updates in physiotherapy education, interprofessional training programs, and increased investment in public health infrastructure. Looking ahead, the field of physiotherapy must adapt to the changing demands of modern workplaces. Incorporating modules on workplace psychology, communication skills, and stress physiology into undergraduate and postgraduate physiotherapy curricula is essential. More empirical research, particularly randomized controlled trials, is needed to evaluate physiotherapy's role in integrated mental health care. Physiotherapists, with their expertise in physical rehabilitation and functional restoration, are uniquely positioned to contribute to mental health promotion, early intervention, and long-term occupational health strategies. Embracing this expanded role will not only enhance clinical outcomes but also position physiotherapists as key stakeholders in the creation of healthier, more resilient workplaces.

3. MANAGING STRESS AND PREVENTING BURNOUT

Stress and burnout have become widespread concerns in modern life, affecting individuals across all professions and age groups. As the demands of daily life increase, individuals are expected to manage multiple roles, meet deadlines, and maintain high levels of productivity, often at the expense of their mental and physical well-being. Chronic stress, when left unmanaged, can evolve into burnout, a state of emotional, physical, and mental exhaustion caused by prolonged exposure to stressful situations. Understanding the mechanisms of stress, its impact, and the strategies to prevent burnout is crucial for maintaining long-term health and optimal functioning. Stress is a natural physiological and psychological response to perceived challenges or threats, activating the body's sympathetic nervous system and triggering the "fight-or-flight" response (McEwen, 1998).

While acute stress can be adaptive and enhance performance in short bursts, chronic stress can have detrimental effects on health, including increased risk of cardiovascular disease, weakened immune function, anxiety, depression, and sleep disturbances (Schneiderman et al., 2005). Burnout, on the other hand, is considered a specific outcome of chronic occupational stress and is characterized by three key dimensions: emotional exhaustion, depersonalization or cynicism, and reduced personal accomplishment (Maslach & Leiter, 2016). Although initially studied in the context of caregiving and human service professions, burnout is now recognized as a broader phenomenon affecting workers across sectors, including students and homemakers. The factors contributing to stress and burnout are multifaceted, involving individual, organizational, and societal dimensions. At the individual level, personality traits such as perfectionism, low resilience, and poor emotional regulation can increase vulnerability to stress. Additionally, negative coping mechanisms like avoidance, substance abuse, or emotional suppression can perpetuate the stress cycle.

On an organizational level, high job demands, low autonomy, lack of recognition, poor management, and unclear expectations are commonly reported stressors (Demerouti et al., 2001). Prolonged exposure to such conditions without adequate support can erode motivation and well-being. Furthermore, the blurring of work-life boundaries, particularly in the era of remote work and digital connectivity, has intensified the pressure to remain constantly available, disrupting recovery and personal time (Derks & Bakker, 2014).

Societally, cultural norms that equate productivity with self-worth and stigmatize rest or vulnerability contribute to a collective environment where stress is normalized and burnout is underreported. The consequences of chronic stress and burnout extend beyond the individual, impacting families, organizations, and communities. Emotionally exhausted individuals may become irritable, disengaged, or less empathetic, which can strain interpersonal relationships and team dynamics. Burnout is associated with reduced job satisfaction, increased absenteeism, and higher turnover rates, all of which affect organizational performance and morale (Shirom, 2005). On a broader scale, stress-related illnesses contribute to the growing burden on healthcare systems and reduce the overall quality of life within societies. At the individual level, cultivating stress management techniques is fundamental. Mindfulness-based practices, such as meditation, body scanning, and breathwork, have been shown to enhance emotional regulation, reduce rumination, and improve psychological resilience (Chiesa & Serretti, 2009).

Establishing healthy lifestyle habits—such as a balanced diet, adequate sleep, and meaningful social connections—further supports emotional well-being. Preventing burnout, however, cannot rest solely on the shoulders of individuals. Organizational responsibility plays a pivotal role. Creating a psychologically safe and supportive workplace culture is essential. Employers should strive to ensure reasonable workloads, offer flexible working arrangements, and encourage employees to take regular breaks and use their vacation time (Leiter & Maslach, 2005). Providing opportunities for professional growth, constructive feedback, and recognizing achievements can foster a sense of purpose and engagement. Open communication channels and accessible mental health resources, including employee assistance programs and counseling, are vital in promoting early intervention and destigmatizing help-seeking behavior. Leadership training on emotional intelligence and stress-sensitive management can also enhance team morale and cohesion. Furthermore, job redesign to increase autonomy, task variety, and alignment with individual strengths and values has been linked to reduced burnout and greater work satisfaction (Bakker & Demerouti, 2007). For institutions such as schools, hospitals, or corporate entities, regular assessment of stress levels and burnout risk among employees through validated tools like the Maslach Burnout Inventory (MBI) can inform targeted interventions.

On a societal level, public health campaigns and education about mental health, work-life balance, and the importance of self-care are necessary to shift cultural attitudes. Policy measures such as regulations on working hours, mandatory rest breaks, and the right to disconnect laws—already implemented in several European countries—can help safeguard mental health and promote sustainable working conditions (Messenger et al., 2017). Additionally, integrating stress management and emotional well-being into educational curricula can equip individuals from an early age with the tools to navigate life's challenges. Social support systems also play a crucial role in buffering stress and enhancing coping. Strong relationships with family, friends, and community networks provide emotional validation, practical help, and a sense of belonging. Research indicates that perceived social support is a significant predictor of psychological resilience and recovery from burnout (Halbesleben, 2006). Encouraging open dialogue about stress and normalizing emotional expression can counteract feelings of isolation and shame.

Group-based interventions, including peer support groups or community wellness programs, can also offer collective coping mechanisms and shared understanding. Technology, while often implicated in increasing stress, can also be harnessed positively. Psychologists, counselors, and therapists can offer tailored support, coping strategies, and therapeutic interventions to prevent the escalation of stress into clinical burnout or depression. While complete elimination of stress is neither possible nor desirable, as moderate stress can foster growth and achievement, the key lies in maintaining a balanced response. Resilience—the capacity to recover and grow from adversity—is a dynamic skill that can be cultivated. Factors that contribute to resilience include optimism, adaptability, a sense of purpose, emotional awareness, and problem-solving skills (Southwick et al., 2014). Cultivating these traits through reflective practices, goal-setting, and experiential learning can equip individuals to navigate complex environments with greater ease. In conclusion, managing stress and preventing burnout require a holistic and sustained effort across personal, organizational, and societal levels. While individuals must take active responsibility for their self-care, the burden cannot rest solely on them. Employers and policymakers must create environments that support mental well-being and promote work-life harmony. As awareness of mental health grows, it is essential to foster a culture where rest, balance, and emotional honesty are valued as much as productivity and achievement. With a collaborative and compassionate approach, it is possible to transform the way stress is perceived and managed, paving the way for healthier, more fulfilling lives.

4. ENHANCING PRODUCTIVITY THROUGH MINDFULNESS

The increasing demands of the modern workplace, constant digital connectivity, and the expectation to multitask have all contributed to heightened stress levels and cognitive fatigue. Amidst these challenges, mindfulness has emerged as a scientifically supported strategy for enhancing productivity and well-being. Mindfulness, defined as intentional and non-judgmental awareness of the present moment, has gained prominence as an evidence-based approach to enhancing well-being and productivity. Initially rooted in contemplative traditions, mindfulness has been widely adapted in organizational and clinical settings due to its positive effects on cognitive functioning, emotional regulation, and work engagement.

Mindfulness training has been shown to activate brain regions associated with executive functions, such as the prefrontal cortex, which is responsible for attention, planning, working memory and cognitive flexibility. Research indicates that even brief mindfulness practices improve sustained attention and working-memory performance, counteracting distraction and mental fatigue (Zeidan et al., 2010). By reducing mental clutter associated with stress and worry, mindfulness enables individuals to focus on priorities, make clearer decisions, and maintain task engagement.

Emotional regulation is another key mechanism through which mindfulness supports productivity. High emotional reactivity and unmanaged stress impair communication, cooperation, and performance. Mindfulness fosters awareness of emotional states and reduces automatic, maladaptive responses. Employees practicing mindfulness report reduced emotional exhaustion and enhanced job satisfaction—predictors of improved performance (Hülsheger et al., 2013). This emotional stability supports teamwork, conflict resolution, and interpersonal functioning within workplace settings.

A substantial body of research supports the role of mindfulness in stress reduction. Chronic stress impairs concentration, memory, and creativity, and contributes to burnout and absenteeism. Mindfulness interrupts the stress response by promoting relaxation and parasympathetic nervous system activation Mindfulness-based interventions (MBIs), such as Mindfulness-Based Stress Reduction (MBSR), lower cortisol levels and alleviate symptoms of anxiety and depression (Khoury et al., 2015). Reduced stress enhances clarity, confidence, and efficiency, enabling employees to re-engage with tasks effectively.

Mindfulness also improves time management and self-regulation. By promoting intentional decision-making and reducing impulsivity, mindfulness decreases tendencies toward procrastination and supports disciplined work habits (Shapiro et al., 2012). It also reduces mind-wandering—a major contributor to reduced accuracy and longer task completion times—helping individuals maintain consistent, goal-directed behaviour.

Creativity and innovation, which are critical for organizational competitiveness, are positively influenced by mindfulness. Open-monitoring meditation enhances divergent thinking and insight-based problem-solving, enabling individuals to generate novel ideas and adapt to new challenges (Colzato et al., 2012).Mindful leaders demonstrate greater clarity, empathy, and responsiveness, fostering trust and psychological safety within teams. Leader mindfulness has been associated with higher employee engagement and job satisfaction, amplifying team and organizational performance (Reb et al., 2014)

Digital mindfulness tools, including apps such as Headspace, Calm, and Insight Timer, have improved accessibility to mindfulness practices. Even brief app-based practices reduce stress and enhance focus, making them easily adaptable to work routines (Bostock et al., 2019). These tools are particularly relevant in hybrid and remote work contexts, where digital fatigue and blurred boundaries increase stress.

At the organizational level, mindfulness contributes to improved job satisfaction, lower absenteeism, and enhanced well-being. Mental health challenges—such as stress, burnout, and emotional exhaustion—are linked to decreased productivity and higher turnover (Riani & Sopiansah, 2023; Ashkanasy & Kay, 2023). When incorporated into comprehensive wellness strategies, mindfulness can reduce burnout, anxiety, and psychological distress among employees (Srivastava et al., 2024; Wang et al., 2024; Lee et al., 2024).

4.1. Mechanisms of Mindfulness in Enhancing Employee Well-Being

Understanding how mindfulness affects individuals within the workplace context elucidates its efficacy. Mindfulness contributes to enhanced self-awareness and emotional regulation. Enhanced self-awareness is crucial for personal and professional development, encouraging proactive behaviors and positive workplace relationships. Additionally, mindfulness is linked to reduced levels of incivility and interpersonal conflicts within teams. Employees practicing mindfulness exhibit lower degrees of emotional reactivity, fostering a more harmonious and collaborative workplace culture (He et al., 2025).

4.2. The Role of Organizational Culture

Organizations that encourage ongoing mindfulness practice, provide training resources, and promote a balance between work and personal life facilitate greater employee engagement and wellness (Huseynova & İslamoğlu, 2024). For instance, organizations can implement digital tools such as mindfulness apps or online workshops that allow for flexible engagement of employees. Given the shift toward remote and hybrid work models, these tools can ensure that mindfulness practices remain accessible (Silva, 2024).

Mindfulness training has been associated with heightened cognitive flexibility, allowing employees to approach challenges with fresh perspectives, which is crucial for maintaining competitive advantage in today's fast-paced business environments (Ioannou, 2023).

However, the implementation of mindfulness must be ethical and context-sensitive. Mindfulness is not a substitute for addressing structural workplace issues such as excessive workloads, poor leadership practices, or inadequate staffing. When introduced appropriately, mindfulness supports goal pursuit by enhancing self-awareness, intrinsic motivation, and value alignment—fostering sustainable productivity rather than promoting passivity.

As workplaces evolve in response to technological and social change, mindfulness is increasingly integrated into professional development, leadership training, and educational settings. Its demonstrated benefits for resilience, adaptability, emotional intelligence, and cognitive agility position it as a valuable skill for navigating complex, high-demand environments.

5. BUILDING HEALTHY WORKPLACES: POLICIES, MEASUREMENT TOOLS, AND SYSTEMIC MENTAL HEALTH INTERVENTIONS

Incorporating established policy frameworks significantly strengthens organizational wellness programs by ensuring that interventions are evidence-based and not merely voluntary add-ons. Such frameworks promote clear leadership accountability, cultural and legal compliance, and standardized approaches to evaluating and mitigating psychosocial risks. Together, they position mental health as an essential component of occupational health rather than an optional organizational service.

Figure 1. Flowchart 1

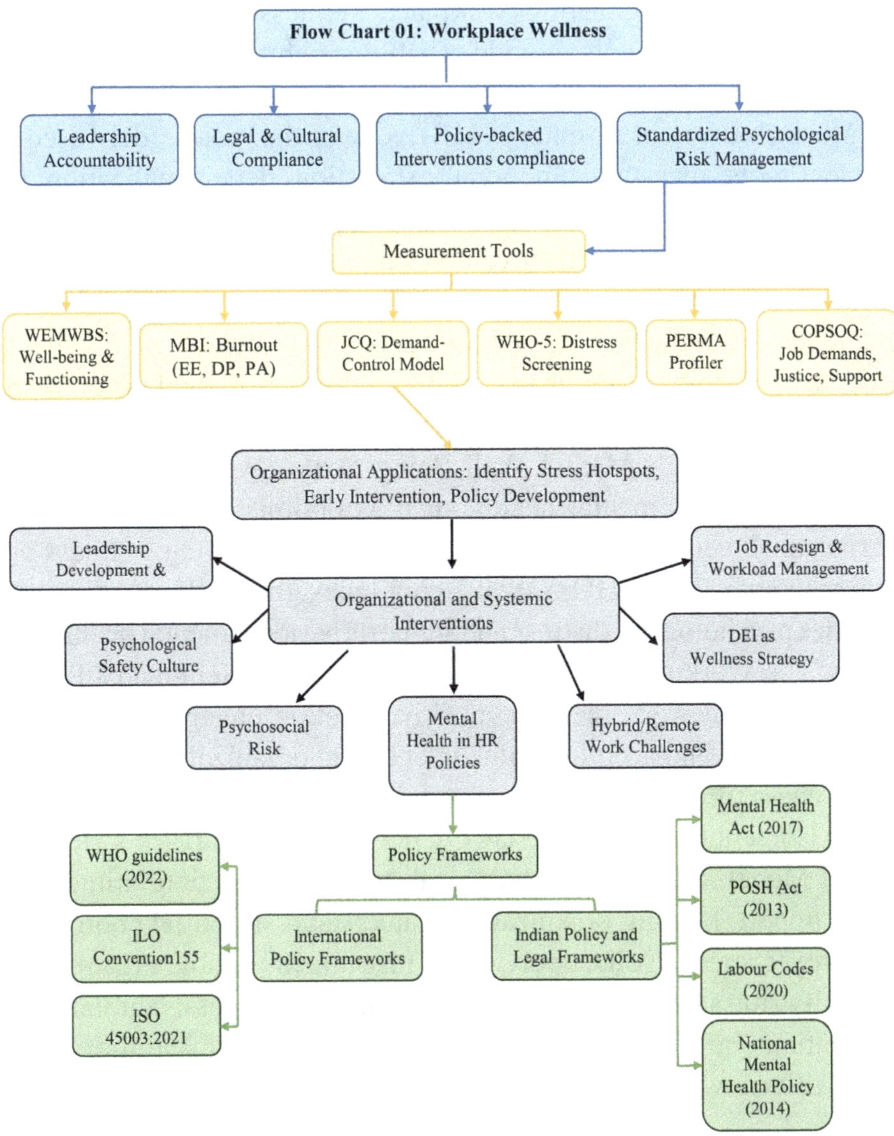

5.1. Measurement Tools for Assessing Workplace Mental Health

Robust mental health assessment is equally crucial for designing, implementing, and evaluating workplace wellness initiatives. Validated measurement instruments provide reliable insights into employee stress levels, burnout risk, psychological well-being, and organizational climate. The Maslach Burnout Inventory (MBI), one of the most widely used assessment tools, measures emotional exhaustion, depersonalization, and reduced personal accomplishment and is applicable across sectors such as healthcare, education, information technology, and corporate environments. The Copenhagen Psychosocial Questionnaire (COPSOQ) offers comprehensive evaluation of psychosocial factors—including job demands, work pace, organizational justice, and social support—and is commonly used in psychosocial risk audits aligned with ISO 45003 guidelines. The Warwick–Edinburgh Mental Well-Being Scale (WEMWBS) assesses positive aspects of mental health, such as optimism, functioning, and interpersonal well-being, making it suitable for evaluating wellness program outcomes. The WHO-5 Well-Being Index, though brief, effectively identifies psychological distress and supports periodic mental health monitoring. The Workplace PERMA-Profiler, based on Seligman's Positive Psychology framework, measures positive emotion, engagement, relationships, meaning, and accomplishment, enabling organizations to track the effectiveness of cultural and developmental interventions. Additionally, the Job Content Questionnaire (JCQ), derived from Karasek's Demand-Control Model, assesses psychological demands, decision latitude, and social support, helping organizations understand structural contributors to employee stress. Collectively, these instruments enable organizations to identify stress hotspots, monitor program effectiveness, facilitate early interventions, inform policy decisions, and transition from intuition-driven to data-driven wellness strategies.

5.2. Organizational and Systemic Interventions for Workplace Mental Health

While individual-level techniques such as mindfulness and yoga offer substantial benefits, sustainable workplace well-being requires systemic, policy-driven, and organizational-level strategies that address structural determinants of stress. Psychosocial risk management is fundamental, requiring regular assessment of hazards such as high workload, unclear roles, poor leadership communication, limited autonomy, workplace conflict, and job insecurity. Addressing these risks helps reduce burn-out, strengthen morale, and enhance overall productivity. Job redesign and workload management further contribute by improving role clarity, aligning tasks with employee strengths, redistributing workload during peak periods, and ensuring adequate staffing. These measures increase job satisfaction and bolster employee resilience.

Leadership development also plays a critical role in promoting workplace mental health. Leaders influence organizational culture and employee well-being, and thus must be equipped with skills in mental health literacy, emotional intelligence, and effective communication. When leaders model healthy behaviors and are evaluated through wellness-related performance indicators, transformational and supportive leadership styles become more prominent, fostering psychological safety and reducing stress. Diversity, Equity, and Inclusion (DEI) initiatives complement these efforts by reducing workplace discrimination—a well-known psychosocial stressor. Anti-discriminatory policies, bias training, inclusive leadership approaches, and employee affinity groups contribute to a psychologically safe environment where equity and belonging are prioritized.

Hybrid and remote work arrangements introduce additional challenges, such as blurred work–life boundaries and digital fatigue. Organizations can address these through "Right to Disconnect" guidelines, rotational offline hours, and clear expectations regarding after-hours communication, and ergonomic as well as mental health support for remote employees. Protecting these boundaries is vital for preventing digital burnout. Creating a culture of psychological safety further strengthens workplace well-being by encouraging open communication, reducing stigma, promoting appropriate risk-taking, and supporting help-seeking behaviors. Practical strategies include anonymous feedback systems, regular check-ins, team-based well-being discussions, and establishing norms that encourage employees to voice concerns without fear.

Embedding mental health considerations into human resource policies ensures long-term consistency and sustainability. Mental health should be integrated into onboarding processes, performance appraisals, promotion criteria, Employee Assistance Programs (EAPs), and return-to-work policies following mental health leave. Such integration supports employees throughout the life cycle of their employment and reinforces mental health as an organizational priority.

5.3. Policy Frameworks Supporting Workplace Mental Health

Policy frameworks further enhance workplace mental health by providing clear guidance on employee rights, organizational responsibilities, and mechanisms for risk management. At the international level, the WHO Guidelines on Mental Health at Work (2022) outline evidence-based recommendations for creating psychologically safe workplaces, emphasizing psychosocial risk assessments, reduction of excessive workload, increased worker autonomy, and mental health training for managerial staff. The ILO Occupational Safety and Health Framework, specifically Convention 155, mandates employers to identify and mitigate hazards affecting physical and psychological well-being, recognizing psychosocial risks—such as stress, harassment, and overwork—as occupational health concerns requiring structured interventions. ISO 45003:2021 provides a comprehensive standard for managing psychosocial risks by identifying stressors related to job demands, role clarity, workload, and leadership style, and by outlining measures for job redesign, flexible scheduling, and improved communication. It is widely regarded as the global benchmark for mental health governance.

In the Indian context, policy frameworks also play a significant role. The National Mental Health Policy (2014) advocates for mental health promotion in workplaces through early identification, de-stigmatization, and capacity building. The Mental Healthcare Act (2017) reinforces the rights of persons with mental illness, requiring workplaces to ensure non-discrimination and reasonable accommodations. The POSH Act (2013) recognizes harassment as a psychosocial hazard and mandates Internal Complaints Committees, thereby directly influencing workplace psychological safety. The Labour Codes (2020) contain provisions concerning work hours, employee welfare, and workplace safety, indirectly shaping key determinants of mental health such as workload, job control, and work–life balance.

6. YOGA-BASED LEADERSHIP AND DECISION-MAKING

The Science and Philosophy of Yoga for Modern Leaders: Yoga, traditionally perceived as a mere physical practice, encompasses a broader philosophical and ethical framework. Central to this philosophy are the Yamas and Niyamas, ethical precepts that offer guidance on personal conduct and interpersonal relations. These two limbs of Ashtanga yoga provide vital insights for modern leadership, emphasizing values such as discipline, compassion, and self-awareness. This multidimensional approach aligns well with the demands for sustainable leadership in organizational settings where empathy and ethical considerations are paramount (Dash, 2024). The distillation of yoga's ethical dimensions into actionable leadership strategies can fundamentally transform decision-making processes.

Research indicates that yoga and mindfulness facilitate improved emotional regulation and stress management, which are crucial for effective leadership. The practice enables leaders to cultivate self-awareness and clarity of thought, allowing for more thoughtful and inclusive decision-making. Mindfulness has been shown to enhance cognitive flexibility and improve executive function, thereby resulting in superior problem-solving capabilities (Garland & Howard, 2018). A multicenter cross-sectional study indicated that leaders promoting work-life balance and self-care resources not only foster resilience within their teams but also enhance their overall effectiveness (Kumar et al., 2023). Incorporating yoga into organizational wellness programs serves as a proactive strategy to mitigate stress while enhancing both physical and mental well-being.

Yoga's holistic philosophy promotes the idea of interconnectedness, fostering collective leadership models that are urgently needed in organizations today. Collaborative leadership, rooted in empathetic engagement and shared responsibility, resonates with the yogic understanding of community and relational ethics. In this respect, yoga becomes a vehicle for empowering leaders to cultivate inclusive environments where diverse perspectives are valued and integrated into the decision-making process.

The leadership landscape increasingly acknowledges the importance of psychological safety as a precursor to effective team performance. Practices derived from yoga emphasize openness, vulnerability, and trust, essential attributes for fostering an environment conducive to innovative thought and collaboration (Wildcroft, 2020). Consequently, the philosophical underpinnings of yoga not only contribute to individual leaders' well-being but also significantly impact collective outcomes within teams and organizations.

Implementing yoga and mindfulness within organizational frameworks also aligns with evidence-based recommendations regarding health promotion and resilience-building practices. Research highlights that regular engagement in mindful activities correlates with improved overall quality of life, mental health, and resilience, thereby enhancing workplace dynamics (Groessl et al., 2015). For modern leaders, espousing these values goes beyond personal transformation, as it directly shapes their organizational culture and fosters a climate of encouragement and growth.

In an age characterized by rapid turnover and shifting organizational structures, yoga-based leadership emerges as a sustainable approach that adapts to change while fostering stability and ethical grounding. The emphasis on self-regulation and self-improvement inherent in yoga translates into leadership practices that prioritize adaptability and ethical decision-making—qualities essential for modern leaders facing unpredictable challenges (Elwy et al., 2014).

Moreover, the practice of yoga encourages a reflective approach to leadership, which reinforces the need for ongoing learning and adaptation. As leaders cultivate personal mindfulness, they inspire a culture that values continuous improvement and professional development. For instance, mindfulness training for school administrators has shown significant positive impacts on well-being and effective leadership, reaffirming the transformative capacity of such practices when integrated into various leadership contexts (Mahfouz, 2018). Through deliberate reflection, leaders are equipped to better navigate their experiences, fostering a more profound connection with their teams and their organizational purpose.

Integrating yoga into leadership training is also associated with improved interpersonal skills. As emphasized by the principles of self-management and relationship management outlined in social-emotional learning frameworks, leaders who practice yoga tend to exhibit enhanced emotional intelligence and empathy (Sanchez & Kazen, 2021). These skills are pivotal in establishing authentic relationships with team members, facilitating collaboration, and generating a culture of support and mutual respect. As leaders embody the philosophical dimensions of yoga, they contribute to a workplace environment that prioritizes human connection and psychological safety.

In essence, yoga provides a repository of tools that modern leaders can draw upon to enhance their decision-making processes. The integration of these practices not only improves individual well-being but also establishes systems of support that benefit the entire organization.

6.1. Yoga and Leadership Qualities: Calmness, Clarity, Empathy, Resilience, and Ethical Decision-Making

Leadership, fundamentally intertwined with interpersonal relationships and decision-making processes, is increasingly aligned with holistic practices such as yoga.

6.1.1. Calmness in Leadership

Calmness is a cornerstone of effective leadership. Leaders often face high-pressure situations, and the ability to maintain composure can significantly influence team dynamics and decision-making processes. Yoga integrates breathing techniques and mindfulness practices that enhance an individual's capacity for calmness. Research suggests that yoga practitioner's exhibit reduced stress levels and increased emotional stability, which is essential for leaders as they often serve as emotional anchors for their teams (Deshmukh et al., 2024)

6.1.2. Clarity

Clarity is another vital leadership quality that is significantly enhanced by yoga practices. Transformational leadership, characterized by its focus on inspiring and motivating followers towards a common vision, depends heavily on the leader's ability to articulate clear goals and provide direction (Ha & Moon, 2023).The practice of yoga, which emphasizes focus and presence, can help leaders develop a clearer vision for their organization and a clearer articulation of expectations. In the context of transformational leadership, goal clarity is crucial as it guides individuals in understanding their roles within the larger framework. Studies have demonstrated that organizations exhibiting high goal clarity foster greater employee engagement and performance (Fürstenberg et al., 2021).

6.1.3. Empathy

Empathy, the ability to understand and share the feelings of others, fosters strong relationships within teams. Yoga practices inherently encourage self-awareness and mindfulness, which are foundational to developing empathetic leadership (Webb, 2022). Yoga emphasizes interconnectedness, enabling leaders to appreciate diverse perspectives and emotions akin to those of team members, facilitating a collaborative and inclusive culture (Cool Cottone, 2017).

6.1.4. Resilience

Resilience, characterized by the ability to recover from setbacks, is crucial for leaders steering organizations through challenging periods. The discipline and balance cultivated through yoga bolster resilience by teaching practitioners to navigate discomfort and challenge (Deshmukh, 2024). The mental fortitude gained through consistent yoga practice empowers leaders to embody resilience, effectively demonstrating to their teams that challenges can be met with persistence and a growth mindset.

6.1.5. Ethical Decision-Making

Ethical decision-making hinges on a leader's ability to balance personal values with organizational goals. Yoga's philosophical underpinnings emphasize ethical living, promoting principles such as truthfulness and non-harming (ahimsa) (Varghese et al., 2017). This commitment to ethical principles can manifest in decision-making processes characterized by integrity and consideration for the implications of their actions. When faced with morally complex situations, leaders trained in ethically mindful practices can evaluate choices more holistically, considering both immediate impacts and long-term ramifications (Wang, 2018).

6.2. Practical Applications - Breathwork, Meditation, Mindful Movement as Tools for Leadership Transformation

Mindfulness is widely recognized for its potential to enhance leadership qualities. Mindfulness practices, which include breathwork, meditation, and mindful movement, serve as tools for leaders to develop self-awareness and emotional intelligence. Leaders who practice mindfulness can navigate complex situations more adeptly, as evidenced by research indicating that mindfulness fosters leadership flexibility and adaptability according to situational demands.

6.2.1. Breathwork and Decision-Making:

Breathwork, a fundamental aspect of yoga, plays a critical role in regulating stress and improving cognitive function, which are vital aspects of effective leadership. In stressful environments, such as corporate settings, leaders often face high-pressure situations that can impair their decision-making abilities. The practice of breathwork aids leaders in overcoming stress-induced paralysis, allowing them to approach decisions with clarity and calmness. The physiological effects of controlled breathing extend to emotional regulation and mental clarity, crucial attributes for effective leadership. The role of breath in enhancing focus and reducing anxiety has been documented. Through controlled and conscious breathing, leaders can maintain composure and ensure that their decisions are not clouded by temporary emotional disturbances. By incorporating breathwork into their daily routines, leaders not only enhance their personal resilience but also model stress management techniques for their teams, promoting a culture of well-being and collective resilience (Simonsson et al., 2023).

6.2.2. Meditation as a Leadership Tool

Meditation serves as another powerful practice within the yogic framework that supports and transforms leadership capacities. The work of Stedham and Skaar (2019) presents a conceptual framework that suggests mindfulness not only improves leader characteristics but also fosters trust-based relationships between leaders and their followers. Mindful leaders are likely to listen actively, respond rather than react, and build stronger, more empathetic connections with their teams. This form of leadership, characterized by a grounded presence and emotional intelligence, aligns closely with the demands of modern organizational contexts, where soft skills are often as crucial as technical abilities.

6.2.3. Mindful Movement: The Physicality of Leadership

Mindful movement, integral to yoga practice, cultivates a heightened awareness of the body, fostering presence and enhancing physical health. Sulastri et al. (2017) emphasize that transformational leadership involves individual consideration and empowerment, akin to the relational dynamics observed in mindful movement. Leaders who embody physical awareness become more conscientious of their team's needs and abilities, fostering an environment where each member feels valued and understood. The practice of embodying mindfulness through movement not only enriches a leader's capacity for empathy but also paves the way for more effective engagement strategies that increase team cohesion and motivation.

6.2.4. The Intersection of Yoga Philosophy and Business Leadership

By blending these ancient philosophies with contemporary business practices, leaders can create frameworks that prioritize ethical decision-making while also enhancing organizational performance. The concept of Karma Yoga, which emphasizes selfless service and duty, suggests that leaders can approach their roles not merely as positions of authority but as opportunities to uplift and empower others. This perspective shifts the focus from self-interest to collective well-being, fostering a culture of collaboration and innovation (Hurst et al., 2018).

7. CASE STUDIES OF ORGANIZATIONAL WELLNESS INITIATIVES

In order to understand the real-world application and effectiveness of integrative yoga-based wellness interventions, it is essential to consider the lived experiences of individuals. The following are the case studies, drawn from compiled assessment data of working professionals who underwent a 3-month structured yoga program under went in the Dept. of Physiotherapy in association with Dept. of Yoga and Holistic Health at Centurion University of Technology And Management, Bhubaneswar, India, illustrate how tailored interventions can foster mental resilience, emotional balance, and overall organizational wellness.

Case Study 1: Swarup Mishra – Animation Professional, Age 31

Swarup worked in the high-demand field of digital animation, frequently facing tight deadlines and client pressure. His pre-intervention assessment revealed frequent feelings of worthlessness, disturbed sleep, excessive worrying, and episodes of sadness or feeling "blue." He often felt overwhelmed without clear cause, and his engagement at work was beginning to decline.

Upon enrolling in the yoga wellness program, Swarup committed to a daily practice that included pranayama, mindfulness-based stress reduction (MBSR), and guided meditations. Initially skeptical, he gradually began noticing changes by the end of the first month. His sleep cycle became more regulated, and he felt less reactive to workplace stressors. By the end of three months, he reported a marked reduction in anxiety, a boost in focus and creativity, and an improved ability to handle interpersonal dynamics at work. His follow-up responses showed a shift from "quite a bit" to "rarely" across most distress markers.

"Yoga helped me create space between stimulus and response," Swarup reflected. "I don't feel consumed by pressure anymore."

Case Study 2: R. Venkatesh – IT Trainee, Age 26

New to his profession, Venkatesh was already showing signs of workplace anxiety and burnout. His assessment responses revealed frequent worry, feelings of being trapped, and disturbed sleep. The digital work culture had intensified his stress, with little physical movement and a lack of mental rest.

The wellness program introduced him to basic Hatha Yoga postures, deep-breathing techniques, and progressive muscle relaxation. Venkatesh responded positively to the body-based mindfulness approach. Over time, he developed greater clarity, emotional regulation, and physical vitality. His after-program scores reflected significant improvement in sleep quality, reduction in overthinking, and enhanced motivation. He even took initiative to lead a tech-yoga club among peers.

"Yoga gave me tools I never had," he said. "Now I breathe through my deadlines."

Case Study 3: Padmalochana Das – Academic Researcher, Age 27

Padmalochana, a researcher in social sciences, struggled with feelings of emotional isolation, low appetite, and mental fatigue. Spending long hours in solitude had affected his self-worth and energy levels. He scored high in areas related to feeling hopeless and drained.

His tailored yoga program focused on energy-building sequences, mindfulness walks, and journaling meditations. Within weeks, he began to notice a lift in his mood. He felt more connected to his purpose and gradually regained his appetite and motivation to engage with colleagues and students.

"The mat became a mirror," he shared. "Every session helped me reconnect with who I am beyond roles and results."

Case Study 4: Manojkumar Dey – Senior HR Manager, Age 52

With decades of experience, Manoj was respected for his discipline but privately battled mental fatigue and emotional disengagement. His assessment reflected high effort-exhaustion and diminished interest in new projects.

He embraced the yoga program wholeheartedly, finding particular resonance with Karma Yoga and its emphasis on selfless action. Breathwork, group chanting, and reflective silence became daily anchors. After three months, Manoj reported feeling reinvigorated and reconnected with his sense of purpose. He also began mentoring junior staff on managing work stress.

"I learned to lead from compassion rather than control," Manoj observed. "Yoga changed my definition of strength."

Case Study 5: Pratibha Rani – Finance Associate, Age 33

Pratibha's role in corporate finance demanded intense attention to detail, which left her with persistent stress and reduced emotional bandwidth. She often felt emotionally numb, had trouble sleeping, and rarely took breaks.

The yoga module designed for her included yoga nidra (deep relaxation), restorative asanas, and body-scan meditations. Pratibha gradually became more attuned to her emotions and physical state. Her stress symptoms declined, and she began practicing 10-minute breathing breaks between work tasks.

"Yoga gave me permission to pause," she said. "Now I approach numbers with more calm and clarity."

Case Study 6: Avinash Behera – Customer Support Executive, Age 29

Avinash managed customer complaints in a telecom firm—a job that often exposed him to irate clients and tense interactions. He admitted to having a short temper and feelings of detachment from his work. His responses showed signs of burnout and internal distress.

His yoga plan emphasized grounding techniques, chanting, and breathe pacing during high-stress moments. He also began using mindfulness reminders through mobile apps. Over three months, Avinash noticed a reduction in emotional reactivity and an increase in patience.

"Now I meet conflict with curiosity instead of anger," he noted. "Yoga turned my triggers into tools."

These cases narratives reveal the profound and multidimensional impact that yoga-based wellness programs can have in diverse professional contexts. By addressing psychological, emotional, and physiological dimensions simultaneously, integrative yoga practices empower individuals to take charge of their mental health while enhancing workplace engagement and productivity. Each of these journeys underscores that healing and resilience are possible—one breath, one posture, one moment at a time

8. CHALLENGES AND FUTURE DIRECTIONS

The undeniable link between mental health and workplace productivity necessitates a critical examination of workplace wellness initiatives and the barriers affecting their effectiveness. Mental health issues significantly impact employees' quality of life, as well as their performance and engagement, shaping the overall health of the organization. The integrative approach to enhancing workplace mental health includes addressing stigma, resource limitations, and measurement issues, alongside fostering cultural competence and equity in workplace wellness. This essay will explore these dimensions, proposing recommendations for fostering sustainable change, including leadership commitment, continuous education, and adaptive strategies.

8.1. Barriers to Workplace Mental Health

Stigma Surrounding Mental Health: One of the most significant barriers to addressing mental health in the workplace is stigma. Individuals facing mental health challenges often encounter stereotypes and prejudice that deter them from seeking help or discussing their issues openly. Research shows that workplaces with stigmatizing cultures see reduced engagement and increased absenteeism among employees experiencing mental health difficulties (De', 2024). Moreover, mental health stigma can take the form of perceived discrimination, which exacerbates feelings of isolation and can lead to further mental health deterioration. Addressing this stigma requires comprehensive educational initiatives aimed at fostering an understanding of mental health issues, promoting a culture of acceptance, and utilizing champions within the organization to advocate for mental health.

Resource Limitations: Resource limitations stand as another formidable barrier. Organizations often struggle to allocate sufficient resources to mental health initiatives, particularly in sectors with tight budgets or in cases where short-term profitability is prioritized over long-term employee well-being. A lack of resources can manifest in insufficient access to mental health services, employee training, and preventive programs. Studies indicate that organizations with higher investments in employee well-being report better worker satisfaction and lower turnover rates (Bartels et al., 2019). Therefore, it is imperative to recognize that investment in mental health resources not only benefits employees but also enhances overall organizational performance.

Measurement Issues: Measuring the effectiveness of mental health initiatives is challenging, compounded by the diverse factors influencing employee well-being (Linton et al., 2016). Existing tools to evaluate workplace wellness often fail to capture the multifaceted nature of mental health or the unique contextual influences of specific work environments. As such, valid and reliable measures are essential for understanding and improving workplace mental health. Recent research emphasizes the need for tailored measures that incorporate subjective well-being scales alongside objective performance metrics, facilitating more robust evaluations of wellness interventions

8.2. Fostering Cultural Competence and Equity in Workplace Wellness

Creating an equitable workplace involves recognizing and addressing the diverse needs of employees, including their cultural backgrounds and individual circumstances. Cultural competence in workplace wellness programs ensures that all employees receive support that is relevant to their unique experiences. Addressing such disparities requires inclusive policies and practices that foster safe reporting mechanisms and responsive interventions tailored to specific employee demographics.

Organizations must also strive for holistic approaches that incorporate diversity, equity, and inclusion (DEI) training into their wellness programs. Practical initiatives such as inclusive leadership training and mentorship programs can help cultivate a supportive environment (Marschke et al., 2011). Moreover, engaging employees in the development of wellness programs can further enhance relevance and accessibility (De', 2024)

8.3. Recommendations for Sustainable Change

Leadership Commitment: Leadership commitment is pivotal in driving cultural change within organizations regarding mental health. Research shows that transformational leadership, which emphasizes vision, employee engagement, and a supportive environment, correlates positively with workplace commitment and overall employee wellness (Kazemipour et al., 2012). Leaders must visibly prioritize mental health, modeling healthy behaviors and advocating for supportive policies within the organization. Moreover, ongoing leadership training focused on emotional intelligence and mental health advocacy can empower leaders to effectively support their teams.

Continuous Education: Continuous education around mental health is essential for sustaining change within organizations. Training programs should encompass not only awareness of mental health issues but also strategies for supporting colleagues in need (De', 2024). Educational initiatives can be complemented by workshops, peer support groups, and resilience training, which create opportunities for employees to learn and share experiences in a safe setting. This approach fosters a proactive culture where mental health is prioritized, and employees feel more equipped to identify and address their wellness needs.

Adaptive Strategies: Flexibility in workplace policies can enhance mental health support, accommodating varied employee needs and external circumstances. Such adaptive strategies may include remote work options, flexible hours, or modified workloads for those experiencing mental health challenges. Evidence suggests that organizations that implement adaptive work strategies report higher levels of employee satisfaction and well-being. Furthermore, regular assessments of workplace mental health initiatives can facilitate iterative improvements, ensuring programs remain effective and relevant over time (Linton et al., 2016).

9. CONCLUSION

Enhancing mental health in the workplace is a shared responsibility requiring integrative, evidence-informed, and compassionate strategies. Yoga and mindfulness offer versatile, accessible tools to build emotionally intelligent, resilient, and ethically grounded workforces. By embracing such holistic approaches, organizations can shift from managing distress to cultivating thriving ecosystems of wellness.

REFERENCES

Ashkanasy, N., & Kay, A. (2023). Mindfulness and emotion: A five-level analysis. *Journal of Management & Organization, 29*(3), 406–424. DOI: 10.1017/jmo.2023.22

Bakker, A. B., & Demerouti, E. (2007). The job demands-resources model: State of the art. *Journal of Managerial Psychology, 22*(3), 309–328. DOI: 10.1108/02683940710733115

Bartels, A., Peterson, S., & Reina, C. (2019). Understanding well-being at work: Development and validation of the eudaimonic workplace well-being scale. *PLoS One*, *14*(4), e0215957. DOI: 10.1371/journal.pone.0215957 PMID: 31022285

BeyondBlue. (2019). *BeyondBlue national mental health and wellbeing study of police and emergency services: Phase 3A—Knowledge translation guide and workbook* (Unpublished report).

Bloom, D. E., Cafiero, E. T., Jané-Llopis, E., Abrahams-Gessel, S., Bloom, L. R., Fathima, S., Feigl, A. B., Gaziano, T., Mowafi, M., Pandya, A., ... (2011). *The global economic burden of noncommunicable diseases.* World Economic Forum.

Bostock, S., Crosswell, A. D., Prather, A. A., & Steptoe, A. (2019). Mindfulness on-the-go: Effects of a mindfulness meditation app on work stress and well-being. *Journal of Occupational Health Psychology, 24*(1), 127–138. DOI: 10.1037/ocp0000118 PMID: 29723001

Chiesa, A., & Serretti, A. (2009). Mindfulness-based stress reduction for stress management in healthy people: A review and meta-analysis. *Journal of Alternative and Complementary Medicine (New York, N.Y.), 15*(5), 593–600. DOI: 10.1089/acm.2008.0495 PMID: 19432513

Colzato, L. S., Ozturk, A., & Hommel, B. (2012). Meditate to create: The impact of focused-attention and open-monitoring training on convergent and divergent thinking. *Frontiers in Psychology, 3*, 116. DOI: 10.3389/fpsyg.2012.00116 PMID: 22529832

Cook-Cottone, C., & Douglass, L. (2017). Yoga communities and eating disorders: Creating safe space for positive embodiment. *International Journal of Yoga Therapy*, *27*(1), 87–93. DOI: 10.17761/1531-2054-27.1.87 PMID: 29131729

Cott, C. A., Finch, E., Gasner, D., Yoshida, K., Thomas, S. G., & Verrier, M. C. (2004). The movement continuum theory of physical therapy. *Physiotherapy Canada. Physiotherapie Canada*, *56*(4), 179–187. DOI: 10.3138/ptc.56.4.179

Dash, B. (2024). Yama and niyama in modern leadership. *JIER*, *4*(3). Advance online publication. DOI: 10.52783/jier.v4i3.1878

De', A. (2024). Approaches to eliminate mental health stigma, sexism, and racism in the workplace. *Journal of Women's Health Care and Management*, *5*(1). Advance online publication. DOI: 10.47275/2692-0948-154

Demerouti, E., Bakker, A. B., Nachreiner, F., & Schaufeli, W. B. (2001). The job demands-resources model of burnout. *The Journal of Applied Psychology*, *86*(3), 499–512. DOI: 10.1037/0021-9010.86.3.499 PMID: 11419809

Derks, D., & Bakker, A. B. (2014). Smartphone use, work-home interference, and burnout: A diary study on the role of recovery. *Applied Psychology*, *63*(3), 411–440. DOI: 10.1111/j.1464-0597.2012.00530.x

. Deshmukh, L., Janghel, U., Sonkuwar, A., & Thakur, R. (2024). Exploring the synergy between yoga and mindfulness sport practices: Enhancing mental and physical well-being. *Indian Journal of Yoga Exercise & Sport Science and Physical Education*, 26–32. https://doi.org/DOI: 10.58914/ijyesspe.2024-9.1.4

Einarsen, S., Hoel, H., Zapf, D., & Cooper, C. L. (2011). *Bullying and harassment in the workplace: Developments in theory, research, and practice* (2nd ed.). CRC Press.

Elwy, A., Groessl, E., Eisen, S., Riley, K., Maiya, M., Lee, J., & Park, C. (2014). A systematic scoping review of yoga intervention components and study quality. *American Journal of Preventive Medicine*, *47*(2), 220–232. DOI: 10.1016/j.amepre.2014.03.012 PMID: 24996759

Fürstenberg, N., Alfes, K., & Kearney, E. (2021). How and when paradoxical leadership benefits work engagement: The role of goal clarity and work autonomy. *Journal of Occupational and Organizational Psychology*, *94*(3), 672–705. DOI: 10.1111/joop.12344

Garland, E., & Howard, M. (2018). Mindfulness-based treatment of addiction: Current state of the field and envisioning the next wave of research. *Addiction Science & Clinical Practice*, *13*(1), 14. Advance online publication. DOI: 10.1186/s13722-018-0115-3 PMID: 29669599

Groessl, E., Maiya, M., Elwy, A., Riley, K., Sarkin, A., Eisen, S., & Park, C. (2015). The essential properties of yoga questionnaire: Development and methods. *International Journal of Yoga Therapy*, *25*(1), 51–59. DOI: 10.17761/1531-2054-25.1.51 PMID: 26667289

Ha, T., & Moon, K. (2023). Distributive justice, goal clarity, and organizational citizenship behavior: The moderating role of transactional and transformational leadership. *Sustainability (Basel)*, *15*(9), 7403. DOI: 10.3390/su15097403

Halbesleben, J. R. B. (2006). Sources of social support and burnout: A meta-analytic test of the conservation of resources model. *The Journal of Applied Psychology*, *91*(5), 1134–1145. DOI: 10.1037/0021-9010.91.5.1134 PMID: 16953774

He, H., Zhao, L., & Liu, B. (2025). Make or break? How positive and negative family experiences affect workplace creativity: The role of energy and mindfulness. *The Journal of Creative Behavior*, *59*(1), e70002. Advance online publication. DOI: 10.1002/jocb.70002

Hülsheger, U. R., Alberts, H. J., Feinholdt, A., & Lang, J. W. (2013). Benefits of mindfulness at work: The role of mindfulness in emotion regulation, emotional exhaustion, and job satisfaction. *The Journal of Applied Psychology*, *98*(2), 310–325. DOI: 10.1037/a0031313 PMID: 23276118

Hurst, S., Maiya, M., Casteel, D., Sarkin, A., Libretto, S., Elwy, A., Park, C. L., & Groessl, E. (2018). Yoga therapy for military personnel and veterans: Qualitative perspectives of yoga students and instructors. *Complementary Therapies in Medicine*, *40*, 222–229. DOI: 10.1016/j.ctim.2017.10.008 PMID: 30219455

Huseynova, G., & İslamoğlu, M. (2024). Mind over matter: Mindfulness as a buffer against workplace incivility. *Frontiers in Psychology, 15*, 1409326. Advance online publication. DOI: 10.3389/fpsyg.2024.1409326 PMID: 39205969

International Labor Organization. (n.d.). *The work stress conundrum.* https://www.ilo.org/safework/events/safeday/33thinkpieces/WCMS_681594/lang--en/index.htm

Ioannou, A. (2023). Mindfulness and technostress in the workplace: A qualitative approach. *Frontiers in Psychology, 14*, 1252187. Advance online publication. DOI: 10.3389/fpsyg.2023.1252187 PMID: 38022994

Kanchibhotla, D., Rao, M. V., & Reddy, P. (2021). The prevalence of musculoskeletal disorders among Indian IT professionals and their association with mental health. *Indian Journal of Occupational and Environmental Medicine, 25*(3), 125–131. DOI: 10.4103/ijoem.ijoem_179_21 PMID: 34759597

Karasek, R., & Theorell, T. (1990). *Healthy work: Stress, productivity, and the reconstruction of working life*. Basic Books.

Kazemipour, F., Amin, S., & Pourseidi, B. (2012). Relationship between workplace spirituality and organizational citizenship behavior among nurses through mediation of affective organizational commitment. *Journal of Nursing Scholarship, 44*(3), 302–310. DOI: 10.1111/j.1547-5069.2012.01456.x PMID: 22804973

Kumar, A., Chawla, K., Mishra, A., Singh, G., Pandey, A., & Rikhari, P. (2023). Are doctors feeling burnout? Multicenter cross-sectional study on burnout syndrome and its determinants during the ongoing pandemic. *Indian Journal of Psychiatry, 65*(5), 541–549. DOI: 10.4103/indianjpsychiatry.indianjpsychiatry_726_22 PMID: 37397848

LaMontagne, A. D., Martin, A., Page, K. M., Reavley, N., Noblet, A., Milner, A., Keegel, T., Allisey, A., Papas, A., & Witt, K.. (2019). Developing an integrated approach to workplace mental health. In Hudson, H. L., & Nigam, J. A. (Eds.), *Total worker health* (pp. 211–227). American Psychological Association. DOI: 10.1037/0000149-013

LaMontagne, A. D., Martin, A., Page, K. M., Reavley, N. J., Noblet, A. J., Milner, A. J., Keegel, T., & Smith, P. M. (2014). Workplace mental health: Developing an integrated intervention approach. *BMC Psychiatry*, *14*(1), 131. DOI: 10.1186/1471-244X-14-131 PMID: 24884425

Lee, J., Lee, K., Lee, J., Hwang, J., & Park, D. (2024). Analysis of job stress, depression, and mindfulness among Korean physical therapists during the COVID-19 pandemic. *Work (Reading, Mass.)*, *80*(2), 741–749. DOI: 10.1177/10519815241289659 PMID: 40172849

Leiter, M. P., & Maslach, C. (2005). *Banishing burnout: Six strategies for improving your relationship with work*. Jossey-Bass.

Linton, M., Dieppe, P., & Medina-Lara, A. (2016). Review of 99 self-report measures for assessing well-being in adults: Exploring dimensions of well-being and developments over time. *BMJ Open*, *6*(7), e010641. DOI: 10.1136/bmjopen-2015-010641 PMID: 27388349

Mahfouz, J. (2018). Mindfulness training for school administrators: Effects on well-being and leadership. *Journal of Educational Administration*, *56*(6), 602–619. DOI: 10.1108/JEA-12-2017-0171

Main, C. J., George, S. Z., & Foster, N. E. (2010). Psychosocial interventions and pain: Implications for physiotherapy. *Manual Therapy*, *15*(6), 486–490. DOI: 10.1016/j.math.2010.07.002

Marschke, E., Preziosi, R., & Harrington, W. (2011). Professionals and executives support a relationship between organizational commitment and spirituality in the workplace. *Journal of Business & Economics Research*, *7*(8). Advance online publication. DOI: 10.19030/jber.v7i8.2320

Maslach, C., & Leiter, M. P. (2016). Understanding the burnout experience: Recent research and its implications for psychiatry. *World Psychiatry; Official Journal of the World Psychiatric Association (WPA)*, *15*(2), 103–111. DOI: 10.1002/wps.20311 PMID: 27265691

McEwen, B. S. (1998). Protective and damaging effects of stress mediators. *The New England Journal of Medicine*, *338*(3), 171–179. DOI: 10.1056/NEJM199801153380307 PMID: 9428819

Messenger, J. C., Ghosheh, N., & Bourne, M. (2017). *Working anytime, anywhere: The effects on the world of work.* International Labour Office.

Murthy, R. S. (2017). National Mental Health Survey of India 2015–2016. *Indian Journal of Psychiatry, 59*(1), 21–26. DOI: 10.4103/psychiatry.IndianJPsychiatry_102_17 PMID: 28529357

OECD. (2015). *Fit mind, fit job: From evidence to practice in mental health and work (Mental Health and Work).* OECD Publishing., DOI: 10.1787/9789264228283-

Paluska, S. A., & Schwenk, T. L. (2000). Physical activity and mental health: Current concepts. *Sports Medicine (Auckland, N.Z.), 29*(3), 167–180. DOI: 10.2165/00007256-200029030-00003 PMID: 10739267

Rajgopal, T. (2020). Mental well-being at the workplace. *Indian Journal of Occupational and Environmental Medicine, 24*(1), 1–5. DOI: 10.4103/0973-2284.276207 PMID: 32435108

Reb, J., Narayanan, J., & Chaturvedi, S. (2014). Leading mindfully: Two studies on the influence of supervisor trait mindfulness on employee well-being and performance. *Mindfulness, 5*(1), 36–45. DOI: 10.1007/s12671-012-0144-z

. Riani, D., & Sopiansah, V. (2023). Design factorial analysis: Identifying the interactions of workplace mindfulness and individual factors in controlling affective commitment. *Jurnal Riset Bisnis dan Manajemen, 16*(2), 196–203. https://doi.org/DOI: 10.23969/jrbm.v16i2.8466

Robertson, M. M., Huang, Y. H., & Lee, J. (2009). Improving computer workstation setup to reduce musculoskeletal disorders. *Journal of Safety Research, 40*(1), 53–59. DOI: 10.1016/j.jsr.2008.12.005 PMID: 19285587

Rugulies, R., Aust, B., Greiner, B. A., Arensman, E., Kawakami, N., LaMontagne, A. D., & Madsen, I. E. H. (2023). Work-related causes of mental health conditions and interventions for their improvement in workplaces. *Lancet, 402*(10410), 1368–1381. DOI: 10.1016/S0140-6736(23)00869-3 PMID: 37838442

Sanchez, B., & Kazen, H. (2021). Qualitative study on at-risk Hispanic adolescents engaged in social emotional learning and mindfulness practices. *International Journal of Educational Methodology*, *7*(4), 615–622. DOI: 10.12973/ijem.7.4.615

Sanderson, K., & Andrews, G. (2006). Common mental disorders in the workforce: Recent findings from descriptive and social epidemiology. *Canadian Journal of Psychiatry*, *51*(2), 63–75. DOI: 10.1177/070674370605100202 PMID: 16989105

Shapiro, S. L., Brown, K. W., & Astin, J. A. (2012). Toward the integration of meditation into higher education: A review of research. *Teachers College Record*, *113*(3), 493–528. DOI: 10.1177/016146811111300306

Shirom, A. (2005). Reflections on the study of burnout. *Work and Stress*, *19*(3), 263–270. DOI: 10.1080/02678370500376649

Silva, A. (2024). Socio-cognitive mindfulness is a well-being booster: A serial mediation model to test the mindfulness reappraisal hypothesis with managers. *Evidence-Based HRM: A Global Forum for Empirical Scholarship, 13*(1), 1–16. https://doi.org/DOI: 10.1108/EBHRM-09-2023-0240

Simonsson, O., Stenfors, C., Goldberg, S., Hendricks, P., & Osika, W. (2023). Altered states of leadership: Mindfulness meditation, psychedelic use, and leadership development. *Frontiers in Psychology*, *14*, 1151626. Advance online publication. DOI: 10.3389/fpsyg.2023.1151626 PMID: 37476092

Sonnentag, S., Binnewies, C., & Mojza, E. J. (2010). Staying well and engaged when demands are high: The role of psychological detachment. *The Journal of Applied Psychology*, *95*(5), 965–976. DOI: 10.1037/a0020032 PMID: 20718528

Southwick, S. M., Bonanno, G. A., Masten, A. S., Panter-Brick, C., & Yehuda, R. (2014). Resilience definitions, theory, and challenges: Interdisciplinary perspectives. *European Journal of Psychotraumatology*, *5*(1), 25338. DOI: 10.3402/ejpt.v5.25338 PMID: 25317257

Sparks, K., Faragher, B., & Cooper, C. L. (2001). Well-being and occupational health in the 21st-century workplace. *Journal of Occupational and Organizational Psychology, 74*(4), 489–509. DOI: 10.1348/096317901167497

Srivastava, S., Khan, M., Kumari, A., & Jain, A. (2024). Does workplace ostracism lead to workplace withdrawal? Testing the moderating–mediating effects of rumination and mindfulness in Indian hospitality industry. *Journal of Organizational Effectiveness: People and Performance, 11*(4), 873–891. DOI: 10.1108/JOEPP-08-2023-0328

Stedham, Y., & Skaar, T. (2019). Mindfulness, trust, and leader effectiveness: A conceptual framework. *Frontiers in Psychology, 10*, 1588. Advance online publication. DOI: 10.3389/fpsyg.2019.01588 PMID: 31354589

Sulastri, S., Andriani, C., & Fitria, Y. (2017). The factors forming formal and non-formal leadership based on Minangkabau culture in Padang. *Asia Pacific Management and Business Application, 6*(1), 15–30. DOI: 10.21776/ub.apmba.2017.006.01.2

Varghese, F., Nolan, J., Bihm, E., Salagame, K., Khanna, R., & Ali, S. (2017). Transformational leadership and Asian Indian values: Duty, selfless service, and nonviolence. *The Counseling Psychologist, 45*(6), 810–829. DOI: 10.1177/0011000017723080

Wang, H., & Guan, B. (2018). The positive effect of authoritarian leadership on employee performance: The moderating role of power distance. *Frontiers in Psychology, 9*, 357. Advance online publication. DOI: 10.3389/fpsyg.2018.00357 PMID: 29628902

Wang, S., Shih, S., & Kuo, L. (2024). Exploring mindfulness interventions for stress resilience in newly graduated nurses: A qualitative study. *Tzu-Chi Medical Journal, 36*(4), 452–459. DOI: 10.4103/tcmj.tcmj_250_23 PMID: 39421497

Webb, J., Padro, M., Thomas, E., Davies, A., Etzel, L., Rogers, C., & Heredia, N. (2022). Yoga at every size: A preliminary evaluation of a brief online size-inclusive yoga and body gratitude journaling intervention to enhance positive embodiment in higher-weight college women. *Frontiers in Global Women's Health, 3*, 852854. Advance online publication. DOI: 10.3389/fgwh.2022.852854 PMID: 35720811

. Wildcroft, T. (2020). *Post-lineage yoga: From guru to #MeToo.* https://doi.org/DOI: 10.1558/isbn.9781781799413

World Health Organization. (2022). *WHO guidelines on mental health at work.* World Health Organization.

Chapter 5
Integrating Cognitive Behavioural Play Therapy, ACT, Mindfulness, and Yoga for Enhancing Psychological Wellbeing in Adolescents:
An Eclectic Clinical Framework

Soumalya Mukherjee
http://orcid.org/0009-0000-3687-8024
University of Calcutta, India

Soheli Datta
http://orcid.org/0009-0004-4690-3560
University of Calcutta, India

ABSTRACT

Adolescence is a pivotal developmental phase characterized by rapid psychological, emotional, and social changes, often accompanied by in-

DOI: 10.4018/979-8-2600-1202-4.ch005

creased vulnerability to internalizing disorders. Traditional therapeutic approaches may not fully address the multifaceted needs of adolescents, necessitating innovative, integrative models. This chapter presents a comprehensive, culturally sensitive, and trauma-informed clinical framework that synergistically combines Cognitive Behavioral Play Therapy (CBPT), Acceptance and Commitment Therapy (ACT), mindfulness-based practices, and yoga-informed interventions. The framework is adaptable to a range of psychopathologies, including anxiety, depression, trauma-spectrum disorders, substance use disorder, suicidal ideation and somatic conditions, and is particularly suited for diverse cultural and neurodevelopmental contexts. Through a structured yet flexible therapeutic process, this model offers mental health professionals a practical, evidence-informed approach to support adolescents in navigating the complexities of their developmental journey.

INTRODUCTION

Adolescence is a dynamic period marked by the interplay of identity formation, emotional maturation, and increasing psychosocial demands. This developmental window, situated at the intersection of childhood dependency and emergent autonomy, is both a site of remarkable growth and heightened vulnerability. When such transitions are met with inadequate coping resources or environmental stressors, adolescents become susceptible to a spectrum of internalizing disorders, including anxiety, depression, somatic symptom-related presentations, dissociative phenomena, and trauma-related conditions (Kessler et al., 2012; Polanczyk et al., 2015).

Epidemiological evidence reveals a troubling escalation in the prevalence of internalizing disorders among adolescents worldwide. A landmark meta-analysis demonstrated that anxiety disorders affect approximately 31.9% and depressive disorders 13.3% of adolescents globally (Polanczyk et al., 2015). These conditions are frequently comorbid with other internalizing presentations such as somatic symptom and related disorders, trauma- and stressor-related disorders, and dissociative symptomatology, particularly in populations exposed to chronic stress or adversity (McLaughlin et al., 2017; Copeland et al., 2018). In the Indian context, the situation is similarly concerning: national mental health surveys indicate that anxiety and depressive disorders constitute a substantial proportion of adolescent psychiatric morbidity, further exacerbated by systemic barriers such as stigma, cultural silence, and a dearth of adolescent-responsive mental health infrastructure (Malhotra & Patra, 2014; Gururaj et al., 2016; Sagar et al., 2020).

Despite the growing clinical burden, conventional psychotherapeutic models often demonstrate significant limitations when applied to adolescent populations. Cognitive Behavioural Therapy (CBT) remains a gold-standard intervention for anxiety and depression (James et al., 2015; Weisz et al., 2017). However, its efficacy is frequently contingent on the presence of advanced cognitive and metacognitive capacities that may not yet be fully developed in younger adolescents or in those who experience affective dysregulation, trauma, or somatization (Kendall et al., 2004). Similarly, traditional insight-oriented or verbal therapies presuppose linguistic fluency, reflective capacity, and tolerance for affective arousal, which can alienate clients whose distress is embodied rather than verbalized (Lieberman & Van Horn, 2011). The overreliance on purely cognitive or linguistic therapeutic mechanisms can inadvertently marginalize adolescents whose psychological suffering is mediated through nonverbal, somatic, or symbolic registers.

In response to these challenges, this chapter introduces a theoretically grounded and clinically flexible eclectic framework that integrates four interrelated modalities: Cognitive Behavioural Play Therapy (CBPT), Acceptance and Commitment Therapy (ACT), mindfulness-based practices, and yoga-informed interventions. This approach is designed to be developmentally sensitive, trauma-informed, and culturally responsive, offering a multidimensional pathway to psychological healing. Drawing from a developmental psychopathology perspective, the framework recognizes that adolescent distress often emerges at the intersection of cognitive distortions, affective dysregulation, disrupted relational patterns, and somatic disconnection. By leveraging the neuroplasticity of the adolescent brain and the malleability of emerging identity structures, this integrative model aims to engage the whole person, mind, body, and self-in-context, in the therapeutic process.

This framework posits that adolescent healing cannot be reduced to cognitive insight or symptomatic relief alone. It necessitates a holistic re-integration of fragmented experiences across somatic, emotional, and symbolic domains. CBPT facilitates cognitive and emotional processing through metaphor, narrative, and play modalities that resonate with adolescents' symbolic thinking and offer a safe distance from overwhelming affect. ACT contributes a process-driven structure for cultivating psychological flexibility, enabling adolescents to engage with difficult thoughts and feelings while pursuing values-based action. Mindfulness practices train attention and visceral awareness, fostering present-moment engagement and emotional regulation. Meanwhile, yoga-informed techniques provide embodied, bottom-up regulation by activating the parasympathetic nervous system, promoting somatic safety, and restoring a felt sense of agency, particularly vital for those with trauma-related dysregulation. Together, these modalities comprise a cohesive therapeutic ecology that can be attuned to the unique developmental profile, cultural context, and symptom expression of each adolescent. The integrative model emphasizes fluidity over rigidity, embodiment over abstraction, and collaboration over prescription. It invites the clinician to move beyond a diagnosis-driven framework toward a more relational, process-oriented, and whole-person approach to care. In doing so, it offers a compelling response to the urgent mental health needs of today's youth, while also aligning with emerging paradigms in trauma-informed and culturally grounded psychotherapy.

The proposed framework aligns with the principles of developmental psychopathology, recognizing that adolescent distress arises from the interplay of biological, psychological and social factors. By integrating evidence-based modalities with holistic practices, the Model offers a flexible, client-centred approach that adapts to the adolescent's readiness for change, cultural context, and unique therapeutic needs. This chapter outlines the theoretical foundations, clinical applications, therapeutic process, and cultural considerations of the framework, providing mental health professionals with a practical guide for implementation.

THEORETICAL FOUNDATIONS

The integrative framework draws on four complementary therapeutic modalities, each contributing unique strengths to address the multifaceted nature of adolescent psychological distress.

Cognitive Behavioural Play Therapy (CBPT)

CBPT is an adaptation of Cognitive Behavioural Therapy (CBT) that incorporates play, which is a natural mode of expression for particularly those adolescents who may struggle with verbal articulation or meta-cognitive reflection, as a medium for therapeutic intervention especially for children and adolescents (Knell, 1993). CBPT uses play to facilitate the expression of thoughts and emotions, allowing therapists to address cognitive distortions, maladaptive behaviours and emotional difficulties in a developmentally appropriate manner. Play provides a safe and non-threatening environment where adolescents can explore their feelings, practice problem-solving and develop coping strategies.

There are three key components of CBPT that includes: *cognitive re-structuring*, which focuses on identifying and challenging the irrational or negative thoughts through play based activities (for instance, role-playing, story-telling etc.); *behavioural activation*, which primarily aims at encouraging adaptive behaviours through structured play (for example, board games to teach impulse control); and finally *skill building* that teaches emotional regulation and problem solving through creative outlets like art or puppets to the adolescents.

CBPT is particularly effective for adolescents who may resist traditional talk therapy due to developmental or emotional barriers. For instance, a teen with anxiety might engage in a game where they "trap" worries in a box, symbolically externalizing and containing distressing thoughts. It allows therapists to engage with adolescents' imaginative and symbolic capacities, making it an ideal foundation for an eclectic framework.

Acceptance and Commitment Therapy (ACT)

ACT is rooted deep down in relational frame theory and functional contextualizm, emphasizing on psychological flexibility through six core processes: acceptance (embracing difficult thoughts and feelings without trying to change them), cognitive defusion (seeing thoughts as mental events, not facts to reduce their control over behaviour), present-moment awareness (staying aware of the current moment to enhance engagement), self-as-context (viewing the self as a perspective, not a fixed identity, for greater adaptability), values clarification (identifying and committing to personal values that guide actions) and committed action (taking consistent steps toward goals aligned with those values, even when faced with obstacles) (Hayes, Strosahl, & Wilson, 2012). Unlike traditional CBT, which focuses on changing negative thoughts, ACT encourages individuals to accept difficult emotions and thoughts while aligning with personal values. It starts with addressing the rigid patterns like avoidance and fusion with thoughts, moving toward adaptive behaviours guided by personal values. Basically, these processes are not linear but iterative, with individuals often working on multiple aspects simultaneously. For example, practicing acceptance can support defusion and clarifying values can enhance committed action. The interconnection is emphasized in the ACT hexa-flex model, which visually represents these processes as mutually reinforcing.

For adolescents, ACT is particularly relevant because it addresses their need for autonomy and identity exploration. It has demonstrated effectiveness in adolescent populations for conditions such as anxiety (Toghiani et al., 2019), depression (Datta & Mukherjee, 2017), and chronic pain (Swain et al., 2015). A randomized controlled trail by Livheim et al. (2015) found that an ACT based group intervention significantly reduced depressive symptoms and stress in adolescents compared to a control group. By fostering acceptance of uncomfortable emotions (for example, anxiety about peer relationships) and encouraging value driven actions (e.g., pursuing meaningful friendships), ACT helps adolescents navigate the complexities of their developmental stage.

Mindfulness

Mindfulness involves cultivating non-judgemental awareness of the present moment, often through practices like meditation, body scans, or mindful breathing (Kabat-Zinn, 1990). The term 'mindfulness' have its origin in Buddhist psychology and comes from the Sanskrit word 'smriti,' which helps us to understand mindfulness as remembering to pay attention to our present moment experience (Shapiro & Carlson, 2009; Black, 2011). It has three basic features that includes: purposefully directing one's attention, being at the present moment and accepting thoughts, sensations and emotions non-judgementally.

In adolescents, mindfulness has shown to reduce stress, improve emotional regulation and enhance attention (Zoogman et al., 2015). From recent researches, it enables us to understand that adolescence is a period where they learn to develop abilities to self-regulate. Such developments mainly take place in the milieu of heightened autonomy, complicated life challenges and exceeding stress reactivity. Mindfulness has the power to address all these concerns. Patricia C. Broderick (2013) developed a program known as Learning to BREATHE (L2B) program, which is a mindfulness-based intervention tailored for adolescents in educational environments. It aims to integrate seamlessly with school curricula, aligning with standards in health and counselling. The program focuses on teaching mindful awareness through group practices, enhancing students' ability to regulate emotions, manage stress, and improve attention and academic performance. Thus, mindfulness is considered to be a standalone concept as well as a component of ACT and Yoga. For instance, a mindfulness exercise might involve guiding an adolescent to focus on their breath while noticing bodily sensations, helping them anchor their attention during moments of anxiety. This practice is particularly effective for adolescents with somatic symptoms or trauma-related dissociation, as it fosters reconnection with the body in a safe, controlled manner.

Yoga

Yoga, as a holistic mind-body discipline, presents a compelling, evidence-based adjunct to conventional therapeutic approaches in promoting adolescent well-being. It broadly encompasses the integration of physical postures (asanas), breath regulation (pranayama) and meditative practices that collectively fosters emotional regulation, attentional control, self-awareness and has gained recognition as a therapeutic tool for mental health. These components align closely with the mechanisms targeted by contemporary psychological interventions such as mindfulness-based therapies, Acceptance and Commitment Therapy (ACT), and Cognitive Behavioural Play Therapy (CBPT), thus positioning yoga as a foundational element in integrative adolescent care.

In adolescents, yoga contributes to improved autonomic regulation, as evidenced by enhanced heart rate variability and reduced cortisol levels, markers associated with decreased stress reactivity (Khalsa et al., 2016). Behaviourally, regular yoga practice has been shown to improve mood, reduce anxiety, and enhance executive functioning in adolescents, which are critical for academic success and interpersonal effectiveness (Felver et al., 2015). Further cognitively, yoga's emphasis on present-moment awareness and non-reactivity mirrors core processes in mindfulness-based interventions. This shared emphasis fosters metacognitive awareness and emotional resilience that are essential during the turbulent period of adolescence (Zoogman et al., 2015). Yoga can also act as a non-verbal play medium through which the internal world of an adolescent is externally observable, which further helps the therapists to understand the areas of distress more accurately.

THE ECLECTIC CLINICAL FRAMEWORK

The eclectic clinical framework integrates CBPT, ACT, mindfulness and yoga into a cohesive therapeutic approach for adolescents. The framework is structured around five phases: assessment, engagement, skill-building, integration and practice and consolidation and termination. Each phase incorporates elements from the four modalities, tailored to the adolescent's needs, cultural background and presenting issues.

Phase 1: *Assessment*

The objective of this phase is to understand the adolescent's psychological needs, strengths and challenges. Here, CBPT uses play based activities (for example, drawing, sand tray) to assess emotional expression, cognitive distortions and coping strategies. For example, a therapist might ask the adolescent to create a 'feeling picture' to identify dominant emotions. ACT explores the adolescent's values and areas of psychological inflexibility using tools like the values card sort, where adolescents identify priorities (e.g., friendship, academic success). Mindfulness further assess the adolescent's ability to focus on the present moment through brief mindful exercises (e.g., a 3-minute breathing space). In this case, yoga observes the adolescent's physical comfort and body awareness during simple yoga poses (e.g., child's pose) to gauge stress levels and somatic awareness. We must ensure that these assessments are culturally sensitive by incorporating culturally relevant metaphors, play materials or yoga practices (for instance, using story-telling traditions from the adolescent's cultural background in CBPT).

Phase 2: *Engagement*

This phase aims at building rapport and establish a safe therapeutic environment for the adolescents to express freely. CBPT here uses play based activities like cooperative games or puppet play to build trust. For example, a therapist might play a board game with the adolescent to foster collaboration and communication. Whereas ACT introduce the concept of acceptance through metaphors (for instance, the 'passengers on the bus' metaphor, where thoughts and feelings are passengers and the adolescent learns to carry without letting them drive). In this phase, we might teach some mindfulness practices, such as, mindful breathing or body scans to help adolescents feel grounded. For example, a 5-minute guided mindful exercise can be introduced during sessions. Here, we incorporate gentle yoga poses (e.g., cat-cow, seated twists) to promote relaxation and body awareness, creating a safe space for emotional exploration. Here, we must allow the adolescents to choose play materials or yoga poses to enhance their sense of autonomy and engagement.

Phase 3: *Skill Building*

The purpose of this phase is to teach coping skills, emotional regulation and psychological flexibility to the adolescents. For that CBPT uses structured play activities to enlighten them with cognitive and behavioural skills. For instance, a role-play activity might help an adolescent practice assertive communication to address peer conflict. ACT guides them in identifying values (e.g., being a supportive friend) and setting value driven goals. The use of cognitive defusion techniques (e.g., labelling thoughts as 'just thoughts') are also introduced to lessen the impact of negative self-talk. Here, we can introduce mindfulness practices to enhance emotional regulation, such as mindful journaling or the 'STOP' technique (Stop, Take a breath, Observe and Proceed). We can also teach yoga sequences that promote emotional regulation, such as a sequence combining warrior poses (to build confidence) and forward folds (to promote calm). Breathing exercises like alternate nostril breathing can enhance focus and concentration. Let us consider a 15-year old boy with social anxiety, we can use CBPT to role play social scenarios, practice ACT based defusion to manage anxious thoughts (e.g., "I'm having the thought that I'll embarrass myself"), engage in mindfulness to stay at the present moment during social interactions, and use yoga to reduce physical tension before social events.

Phase 4: *Integration and Practice*

The ultimate objective of this phase is to combine skills from all modalities into a cohesive practice. Here, we can use a 'coping toolbox' through play, where adolescents select play based strategies (e.g., drawing, story-telling) to manage stress. Further we can encourage committed action by helping them set small value driven goals (e.g., joining a school club to align with the value of connection). Integrating mindfulness into daily routine becomes necessary at this phase. It can be incorporated by practicing mindful eating or walking to reinforce present moment awareness. At this stage, we need to develop a personalized yoga practice that adolescents can use outside therapy sessions, such as, a 10-minute sequence for stress relief. At this stage, we can think of a group-settings, where we can combine modalities in activities like mindfulness-based yoga session followed by a CBPT group game to practice social skills, reinforcing ACT values through group discussions.

Phase 5: *Consolidation and Termination*

This is the last phase which aims to reinforce skills that have already learned, evaluate the progress and prepare the adolescent for therapy termination. We can use play to reflect on progress, such as creating a 'growth story' where adolescents narrate their therapeutic journey through art or story-telling. On the other hand, we can review value driven actions and celebrate achievements, using tools like the 'life compass' to map future goals. Further we might encourage adolescents to maintain practices as part of their daily routine, providing resources like mindfulness apps or guided recordings. And finally we can create a take-home yoga plan, including simple poses and breathing exercises, to support ongoing well-being. Before terminating the therapeutic intervention, we must ensure that termination activities respect cultural values such as incorporating family or community rituals to mark the end of the therapy.

Thus, the eclectic clinical framework presented here offers a comprehensive and developmentally nuanced model for adolescent psychotherapy. By systematically integrating Cognitive Behavioural Play Therapy, Acceptance and Commitment Therapy, mindfulness, and yoga across five therapeutic phases: Assessment, Engagement, Skill-Building, Integration and Practice, and Consolidation and Termination, the framework provides a cohesive roadmap for clinicians seeking to address the multifaceted dimensions of adolescent distress. Each phase is deliberately designed to support the adolescent's evolving therapeutic needs, drawing on diverse modalities to enhance emotional regulation, cognitive flexibility, somatic awareness, and values-based living. Crucially, this model is not only empirically grounded but also adaptable to varying cultural contexts, incorporating culturally resonant metaphors, rituals, and practices to foster relevance and resonance in diverse clinical settings. While this phase-based framework offers the scaffolding for longitudinal therapeutic progress, its efficacy is ultimately determined by how interventions are delivered within each session. The therapeutic encounter itself serves as the primary site where safety, regulation, insight, and integration converge. In the following section, we shift from a macro-level overview of the framework to a micro-level analysis of session structure. This detailed breakdown will outline the flow, rhythm, and key components of a typical session within the eclectic model, providing clinicians with practical guidance on sequencing interventions, facilitating transitions between modalities, and maintaining attuned therapeutic presence across stages of the session.

SESSION STRUCTURE: A FOUR PHASE THERAPEUTIC ARCHITECTURE

The session structure within this eclectic clinical framework is designed to provide a structured yet flexible approach to therapy, supporting adolescents through their emotional and psychological voyages. Each 60-minute session is organised into four main phases: opening attunement, somatic grounding, core therapeutic engagement and reflective closure. These phases work together to ensure that the session's flow remains adaptive, client-centred and tailored to the individual needs of the adolescent. The therapeutic approach emphasizes emotional safety, regulatory balance, and consistency, all while leaving room for creativity and clinical intuition.

(1) Opening Attunement (5-10 minutes)

The first phase of the session is designed to establish the emotional tone and foster relational alignment between the therapist and the adolescent. During this time, the therapist works to ensure that the adolescent feels emotionally safe and is ready to engage in the therapeutic process. The opening attunement involves a check-in where the adolescent can express their emotional state using metaphors or symbolic language, such as describing their mood as the 'weather,' identifying colours that represent how they feel, or using objects that may help articulate their internal experience. Transitional objects or sensory tools, like tactile items or sand trays, can also serve as a bridge to deeper emotional engagement. The therapist may lead guiding breathing exercises or body-mind scans to help the adolescents tune into their present state that primarily focuses on physical sensations or emotions that otherwise go unheeded. This phase plays a crucial role in co-regulation, particularly for adolescents who may have histories of trauma or emotional dysregulation. By offering a non-threatening and creative entry into the session, the therapist helps the adolescent to enter a receptive and grounded emotional state, setting the stage for deeper therapeutic works that further follows.

(2) Somatic Grounding (10 minutes)

In the next phase, the therapist focuses on somatic grounding, using yoga-informed movement and breathing techniques to regulate adolescent's physiological state and support emotional balance. This phase serves as a foundational tool for fostering autonomic regulation, which is especially beneficial for adolescents dealing with heightened emotional states, anxiety, or trauma related symptoms. Through gentle and intentional breathing practices, such as square box breathing, the adolescent is encouraged to reconnect with their body and bring attention to the present moment, helping them to mitigate hyper-arousal or dissociation. This sets the stage for the adolescent to deviate from the traditional talk therapy and engage in several creative activities further developing their interest to continue the therapy session. Here, in addition to the breath-work, the therapist may guide the adolescent through gentle movement sequences, such as cat-cow stretches or variations of child's pose, designed to activate both the sympathetic and parasympathetic nervous systems in a balanced way. These movements help to restore a sense of calm and focus, especially for those adolescents who may struggle with chronic anxiety symptoms. The use of proprioception and kinaesthetic awareness through these practices enhances the adolescent's ability to notice and regulate physical sensations, laying the groundwork for more profound emotional exploration during the session.

(3) Core Therapeutic Engagement (30 minutes)

Now we step into the core therapeutic phase of the session which is dedicated to the primary therapeutic work, involving the integration of CBPT, ACT, mindfulness and yoga based interventions. This phase serves as the heart of the therapeutic encounter, where the clinician draws from a variety of techniques and modalities based on the adolescent's emotional and cognitive readiness. For instance, CBPT interventions such as role-play, story completion or puppet dialogues provide a safe and engaging way to explore maladaptive cognitive patterns and emotional blocks. Metaphor-based exercises like the 'tug-of-war with a monster' or the 'worry-box,' allow the adolescent to externalize their internal conflicts and explore new perspectives. Again the mindful exercises like body scans or guided imagery, are used to deepen the present moment awareness of their internal world. Here, ACT based interventions include the application of values clarification that further helps adolescents to articulate what truly matters to them and motivating committed action toward living in alignment with their core values, even in the presence of discomfort. The therapist maintains a flexible approach, adjusting interventions based on the adolescent's real time cues which indicates whether that's an emotional shift, a sudden insight or an internal resistance. The adolescent is encouraged to engage fully in this phase, using creative expressions or symbolic actions to address internal struggles. The therapist's role is to maintain an attuned and responsive presence, providing a container for emotional exploration while also guiding the adolescent towards new ways of thinking, feeling and behaving.

(4) Reflective Closure (10-15 minutes)

The final phase of the session highlights the reflection and closure that helps the adolescents to process and consolidate the therapeutic experience. While conducting this phase, the therapist supports the adolescent in reflecting on the key insights and breakthroughs they gained from the session. The adolescent may be invited to share their views using some creative means for example, through story-telling, journaling or may be drawing. This further helps the therapist to understand the adolescent's interpretation of the session. The goal of this phase is to foster a sense of integration and closure, ensuring that the adolescent leaves the session with a clear sense of accomplishment, commitment and emotional balance. The therapist may introduce a grounding ritual, such as deep breathing or a physical stretch, to help the adolescent reorient to the present moment and prepare for their transition out of the therapeutic space. Additionally, micro-goals or action steps can be set for the adolescent to focus on before the next session, further reinforcing the commitment to growth and change. This reflective closure ensures that the adolescent's emotional state is stabilized before leaving the session, offering a sense of continuity and safety.

Thus, throughout the session, the therapist's approach remains relational, attuned and process focused. The clinician does not follow a rigid protocol but instead uses clinical intuition and moment-to-moment assessment to guide the adolescent through the various stages of the session. A non-directive stance is maintained, where the adolescent is viewed as an active partner in their healing journey. The therapist's embodiment practice, such as mindfulness or yoga, is essential in enhancing the therapeutic presence and fostering a connection of co-regulation with the adolescent. This four-phase structure provide a balanced, adaptive and client-centred approach that allows for both flexibility and consistency in addressing the complex needs of adolescents. By combining cognitive, emotional, somatic and relational interventions, the session structure fosters an environment where the adolescent can safely explore and navigate their psychological experiences, ultimately supporting their overall well-being and developmental growth.

CLINICAL APPLICATIONS

The integrative framework outlined in this chapter offers a versatile and developmentally responsive approach to treating a wide range of psychological difficulties in adolescents. By combining elements from CBPT, ACT, mindfulness and yoga informed interventions, the model provides a multi-modal platform capable of addressing the cognitive, emotional and somatic dimensions of adolescent distress. Its flexibility makes it applicable across various clinical presentations and diagnostic categories, while its client centred and culturally sensitive stance ensures alignment with diverse lived experiences.

In the treatment of *anxiety disorders*, this model targets both the cognitive and physiological components of the condition. ACT's focus on cognitive defusion allows adolescents to relate differently to their anxious thoughts, reducing the tendency to catastrophize or avoid internal experiences. Simultaneously, mindfulness practices help to cultivate attentional control and visceral awareness, enabling adolescents to become more anchored in the present moment rather than consumed by worry. Yoga-based interventions offer bottom-up regulation by soothing the hyper aroused nervous system through structured breathing practices and calming movement. CBPT adds an experiential layer that help to dig deeper into the roots of the thoughts by using symbolic play, story-telling and exposure techniques embedded in narrative frameworks which gently confront and reframe fears.

For adolescents grappling with *depressive symptoms*, this framework offers a layered and compassionate approach to activation and meaning-making. Depression in adolescents often manifests through anhedonia, low motivation, and persistent negative self-talk. ACT helps to address these patterns by introducing value-based action and shifting the focus from symptom elimination to meaningful engagement with life. This in turn uses the metaphor to substitute the correspondence of the thought with the adolescent rather than alternating and restructuring the thought itself. Mindfulness further interrupts the cycle of rumination and supports emotional clarity, while yoga reintroduces vitality through movement and breathing exercises, contradicting the physiological lethargy and disconnection associated with depressive states. CBPT contributes by creating space for gentle restructuring of depressive narratives, allowing for self-compassion and hope to emerge through metaphor and play.

In cases of *trauma related to abuse and dissociative disorders*, the integrative model is especially powerful due to its trauma-sensitive orientation. Adolescents with trauma histories often struggle with body-based symptoms, fragmented identity and emotional dysregulation. Yoga and mindfulness help to restore disrupted somatic awareness and provide grounding experiences that support nervous system stabilization. ACT supports identity consolidation through processes like self-as-context, further allowing the adolescents to view traumatic memories as experiences rather than defining truths, thus decoupling their identity from trauma narratives and finally regaining sense of agency. CBPT offers a safe container for symbolic re-narration of trauma stories, often using imaginative play or metaphor to facilitate integration in ways that feel less threatening and more accessible. This model ensures that all interventions are delivered with pacing, consent and attention to emotional safety.

For adolescents presenting with *suicidal ideation and behaviours*, the framework offers a compassionate and clinically rigorous pathway for intervention. Suicidality is rarely a singular symptom; it often reflects underlying trauma, unrelenting distress, existential despair and disrupted attachment. The integrative model addresses these complexities by incorporating ACT-based interventions that help adolescents shift from experiential avoidance to values-guided living. Through several metaphors, out of which is 'carrying your pain while moving toward is what matters,' clients begin to reframe their sufferings and rediscover their meaning and purpose in life even in the presence of psychological pain. Mindfulness and yoga based interventions serve as a crucial tool for managing acute affective arousal and supporting emotional containment. These practices allow adolescents real time access to grounding techniques, thereby enhancing distress tolerance and reducing impulsivity. Importantly, CBPT facilitates indirect, developmentally appropriate conversations about suicidality through symbolic expression and narratives that externalize despair or helplessness may create emotional distance that further allows the therapeutic exploration of those deeply painful experiences. The therapist's stance throughout remain attuned and relational, with safety planning, collaborative alliance and containment forming the ethical and clinical scaffolding. Rather than pathologizing suicidal ideation or behaviour, this model seeks to validate the adolescent's suffering while offering a concrete, embodied and meaningful course of actions for navigating it.

This framework also proves highly effective in treating *somatic symptom and related disorder*, in which psychological distress is expressed primarily through physical complaints. These adolescents often struggle to make sense of their physical sensations and may lack the language to articulate underlying emotional pain. Yoga fosters reconnection with the body and helps desensitize the somatic hypervigilance, while mindfulness promotes awareness of the mind-body connection. ACT gently confronts the experiential avoidance and introduces acceptance as a way to relate to discomfort without becoming overwhelmed. CPBT facilitates exploration of somatic metaphors that allows adolescents to give symbolic form to their symptoms and further helps to reframe them as meaningful expressions rather than purely pathological phenomenon.

Now-a-days, the increasing prevalence rates of *adolescent substance use* have successfully grabbed our attention, which often indicates the presence of complex psychological profiles, including trauma histories, emotional dysregulation, identity confusion, peer-related stress and family dysfunction among adolescents. Substance use may also function as an escape, a form of self-medication or a social survival strategy. This eclectic model helps to address these patterns from multiple entry points. ACT's emphasis on values clarification and acceptance is particularly effective in helping adolescents explore the functions of their substance use and recognize its misalignment with deeper life goals. Rather than solely focusing on abstinence or symptom control, this model invites adolescents to reconnect with intrinsic motivations and explore value congruent alternatives. Simultaneously, mindfulness will enhance the impulse control, improve present moment awareness and equip adolescents to observe cravings without acting on them, which is an evidence-supported technique known as 'urge surfing' (Marlatt & Gordon, 1985). Yoga informed interventions further support emotional regulation by recalibrating the nervous system and fostering a positive, embodied sense of self that is often absent in youth with prolonged substance involvement. Meanwhile, CBPT provides a safe, symbolic space to explore the emotional and relational drivers of addiction, using stories, metaphors and play to give voice to internal conflicts and ambivalence. Taken together, this model moves beyond reductionist approaches to substance use and instead offers a holistic, trauma-informed and developmentally resonant pathway to recovery.

Besides this, the integrative model also suits well for adolescents with *neurodevelopmental divergence*, *attachment disruptions* or *subclinical emotional difficulties*. Adolescents with autism spectrum traits or attentional challenges may find the traditional verbal psychotherapy difficult to engage in. However, the sensory tools, symbolic methods and experiential practices embedded in this framework offer alternative entry points into the therapeutic process. Likewise, adolescents who present with sub-threshold mood or anxiety symptoms benefit from the preventive and skill-building aspects of this model, which fosters self-awareness, emotional literacy and resilience. This model too works well with those who do not have a diagnosed clinical psychopathology as it allows to consider the values driven approach along with the play therapy techniques that help them to dive deeper into their internal orb. Further allowing them to engage in mindfulness exercises and yoga postures which encourages them to continue the therapy session rather than terminating abruptly.

Beyond its diagnostic applications, this framework is designed to operate within diverse cultural contexts. The inclusion of yoga and mindfulness honours the indigenous and eastern healing traditions, positioning the therapy within a broader spiritual or holistic framework when appropriate. This makes it particularly relevant in collectivist cultures, where psychological distress may be expressed through somatic idioms, or metaphysical language. Rather than pathologizing these expressions, the framework respects them, embedding psychotherapeutic interventions in a culturally congruent form. This enhances engagement, fosters trust and supports deeper therapeutic alliance. Hence, this eclectic framework demonstrates strong adaptability across clinical presentations, cultural backgrounds, and individual differences. Its developmental sensitivity, trauma-informed stance and integration of body, mind and meaning offer a rich, effective and compassionate pathway for supporting adolescents through psychological distress. Whether the challenges stem from acute clinical disorders, relational trauma or more diffuse emotional struggles, this model provides a multidimensional map toward healing and growth.

LIMITATIONS AND FUTURE DIRECTIONS

While the proposed eclectic clinical framework offers significant promise in addressing the multifaceted nature of adolescent psychological distress, it is important to acknowledge its limitations to ensure balanced understanding and responsible application. Like all integrative models, this approach must navigate the inherent tension between breadth and depth. Although the integration of CPBT, ACT, mindfulness and yoga enhances flexibility and adaptability, it also risks theoretical diffusion if not grounded in a clear clinical rationale. Therapists who lack formal training in one or more of these modalities may struggle to maintain fidelity to core principles, potentially diluting therapeutic effectiveness or leading to inconsistent application. One key limitation lies in the training burden placed on practitioners. Effective implementation of this model requires a high level of competency across diverse domains that range from play therapy and ACT processes to trauma-sensitive yoga and mindfulness facilitation. Many clinicians, particularly those in resource limited or high demand settings, may not have multidisciplinary training or supervision required to implement the full scope of the model with integrity. There are logistical and systemic challenges too. Incorporating somatic practices, movement, and experiential play into psychotherapy sessions requires flexibility in physical space, session length and institutional support. In more rigid clinical environments such as hospital systems or standardized school settings, therapists may find it difficult to fully operationalize the model due to environmental constraints or productivity pressures. Even from a research standpoint, the current framework remains largely theoretical and clinical in nature. Thus, there is a need for systemic studies that assess the integrated model's efficacy, both qualitatively and quantitatively, across different diagnostic categories, developmental profiles and sociocultural contexts.

Now looking ahead, there are several future directions that can enhance the relevance, reach and impact of this integrative framework. To begin with, the development of structured yet flexible intervention manuals or treatment guidelines would support consistent implementation while preserving clinical creativity. These resources could provide session templates, metaphor inventories, and culturally adapted practices that make the model more accessible for a wide range of practitioners. Secondly, multimodal research that includes randomized controlled trials, longitudinal outcome studies and mixed method designs, can help to establish an empirical foundation for the model. Additionally, cross-cultural research is vital to ensure the model's adaptability and respect for diverse expressions of distress and healing. Another important direction involves integrating the framework into school-based and community mental health settings, where preventive and early intervention strategies can reach adolescents who may not otherwise access formal therapy. Group formats, peer based delivery models and hybrid digital adaptations (e.g., apps or teletherapy modules) may further expand access while retaining therapeutic integrity. Finally, therapist self-care and embodiment practices must be emphasized as a foundational component of the model's sustainability. Therapists who regularly engage in mindfulness, yoga or creative reflection are better positioned to model regulation, remain attuned and deliver interventions with authenticity and presence. Thus, while the eclectic integrative framework holds considerable potential as a holistic, flexible and culturally responsive model of adolescent therapy, its full realization depends on ongoing training, ethical application, empirical validation and system level adaptation. Addressing these limitations and pursuing these future directions will help ensure that the model evolves with rigor, inclusivity and effectiveness at its core.

CONCLUSION

This chapter has presented an integrative, developmentally sensitive framework that unites cognitive behavioural play therapy (CPBT), acceptance and commitment therapy (ACT), mindfulness and yoga informed interventions into coherent and flexible clinical model tailored for adolescents. This eclectic framework has been designed to address the complexity of psychological distress among youths, further recognizing that no single modality can fully capture the layered interplay of cognitive, emotional, somatic, relational and cultural factors influencing adolescent mental health.

The recent developments in clinical psychology, neuroscience and trauma studies affirm the necessity of moving beyond narrowly focused, symptom-reduction paradigms. Contemporary researches have demonstrated that interventions incorporating bottom-up regulation (e.g., yoga, somatic awareness), experiential processing (e.g., play metaphor) and psychological flexibility (e.g., ACT and mindfulness) are particularly effective in promoting sustainable well-being among adolescents. Noting these advances, the current framework offers a timely response to the developmental realities of adolescence that is marked by neuroplasticity, identity formation and evolving emotional complexity (Casey, Jones, & Hare, 2008; Dahl et al., 2018). Emerging findings from affective neuroscience and polyvagal theory further support this integrative direction. The recognition of the adolescent brain's heightened sensitivity to social threats and affective experiences underscores the importance of interventions that engage body as much as the mind. Trauma informed somatic practices such as, trauma sensitive yoga, breath based grounding, directly influence autonomic functioning, allowing the adolescents to build internal safety before engaging in more cognitively demanding therapeutic work (Emerson & Hopper, 2011; Khalsa et al., 2012). Similarly, research in interoception and embodiment has revealed that cultivating awareness of internal bodily signals which is often underdeveloped in trauma affected youth, is central to emotional regulation and identity integration.

Thus, these modern developments align with a broader paradigm shift in adolescent psychotherapy that deviates from rigid, protocol driven models and appreciates process based, culturally grounded and relationship centred approaches. The clinicians and researchers alike are advocating for therapeutic models that are responsive not only to diagnostic labels but to individual development, cultural worldview, somatic experience and personal meaning making. This framework embodies that shift by offering a modular yet cohesive structure that can be adapted to each adolescent's evolving readiness, needs and cultural context. Exigently, the model too reflects a reorientation in mental health care that values well-being and resilience as much as symptom relief. Through practices that foster mindfulness, creativity, bodily presence, and value guiding living, the framework moves beyond a problem-centred lens to support adolescents in cultivating agency, coherence and purpose. This vision is increasingly echoed in public health and global mental health initiatives that call for integrative, preventive and scalable interventions grounded in both scientific evidence and humanistic care.

To conclude this chapter, we can say that this eclectic framework stands at the intersection of tradition and innovation that offers a robust therapeutic map attuned to the realities of adolescent life. It supports clinicians and mental health professionals in meeting young people who are developmentally, emotionally, culturally and somatically sensitive and further guiding them toward growth, integration and well-being. As modern mental health care evolves to embrace complexity, incarnation and contextual sensitivity, frameworks like this are not merely relevant but are quintessential.

REFERENCES

Black, D. S. (2011). *A brief definition of mindfulness.* Mindfulness Research Guide.

Broderick, P. C. (2013). *Learning to Breathe: A Mindfulness Curriculum for Adolescents to Cultivate Emotion Regulation, Attention, and Performance*. New Harbinger Publications.

Casey, B. J., Jones, R. M., & Hare, T. A. (2008). The adolescent brain. *Annals of the New York Academy of Sciences, 1124*(1), 111–126. DOI: 10.1196/annals.1440.010 PMID: 18400927

Copeland, W. E., Shanahan, L., Hinesley, J., Chan, R. F., Aberg, K. A., Fairbank, J. A., van den Oord, E. J. C. G., & Costello, E. J. (2018). Association of childhood trauma exposure with adult psychiatric disorders and functional outcomes. *JAMA Network Open, 1*(7), e184493. DOI: 10.1001/jamanetworkopen.2018.4493 PMID: 30646356

Dahl, R. E., Allen, N. B., Wilbrecht, L., & Suleiman, A. B. (2018). Importance of investing in adolescence from a developmental science perspective. *Nature, 554*(7693), 441–450. DOI: 10.1038/nature25770 PMID: 29469094

Datta, S., & Mukherjee, T. (2017). A clinical case study using acceptance and commitment therapy. *Indian Journal of Clinical Psychology, 44*(1), 68–74.

Emerson, D., & Hopper, E. (2011). *Overcoming Trauma through Yoga: Reclaiming Your Body*. North Atlantic Books.

Felver, J. C., Butzer, B., Olson, K. J., Smith, I. M., & Khalsa, S. B. S. (2015). Yoga in public school improves adolescent mood and affect. *Contemporary School Psychology, 19*(4), 184–192. DOI: 10.1007/s40688-014-0031-9 PMID: 26478825

Gururaj, G., Varghese, M., Benegal, V., Rao, G. N., Pathak, K., & Singh, L. K.NMHS collaborators group. (2016). *National Mental Health Survey of India, 2015–16: Summary*. NIMHANS Publication.

Hayes, S. C., Strosahl, K. D., & Wilson, K. G. (2012). *Acceptance and Commitment Therapy: The Process and Practice of Mindful Change.* Guilford Press. DOI: 10.1037/17335-000

James, A. C., James, G., Cowdrey, F. A., Soler, A., & Choke, A. (2015). Cognitive behavioural therapy for anxiety disorders in children and adolescents. *Cochrane Database of Systematic Reviews*, 2. PMID: 25692403

Kabat-Zinn, J. (1990). *Full Catastrophe Living: Using the Wisdom of Your Body and Mind to Face Stress, Pain, and Illness.* Delacorte Press.

Kendall, P. C., Safford, S., Flannery-Schroeder, E., & Webb, A. (2004). Child anxiety treatment: Outcomes in adolescence and impact on substance use and depression at 7.4-year follow-up. *Journal of Consulting and Clinical Psychology*, *72*(2), 276–287. DOI: 10.1037/0022-006X.72.2.276 PMID: 15065961

Kessler, R. C., Avenevoli, S., & Merikangas, K. R. (2012). Mood disorders in children and adolescents: An epidemiologic perspective. *Biological Psychiatry*, *49*(12), 1002–1014. DOI: 10.1016/S0006-3223(01)01129-5 PMID: 11430842

Khalsa, S. B. S., Hickey-Schultz, L., Cohen, D., Steiner, N., & Cope, S. (2012). Evaluation of the mental health benefits of yoga in a secondary school: A preliminary randomized controlled trial. *The Journal of Behavioral Health Services & Research*, *39*(1), 80–90. DOI: 10.1007/s11414-011-9249-8 PMID: 21647811

Knell, S. M. (1993). *Cognitive-Behavioral Play Therapy*. Jason Aronson.

Lieberman, A. F., & Van Horn, P. (2011). *Psychotherapy with infants and young children: Repairing the effects of stress and trauma on early attachment*. Guilford Press.

Livheim, F., Hayes, L., Ghaderi, A., Magnusdottir, T., Högfeldt, A., Rowse, J., Turner, S., Hayes, S. C., & Tengström, A. (2015). The effectiveness of acceptance and commitment therapy for adolescent mental health: Swedish and Australian pilot outcomes. *Journal of Child and Family Studies*, *24*(4), 1016–1030. DOI: 10.1007/s10826-014-9912-9

Malhotra, S., & Patra, B. N. (2014). Prevalence of child and adolescent psychiatric disorders in India: A systematic review and meta-analysis. *Child and Adolescent Psychiatry and Mental Health*, *8*(1), 22. DOI: 10.1186/1753-2000-8-22 PMID: 25071865

McLaughlin, K. A., Koenen, K. C., Hill, E. D., Petukhova, M., Sampson, N. A., Zaslavsky, A. M., & Kessler, R. C. (2017). Trauma exposure and posttraumatic stress disorder in a national sample of adolescents. *Journal of the American Academy of Child and Adolescent Psychiatry*, *52*(8), 815–830. DOI: 10.1016/j.jaac.2013.05.011 PMID: 23880492

Polanczyk, G. V., Salum, G. A., Sugaya, L. S., Caye, A., & Rohde, L. A. (2015). Annual research review: A meta-analysis of the worldwide prevalence of mental disorders in children and adolescents. *Journal of Child Psychology and Psychiatry, and Allied Disciplines*, *56*(3), 345–365. DOI: 10.1111/jcpp.12381 PMID: 25649325

Shapiro, S. L., & Carlson, L. E. (2009). *The Art and Science of Mindfulness: Integrating Mindfulness into Psychology and the Helping Professions*. American Psychological Association. DOI: 10.1037/11885-000

Swain, J., Hancock, K., Hainsworth, C., & Bowman, J. (2015). Mechanisms of change: Exploratory outcomes from a randomised controlled trial of acceptance and commitment therapy for anxious adolescents. *Journal of Contextual Behavioral Science*, *4*(1), 56–67. DOI: 10.1016/j.jcbs.2014.09.001

Toghiani, M., Ghasemi, F., & Sharifi, T. (2019). The effectiveness of acceptance and commitment group therapy on social anxiety in female dormitory residents in Isfahan University of Medical Sciences. *Journal of Education and Health Promotion*, *8*(1), 41. DOI: 10.4103/jehp.jehp_111_18 PMID: 30993134

Weisz, J. R., Kuppens, S., Ng, M. Y., Eckshtain, D., Ugueto, A. M., Vaughn-Coaxum, R., Jensen-Doss, A., Hawley, K. M., Krumholz Marchette, L. S., Chu, B. C., Weersing, V. R., & Fordwood, S. R. (2017). What five decades of research tells us about the effects of youth psychological therapy: A multilevel meta-analysis and implications for science and practice. *The American Psychologist*, *72*(2), 79–117. DOI: 10.1037/a0040360 PMID: 28221063

Zoogman, S., Goldberg, S. B., Hoyt, W. T., & Miller, L. (2015). Mindfulness interventions with youth: A meta-analysis. *Mindfulness*, *6*(2), 290–302. DOI: 10.1007/s12671-013-0260-4

Chapter 6
Rainbow Mindfulness: Integrating Mindfulness-Based Interventions for the LGBTQIA+ Community

Utkarsh Srivastava
http://orcid.org/0009-0003-2026-1718
University of Delhi, India

Aditi Dhoundiyal
http://orcid.org/0009-0006-9085-5986
University of Delhi, India

ABSTRACT

The psychosocial and mental health issues indicating that the LGBTQIA+ individuals faces are thoroughly examined in this chapter, with particular attention paid to ideas like gender identity, gender dysphoria, minority stress, anxiety disorders, and mood disorders. It looks at how institutional discrimination, stigma, and intersectionality affect mental health outcomes, emphasizing the particular vulnerabilities faced by LGBTQIA+ people in India. By discussing evidence-based interventions that have the potential to lessen psychological distress, increase resilience, and promote identity integration, such as mindfulness-based therapies, yoga, and meditation, the chapter expands the conversation while drawing on contemporary empirical research. The role of mindfulness in reducing stress, anxiety, and

DOI: 10.4018/979-8-2600-1202-4.ch006

depression symptoms is specifically discussed, with a focus on transgender and gender-diverse youth. This highlights the importance of affirmative care models that are sensitive to cultural differences in order to effectively address the complex vulnerabilities that LGBTQIA+ people face.

INTRODUCTION

The LGBTQIA+ community encompasses a wide and inclusive spectrum of individuals who identify as lesbian, gay, bisexual, transgender, queer or questioning, intersex, asexual, and others whose gender or sexual identities diverge from cisnormative and heteronormative expectations. The acronym itself signifies not only the breadth of human diversity but also a symbolic act of resistance against social systems that have historically constrained identity and sexuality (Connell, 2015; Morris, 2023). Over the decades, the LGBTQIA+ movement has profoundly shaped sociocultural and political discourses across the globe, advancing broader struggles for equity, recognition, and human rights.

A key construct in understanding this diversity is gender identity, which refers to an individual's internal and deeply felt sense of self as male, female, both, neither, or positioned somewhere along the gender continuum. This self-concept is distinct from the biological sex assigned at birth. For many transgender and gender-nonconforming individuals, the journey of self-realization is profoundly personal and may involve social, psychological, or medical transitions aimed at aligning lived experiences with internal identities (Sansfaçon et al., 2020). Research in neuroendocrinology has demonstrated that gender identity may be shaped by neurobiological mechanisms, challenging traditional binary frameworks of sex and gender (Roselli, 2018). Complementary to these scientific perspectives, philosophical and social theorists conceptualize gender as a fluid and evolving experience that arises through dynamic interactions between social expectations and personal agency (Cosker-Rowland, 2023).

Parallel to gender identity, sexual orientation refers to an individual's enduring pattern of emotional, romantic, or sexual attraction toward others. Orientation may be heterosexual, homosexual, bisexual, pansexual, asexual, or fluid, reflecting an identity that can evolve over time. While early models described sexual orientation development as linear or milestone-based, contemporary research emphasizes its fluidity and its interplay of biological, psychological, and sociocultural influences (Saewyc, 2011; Cook, 2020; Bogaert & Skorska, 2020). Studies have identified potential biological correlates, such as prenatal hormonal exposure linked with same-sex attraction, while also acknowledging the significant role of environmental, familial, and cultural factors in shaping sexual orientation (Baams & Kaufman, 2023).

Despite notable progress in legal and social recognition, the LGBTQIA+ population continues to face systemic discrimination within institutions such as healthcare, education, and law. However, growing academic and public acknowledgment of the community's legitimacy has fostered policy reforms, inclusive healthcare initiatives, and increasing social acceptance (Mishra, 2022; Shaikh et al., 2024). A deeper understanding of gender identity and sexual orientation thus enables researchers, practitioners, and policymakers to develop more inclusive frameworks that promote equality and empathy in addressing human diversity.

PSYCHOSOCIAL CHALLENGES AMONG LGBTQIA+ INDIVIDUALS

Psychosocial challenges encompass the intertwined psychological and social factors that shape emotional well-being, behavioral regulation, and interpersonal functioning. For individuals identifying as LGBTQIA+, these challenges are often intensified by persistent stigma, marginalization, and social exclusion embedded within heteronormative and cisnormative structures (Meyer, 2003). Family rejection remains one of the most profound sources of distress. Snapp et al. (2015) found that LGBTQIA+ youth frequently encounter familial hostility or alienation, resulting in emotional isolation and, in severe cases, homelessness. Concealing one's authentic identity often becomes a coping mechanism to avoid social rejection but simultaneously generates internalized shame and deteriorates self-esteem (Ryan et al., 2010; Pachankis, 2007).

Social discrimination and marginalization further exacerbate psychological strain. According to Russell and Fish (2016), LGBTQIA+ individuals experience higher levels of loneliness and reduced social support, both closely associated with adverse mental health outcomes. Meyer's (2003) Minority Stress Model provides a theoretical framework for understanding these phenomena, emphasizing that external prejudice, anticipated rejection, and internalized stigma cumulatively heighten psychological distress. Discrimination also permeates educational and workplace settings, leading to exclusion, career stagnation, and harassment (Kosciw et al., 2018; Goldberg et al., 2020). Such systemic inequities cultivate chronic stress and diminish emotional resilience. Bullying and violence remain significant concerns, particularly among LGBTQIA+ adolescents. Toomey and Russell (2013) demonstrated that these youth experience markedly higher rates of school-based victimization, correlating with depression, anxiety, and academic disengagement. Continuous exposure to such hostility normalizes avoidance and self-silencing behaviors. Furthermore, healthcare disparities compound these psychosocial challenges. Despite increased awareness, many healthcare professionals remain inadequately trained to address LGBTQIA+ needs, resulting in substandard or biased care (Kattari et al., 2016; Cahill & Makadon, 2014). This lack of competence discourages care-seeking and perpetuates cycles of neglect. Empirical evidence indicates significantly elevated rates of depression, anxiety, substance use, and suicidality among LGBTQIA+ populations (Marshal et al., 2011; Plöderl & Tremblay, 2015). These outcomes stem from cumulative experiences of rejection, discrimination, and invisibility, emphasizing the need for inclusive policies and culturally sensitive psychosocial interventions.

INTERSECTIONALITY, SOCIAL CONTEXT, AND PERSPECTIVES

The lived realities of LGBTQIA+ individuals are profoundly shaped by intersectionality, which recognizes how overlapping social identities—such as race, religion, class, and disability—combine to create distinct experiences of privilege and oppression. For LGBTQIA+ individuals belonging to multiple marginalized groups, such as sexual minorities of color or those from conservative religious backgrounds, discrimination often operates on multiple levels, exacerbating exclusion and limiting access to safety and resources (Shaikh et al., 2024; Mishra, 2022). These intersecting inequities manifest across domains such as healthcare, employment, and education. Social rejection, bullying, and familial estrangement are major predictors of adverse mental health outcomes, contributing to higher prevalence rates of anxiety, depression, and suicidality (Schnabel, 2018; Sharma, 2021). Prolonged exposure to stigma fosters hypervigilance and erodes trust in institutions (Shaikh et al., 2024).

Conversely, social environments that promote inclusivity, representation, and open dialogue can mitigate minority stress and enhance psychological well-being. Research highlights that affirming care models, peer-support networks, and community engagement significantly foster belonging and resilience (Matsuzaka et al., 2021; Pullen Sansfaçon et al., 2020). Historically, gender and sexual variance were criminalized or pathologized, perpetuating stigma and exclusion. Yet, sustained activism and scholarship have driven notable progress in legal and cultural recognition (Morris, 2023; Sharma, 2021). Legal reforms such as anti-discrimination acts, same-sex partnership recognition, and gender-affirming healthcare represent key milestones, although their implementation remains uneven globally (Schnabel, 2018; Connell, 2015). Understanding intersectionality is thus essential for developing inclusive policies and equitable systems that reflect the multifaceted nature of human experience.

STRESS AND THE IMPORTANCE OF STRESS MANAGEMENT IN THE LGBTQIA+ COMMUNITY

Stress is a universal physiological and psychological response to perceived threats or challenges. However, for LGBTQIA+ individuals, stress frequently arises from minority status and identity-based stigma. Meyer's (2003) Minority Stress Theory distinguishes between distal stressors—such as discrimination and violence—and proximal stressors, including internalized stigma, concealment, and fear of rejection. These factors collectively contribute to the elevated incidence of depression, anxiety, and suicidality reported within the community (Hatzenbuehler et al., 2009; Feinstein et al., 2012). Classical frameworks, including Selye's

(1956) General Adaptation Syndrome and Folkman's (1984) Transactional Model of Stress and Coping, contextualize the physiological and cognitive mechanisms underlying stress responses. Prolonged exposure to identity-based stress undermines adaptive capacities, leading to psychological and physical exhaustion (Meyer, 2015; Pachankis et al., 2015). Intersectional analyses further reveal that individuals navigating multiple forms of marginalization—such as race, caste, or disability—face intensified vulnerability to minority stress (Balsam et al., 2011; Ghabrial, 2025).

Manifestations of chronic stress among LGBTQIA+ individuals include internalized homophobia or transphobia, social withdrawal, and emotional dysregulation (Craney et al., 2018; Wandrekar & Nigudkar, 2020). These stressors form cyclical patterns that reinforce vulnerability and deteriorate mental health over time. Nonetheless, protective factors such as social support, community connectedness, and resilience substantially buffer against these effects. Empirical studies have demonstrated that engagement in advocacy, peer-support groups, and affirming communities enhances self-acceptance and psychological well-being (Mereish & Bradford, 2014; Kwon, 2013; McConnell et al., 2018). Adaptive coping mechanisms—such as mindfulness, cognitive reframing, and emotional regulation—also reduce distress and foster life satisfaction (Railley, 2023; Ferbežar et al., 2024).

In India, mental health institutions and organizations like NIMHANS and UNDP have developed culturally sensitive psychosocial life-skills programs aimed at strengthening LGBTQIA+ individuals' coping capacities through group-based resilience and peer engagement (Railley, 2023). These initiatives are critical in contexts where stigma and familial or institutional exclusion persist. Unaddressed minority stress can perpetuate cycles of mental illness, social marginalization, and reduced life satisfaction. Hence, it is essential for mental health professionals to integrate affirmative, evidence-based, and culturally grounded interventions in their practice (Choi et al., 2020; American Psychiatric Association, n.d.). Such approaches not only enhance individual well-being but also advance the broader objectives of health equity and social justice for the LGBTQIA+ community.

MENTAL HEALTH CHALLENGES FACED BY LGBTQIA+ COMMUNITY IN INDIA

The LGBTQIA+ population in India endures a disproportionately high burden of mental health challenges, primarily due to deep-rooted stigma, social exclusion, and institutional neglect. Empirical research indicates that LGBTQIA+ individuals are significantly more likely to suffer from depression, anxiety, and suicidal ideation compared to cisgender heterosexual peers (Wandrekar & Nigudkar, 2020). Until the decriminalization of Section 377, legal structures reinforced societal discrimination, contributing to a culture of silence, guilt, and rejection. Even post-decriminalization, familial and community rejection remains a prominent source of psychological distress (Wandrekar & Nigudkar, 2020; Grigoreva & Szaszkó, 2024). Moreover, healthcare systems are often ill-equipped to handle LGBTQIA+ concerns, with individuals reporting invalidation and prejudice from professionals (Ghabrial, 2025).

The application of minority stress theory in Indian studies reveals how chronic exposure to discrimination leads to mental health deterioration (Meyer, 2003; Ferbežar et al., 2024). Many LGBTQIA+ individuals resort to avoidant coping strategies, including substance use, because of a lack of accessible support systems (Craney et al., 2018). Intersectionality complicates these challenges—those from Dalit, Adivasi, or Muslim backgrounds face additional discrimination in access to healthcare, employment, and education (McConnell et al., 2018; Ghabrial, 2025). The compounding effect of multiple marginalized identities results in higher psychological vulnerability and limited resource access. Some progress has been made through community-driven interventions that provide safe spaces, peer counseling, and life-skills training (Railley, 2023). However, there remains a critical need for culturally attuned, trauma-informed, and LGBTQIA+ affirmative mental health services to address these disparities (Choi et al., 2020)

GENDER IDENTITY & GENDER DYSPHORIA

Gender identity-related distress is one of the most significant and under-addressed mental health concerns within the LGBTQIA+ spectrum. Gender dysphoria, as defined in clinical contexts, is the profound distress experienced by individuals whose gender identity does not align with their sex assigned at birth. This mismatch often leads to psychological suffering, especially in societies lacking affirmation and support (Grigoreva & Szaszkó, 2024). Frequent experiences of misgendering, invalidation, or outright rejection from family and institutions compound distress (Ghabrial, 2025). These challenges are often intensified by lack of access to gender-affirming healthcare, such as hormone therapy or surgical procedures, which are essential for many transgender individuals' mental well-being (Wandrekar & Nigudkar, 2020). Bockting's earlier findings (referenced in Ghabrial, 2025) highlight a strong association between gender-based discrimination and elevated levels of anxiety, depression, and suicidality. Additionally, qualitative research confirms that transgender individuals often internalize stigma, further heightening distress (Ferbežar et al., 2024). Effective intervention strategies emphasize the importance of affirming therapy, peer support, and legal protection. Mental health professionals must create inclusive therapeutic spaces where gender identity can be safely explored without judgment (Meyer, 2003). Moreover, legal and policy-level support for gender-affirming care—along with societal sensitization—can reduce dysphoria and promote psychological well-being (Railley, 2023; Craney et al., 2018).

Gender Dysphoria and Mental Health Among Transgender Youth in India

Emerging research in India reveals severe mental health challenges among transgender and gender-diverse youth. A clinic-based study in Chennai found 24–25% of help-seeking transgender individuals experience moderate to severe anxiety and depression, highlighting their psychological vulnerability (Srinivasan & Chandrasekaran, 2025). A community study in Karnataka reported over 30% of transgender adolescents had active suicidal ideation and over 50% attempted suicide by age 20 (Halli et al., 2021).

These findings align with broader assessments showing underutilization of mental health care, trauma exposure, and pervasive stigma (Gaur et al., 2023; Ranade et al., 2025). While gender dysphoria remains a core issue, social stressors such as familial rejection and community violence contribute more significantly to distress (Arvind et al., 2021; Ranade et al., 2025). Psychosocial adversity is widespread; over 60% reported verbal abuse, and more than 20% faced physical or sexual assault, correlating strongly with poor mental health and low self-esteem (Srinivasan & Chandrasekaran, 2020). Protective interventions remain underexplored, though peer support networks show promise in reducing isolation (Khapre et al., 2024). Most Indian research focuses on adults or HIV, with limited data on adolescents or psychological care models (Raj & Dubey, 2024). Internationally recognized therapies like affirmative CBT or mindfulness lack adaptation and implementation in Indian settings, compounded by insufficient school support and provider training (Wandrekar, 2020; Gaur et al., 2023). Addressing these gaps is crucial to improving transgender youth mental health care in India.

ANXIETY DISORDERS AND LGBTQ COMMUNITY

Anxiety disorders include a range of symptoms characterized primarily by excessive or abnormal feelings of anxiety, which significantly affect an individual's emotional state or mood. Anxiety disorders involve excessive fear or anxiety that is difficult to control and negatively impacts daily activities (APA, 2022)." There are various sub categories of anxiety disorders, each with its own set of diagnostic criteria, according to the Diagnostic and Statistical Manual of Mental Disorders, Fifth Edition. These include "selective mutism", "generalized anxiety disorder", "separation anxiety disorder", "panic disorder", "agoraphobia", "social anxiety", and "specific phobia". The common signs and symptoms of anxiety disorders involve experience of distress accompanied with disturbances of sleep, attention, social and occupational functioning (Chand & Marwaha, 2023; Hague, 2022).

According to the "World Health Organization", about 3.6% of the global population suffers from anxiety disorders. A systematic review by Remes et al. (2016) indicates the prevalence of anxiety disorders in adults ranging from 3.8% to 25%, with generalized anxiety disorder being the most commonly diagnosed in the population. However, a recent meta-analysis of 26 articles reports that LGB individuals have higher risks of various mental disorders than do heterosexual individuals (Wittgens et al., 2022). In support of this, another meta-analysis of Chinese studies indicates the prevalence of anxiety symptoms in LGB individuals to be found around 32.2%, (Wei et al., 2020).

Therefore, anxiety disorders are becoming increasingly prevalent in the LGBTQI+ population. It can be attributed to the repeated exposure to threats faced by the minority on a regular basis (Herek & Garnets, 2007; Meyer, 2003). Such threat can include childhood maltreatment, bullying, and physical and sexual assault at rates much higher than heterosexual peers (Balsam et al., 2011) as well as discrimination and rejection (Meyer, 2003, 2013). This exposure to violence, discrimination, and rejection often occurs in social contexts that lack legal protection (Hatzenbuehler, Keyes, & Hasin, 2009). Casey et al., (2019) have further shed light on kinds of discrimination faced by LGBTQ adults across the U.S. The study found that discrimination against LGBTQ adults is widespread across various domains, including healthcare, employment, and interpersonal interactions. Over half reported experiencing slurs, microaggressions, harassment, or violence. Many also avoided healthcare due to anticipated discrimination, especially transgender individuals. LGBTQ racial/ethnic minorities faced higher levels of discrimination in legal and employment settings. LGBTQ youth are more likely to be victims of bullying (Juvonen and Graham, 2014; Earnshaw et al., 2017). LGBTQ victims of bullying in school report higher levels of absenteeism and lower academic achievement (Nishina et al., 2005). Therefore, increasing the prevalence of significant increase in the symptoms of anxiety and mood disorders

MOOD DISORDERS AND LGBTQ COMMUNITY

The co-occurrence of mood disorders and anxiety disorders is a widely recognized phenomenon in clinical practice and research (Saha et al., 2020). Mood refers to a persistent emotional state that influences an individual's internal experience and external behavior across various contexts. Mood or affective disorders are characterized by significant disturbances in emotional functioning, marked by prolonged periods of low mood (depression) or elevated mood states (hypomania or mania) (Spijker & Claes, 2014). According to the Diagnostic and Statistical Manual of Mental Disorders (DSM-5), mood disorders fall under two broad categories: bipolar disorders and depressive disorders). Depressive disorders can be predominantly categorized into "Major Depressive Disorder", "Persistent Depressive Disorder" (dysthymia), "Disruptive Mood Dysregulation Disorder", and "Premenstrual Dysphoric Disorder" (Sekhon & Gupta. 2023). Bipolar disorders are also classified into bipolar I, bipolar II and cyclothymic disorder. The main feature of bipolar I disorder is at least one manic episode that lasts for at least a week, followed by significant depressed or hypomanic episodes. These manic episodes can seriously impede functioning or perhaps necessitate hospitalization. On the other hand, Bipolar II disorder is characterized by at least one episode of hypomanic and one episode of major depression, with no history of a full blown mania.

Hypomania is less severe and it typically lasts for a minimum of four consecutive days. It does not significantly impair one's social or occupational functioning. Cyclothymia is considered as a subclinical form of bipolarity, followed by persistent mood fluctuations involving mild depressive symptoms and brief episodes of elevated mood that do not meet the full criteria for major depression or hypomania (Kurumaji, 2013). Individuals diagnosed with mood disorder may experience times of apathy, melancholy or hopelessness, lack of sleep and appetite, interest in previously enjoyable activities, as well as periods of elevated mood, increase in level of energy, and engagement in risky and impulsive behavior during manic episodes (Harrison, 2007).

Sexual minorities are at least 1.5 times more likely to suffer mood disorders, anxiety, and substance use disorders (Plöderl & Tremblay, 2015; Semlyen et al., 2016). Studies have also shown that among the LGB community, there are gender-specific trends in mental health. For example, compared to heterosexual people, gay and bisexual males have been found to have a much greater prevalence of mood disorders (Sandfort et al., 2014). Similar patterns have been found in India, where recent study has also revealed a significant prevalence of mood disorders among LGBTQIA+ community. For example, Das and Govindappa (2023) found that, especially during the COVID-19 pandemic, 44.3% of their sample in northern Kerala reported having depression and 41.5% reported having anxiety. Several psychosocial stressors and systemic disadvantages are responsible for the rising prevalence of mood disorders among LGBTQ people. For example, D'Augelli (2002) found that adolescents who identify as LGBT had far greater rates of somatization and depression than their counterparts who do not. More than 75 percent of participants in his study reported verbal abuse, and 15 percent reported physical assault. Those who experienced more victimization were also more likely to report mental health issues. LGBTQ youth who endure continuous victimization throughout adolescence and early adulthood are more likely to suffer from depression and PTSD (Mustanski et al., 2016). Regular experiences with discrimination are also found to be substantially associated with social anxiety, internalized homonegativity, rejection sensitivity, and depressive symptoms (Feinstein et al., 2012). This regular form of discrimination can be seen in the form of "persistent discrimination," which refers to an ongoing systemic bias that LGBTQ individuals encounter in education, employment, healthcare, and interpersonal relationships, factors that collectively foster a hostile social environment and increase mental health risk (Yarns et al., 2016).

Di Marco et al. (2021) also pointed out that this exclusion might manifest in a variety of ways, such as institutional discrimination, marginalization at work, and rejection from family, all of which exacerbate feelings of loneliness. The difficulties LGBTQ people encounter in negotiating heteronormative societal norms have also been highlighted by Jakobsen et al. (2023). These difficulties frequently result in internal conflict and stress, which exacerbates mood disorders. In addition, earlier research has emphasized how a person's sexual orientation influences their mental health. For example, two Canadian studies found that the prevalence of mood and anxiety disorders in gay/bisexual males and lesbian/bisexual women was significantly correlated with sexual orientation (Steele et al., 2009). Therefore, due to their minority status, people who identify as lesbian, gay, or bisexual (LGB) may face particular psychological pressures (Matthews et al., 2002) as compared to their heterosexual counterparts making them far more susceptible to mental health issues (Kidd et al., 2016). LGBTQ people frequently reported reduced perceived support, especially from family members, which makes these difficulties much worse. The detrimental impacts of minority stress may be exacerbated by this decreased support, which may also result in less resilience. For instance, More than 75% of participants in the Gmelin et al. (2022) study reported verbal abuse, and 15% reported physical assault. Those who experienced more victimization were also more likely to report mental health issues.

ROLE OF MINDFULNESS IN REDUCING THE SYMPTOMS OF MENTAL DISORDERS IN LGBTQIA+ COMMUNITY

Mindfulness can be referred to as a process that cultivates a mental state characterized by nonjudgmental awareness of one's present-moment experiences including one's thoughts, emotions, bodily sensations and the environment (Bishop et al., 2004). Recent research has shown that intervention based on mindfulness can effectively reduce symptoms of mood and anxiety disorders through several interconnected psychological and neurobiological mechanisms. It is found to strengthen attention regulation as mindfulness helps individuals to shift focus away from ruminative or worry based thought patterns towards objective, non-judgemental observation of emotions as they arise. This process results in reduced negative self-evaluation and greater tolerance of unpleasant affective states. On a neurobiological level, practicing mindfulness can enhance the activities and connectivity of brain regions associated with emotional regulation and cognitive control, particularly the anterior cingulate cortex and lateral prefrontal cortex. These changes can further support the improvement in the capacity to notice early emotional cues.(Farb et al., 2012; Pruessner et al., 2024). Moreover, mindfulness also promotes cognitive reappraisal i.e. the ability to reinterpret negative events in more adaptive ways and self-compassion, showing kindness towards oneself during distress. Together, these two processes can help in alleviating the depressive symptoms linked to harsh self-criticism and internalized stigma, which are especially prevalent among LGBTQ individuals facing identity-based stressors. By nurturing a more accepting and compassionate relationship with oneself, mindfulness offers a protective buffer against the cumulative effects of minority stress, thereby supporting recovery(Mamede et al., 2022).

Mindfulness-based interventions (MBIs) have gained significant recognition as effective approaches for alleviating symptoms of mood and anxiety disorders. Among the most widely studied MBIs are Mindfulness-Based Stress Reduction (MBSR) and Mindfulness-Based Cognitive Therapy (MBCT). The MBSR method incorporates regular mindfulness exercises such as body scans and mindful breathing that use present-moment and nonjudgmental strategies to increase awareness of one's thoughts and bodily sensations. This approach enhances individuals' capacity to notice internal experiences without reacting impulsively (Smith et al., 2015). On the other hand, MBCT integrates the principles of Cognitive Behavioral Therapy (CBT) with mindfulness techniques. It not only reduces the acute symptoms of major depression disorder but lowers the risk of relapses by helping individuals to identify early signs of negative thinking. Therefore, reducing automatic rumination (Wong et al., 2011). These methods enable people to observe worrisome thoughts without responding to them, which gradually lessens the influence of these ideas on emotional wellness. They also break the cycles of worry and rumination, which are the two processes most closely linked to anxiety and depression.

These treatments have shown effectiveness in reducing the symptoms of anxiety and mood disorders in larger LGBTQ+ communities (Goldberg et al., 2018, 2021). For instance, Klimo et al. (2024) used a pilot study on LGBTQ+ teenagers to lower the symptoms of anxiety and depression using an intervention called "Learning to Breathe-Queer." This intervention was based on mindfulness principles like acceptance, nonjudgmental attention, and present-moment awareness, and it included content specifically designed for the experiences of sexual and gender minorities. The individuals reported moderate to significant decreases in their anxiety and depression symptoms. Additionally, they reported increased self-awareness, intuitive eating, and physical activity.

Extending beyond clinical populations, Mindfulness based therapies have been found effective for individuals experiencing gender dysphoria which often co-occurs with symptoms of anxiety, depression, trauma, and social exclusion among transgender and gender-diverse individuals (Buckner, 2020). For example, Bigelow (2023), in a study involving transgender and gender-diverse youth aged 14–24, implemented guided mindfulness sessions and observed a statistically significant reduction in anxiety scores. Participants described the meditative experience as one that "calms and connects," and emphasized that such practices helped them better regulate their emotions and feel grounded in their bodies. These findings suggest that mindfulness, when adapted to LGBTQIA+ experiences, may offer psychosocial relief and enhance self-acceptance. Similarly, Iacono et al. (2022) co-developed an LGBTQ+ affirmative mindfulness curriculum with sexual and gender minority youth. Participants reported that an affirming context, safe facilitation, and attention to body dysphoria were essential in making mindfulness both accessible and healing. They highlighted self-compassion as particularly beneficial, echoing existing literature that connects self-acceptance and present-moment awareness with reductions in internalized transphobia. A quasi-experimental study by Savafi et al. (2024) in Tehran evaluated a mindfulness training program among transgender adults and found significant post-intervention improvements in social adjustment, hope, and self-esteem. These psychosocial outcomes are especially relevant in cultures where gender nonconformity remains stigmatized. The study further indicated that mindfulness may indirectly help mitigate symptoms of dysphoria by improving one's sense of agency, emotional regulation, and connection with community.

Despite such positive outcomes, scholars have raised caution that mindfulness practices must be implemented within trauma-informed and context-sensitive frameworks. For example, Buckner (2020) emphasized that for individuals experiencing gender dysphoria, meditation can initially intensify distress by increasing bodily awareness which may often be a primary site of discomfort and dysphoria. Viewing gender dysphoria through a trauma lens, Buckner has further argued for the gradual and supported introduction of mindfulness practices, ideally facilitated in affirming environments with grounding techniques and flexible participation options. Additionally, adverse experiences associated with mindfulness have also been reported in broader clinical literature. Individuals may encounter increased anxiety, emotional numbing, or resurfacing of traumatic memories, particularly in unsupervised or intensive practice contexts (Baer et al., 2019; Lindahl et al., 2017). These risks appear more pronounced among individuals with pre-existing conditions such as psychosis or bipolar disorder, where mindfulness interventions may transiently exacerbate symptoms (Baer et al., 2019; Van Dam et al., 2018). Practical barriers further limit accessibility for formal mindfulness-based programs such as MBCT and MBSR often demand significant time, financial resources, and sustained commitment, which may be challenging for individuals facing chronic stressors or economic marginalization (Kuyken et al., 2015). These findings collectively highlight the importance of screening individual vulnerability, ensuring skilled facilitation, and embedding mindfulness within supportive therapeutic contexts when working with diverse or high-risk populations (Van Dam et al., 2018).

However, empirical studies have documented the psychosocial benefits of culturally aligned practices such as meditation and yoga for LGBTQIA+ individuals. For instance, Joshi et al. (2022) examined Meditation on Twin Hearts, a pranic healing-based guided meditation among hijra (transgender) women in Mysuru. After a single session, participants reported substantial reductions in anxiety, depression, and suicidal ideation, alongside subjective relief and increased emotional calm. The authors highlighted the cultural resonance and accessibility of such practices within South Asian spiritual traditions. Bazzano et al. (2022) have also discussed incorporating yoga and pranayama within psychosocial programs for transgender youth, observing improvements in affect regulation, body-related distress, and sleep quality. Similarly, Subhash et al. (2024) have highlighted a case study of a 16-year-old transgender adolescent in Kerala who underwent a combined intervention of yoga, Ayurveda, and counseling, showing marked improvement in mood, sleep, and behavioral functioning. Therefore, these findings underscore the therapeutic potential of blending mindfulness with culturally grounded healing modalities, offering holistic support for gender-diverse individuals.

Overall, the emerging body of empirical, theoretical, and qualitative research indicates that mindfulness and meditation can serve as valuable adjuncts to psychological care for LGBTQIA+ individuals experiencing gender dysphoria, anxiety, and depression. These interventions appear to reduce distress, enhance emotional regulation, foster self-compassion, and promote identity integration across youth and adult populations (Iacono et al., 2022; Klimo et al., 2024). Importantly, studies from India and other non-Western contexts demonstrate that brief and culturally contextualized mindfulness practices such as pranic or yoga-based meditation can meaningfully support well-being among marginalized groups while maintaining cultural authenticity (Joshi et al., 2022). Nonetheless, the current evidence base remains preliminary. To strengthen confidence in these approaches, longitudinal and randomized controlled studies are needed to assess long-term outcomes, clarify mechanisms of change, and refine trauma-informed, gender-affirmative mindfulness protocols suitable for diverse cultural contexts.

CONCLUSION

A field that is undergoing considerable change, moving away from historical pathologization and toward approaches that emphasize inclusiveness, resilience, and rights-based care, is reflected in the research focus on LGBTQIA+ mental health in India. Elevated incidence of mood and anxiety disorders among LGBTQIA+ people are continuously driven by enduring issues such intersectional discrimination, minority stress, and structural exclusion. Although mindfulness and meditation provide significant, culturally relevant benefits, such as symptom relief and positive self-integration, especially in trauma-informed, affirming environments, their influence is reduced if more widespread structural injustices continue. Coordination of reforms in the legal, policy, community, and clinical spheres is necessary for sustainable success, directly addressing problems including societal stigma, healthcare exclusion, and familial rejection. Expanding empirical research is crucial for evidence-based practices, particularly through localized, longitudinal, intervention-focused investigations. Finally, the only way for LGBTQIA+ people to fully flourish in society is through the merger of social justice and affirmative mental health care.

REFERENCES

American Psychiatric Association. (2022). *DSM-5 TM guidebook the essential companion to the diagnostic and statistical manual of mental disorders* (5th ed.). Dc American Psychiatric Publishing.

Arvind, A., Pandya, A., Amin, L., Aggarwal, M., Agrawal, D., Tiwari, K., Singh, S., Nemkul, M., & Agarwal, P. (2021). Social strain, distress, and gender dysphoria among transgender women and Hijra in Vadodara, India. *International Journal of Transgender Health, 23*(1-2), 149–163. DOI: 10.1080/26895269.2020.1845273 PMID: 35403111

Baams, L., & Kaufman, T. M. L. (2023). Sexual Orientation and Gender Identity/Expression in Adolescent Research: Two Decades in Review. *Journal of Sex Research, 60*(7), 1004–1019. DOI: 10.1080/00224499.2023.2219245 PMID: 37307300

Baer, R., Crane, C., Miller, E., & Kuyken, W. (2019). Doing no harm in mindfulness-based programs: Conceptual issues and empirical findings. *Clinical Psychology Review, 71*(1), 101–114. DOI: 10.1016/j.cpr.2019.01.001 PMID: 30638824

Balsam, K. F., Molina, Y., Beadnell, B., Simoni, J., & Walters, K. (2011). Measuring multiple minority stress: The LGBT People of Color Microaggressions Scale. *Cultural Diversity & Ethnic Minority Psychology, 17*(2), 163–174. DOI: 10.1037/a0023244 PMID: 21604840

Bazzano, A. N., Sun, Y., Chavez-Gray, V., Akintimehin, T., Gustat, J., Barrera, D., & Roi, C. (2022). Effect of Yoga and Mindfulness Intervention on Symptoms of Anxiety and Depression in Young Adolescents Attending Middle School: A Pragmatic Community-Based Cluster Randomized Controlled Trial in a Racially Diverse Urban Setting. *International Journal of Environmental Research and Public Health, 19*(19), 12076. DOI: 10.3390/ijerph191912076 PMID: 36231378

Bigelow, L. B. (2023). Mindfulness Meditation Programs Informed by Transgender Youth. *Mindfulness, 14*(1), 128–140. DOI: 10.1007/s12671-022-02048-6 PMID: 36590761

Bishop, S. R., Lau, M., Shapiro, S., Carlson, L., Anderson, N. D., Carmody, J., Segal, Z. V., Abbey, S., Speca, M., Velting, D., & Devins, G. (2004). Mindfulness: A proposed operational definition. *Clinical Psychology : a Publication of the Division of Clinical Psychology of the American Psychological Association, 11*(3), 230–241. DOI: 10.1093/clipsy.bph077

Bogaert, A. F., & Skorska, M. N. (2020). A short review of biological research on the development of sexual orientation. *Hormones and Behavior, 119*, 104659. DOI: 10.1016/j.yhbeh.2019.104659 PMID: 31911036

Buckner, R. (2020). Zen in distress: Theorizing gender dysphoria and traumatic remembrance within Sōtō Zen meditation. *Religions, 11*(11), 582. DOI: 10.3390/rel11110582

Cahill, S., & Makadon, H. (2014). Sexual orientation and gender identity data collection in clinical settings and in electronic health records: A key to ending LGBT health disparities. *LGBT Health, 1*(1), 34–41. DOI: 10.1089/lgbt.2013.0001 PMID: 26789508

Casey, L. S., Reisner, S. L., Findling, M. G., Blendon, R. J., Benson, J. M., Sayde, J. M., & Miller, C. (2019). Discrimination in the United States: Experiences of lesbian, gay, bisexual, transgender, and queer Americans. *Health Services Research, 54*(S2), 1454–1466. DOI: 10.1111/1475-6773.13229 PMID: 31659745

Chand, S. P., & Marwaha, R. (2023). *Anxiety*. National Library of Medicine; StatPearls Publishing. https://www.ncbi.nlm.nih.gov/books/NBK470361/

Choi, S. K., Divsalar, S., Flórez-Donado, J., Kittle, K., Lin, A., Meyer, I. H., & Torres-Salazar, P. (2020). Stress, health, and well-being of LGBT people in Colombia.

Connell, R. W. (2015). Pride and prejudice and professionalism: The right to be out—Sexual orientation and gender identity in America's public schools. *Contexts, 12*(4), 371–391. DOI: 10.1177/1536504215611898

Cook, C. C. H. (2020). The causes of human sexual orientation. *Theology and Sexuality, 27*(1), 1–19. DOI: 10.1080/13558358.2020.1818541

Cosker-Rowland, R. (2023). Recent work on gender identity and gender. *Analysis, 83*(4), 801–820. DOI: 10.1093/analys/anad027

Craney, R. S., Watson, L. B., Brownfield, J., & Flores, M. J. (2018). Bisexual women's discriminatory experiences and psychological distress: Exploring the roles of coping and LGBTQ community connectedness. *Psychology of Sexual Orientation and Gender Diversity*, *5*(3), 324–337. DOI: 10.1037/sgd0000276

D'augelli, A. R. (2002). Mental health problems among lesbian, gay, and bisexual youths ages 14 to 21. *Journal of Technological Advancements*, *7*(3), 433–456. DOI: 10.1177/1359104502007003039

Das, H. K., & Govindappa, L. (2023). Anxiety, depression and social support of LGBTIQ during COVID-19 in Kerala, India. *The International Journal of Social Psychiatry*, *69*(8), 1971–1978. DOI: 10.1177/00207640231183913 PMID: 37353961

Di Marco, D., Hoel, H., & Lewis, D. (2021). Discrimination and Exclusion on Grounds of Sexual and Gender Identity: Are LGBT People's Voices Heard at the Workplace? *The Spanish Journal of Psychology*, *24*, e18. Advance online publication. DOI: 10.1017/SJP.2021.16 PMID: 33745498

Earnshaw, V. A., Reisner, S. L., Juvonen, J., Hatzenbuehler, M. L., Perrotti, J., & Schuster, M. A. (2017). LGBTQ Bullying: Translating Research to Action in Pediatrics. *Pediatrics*, *140*(4), e20170432. DOI: 10.1542/peds.2017-0432 PMID: 28947607

Farb, N. A. S., Anderson, A. K., & Segal, Z. V. (2012). The Mindful Brain and Emotion Regulation in Mood Disorders. *Canadian Journal of Psychiatry*, *57*(2), 70–77. DOI: 10.1177/070674371205700203 PMID: 22340146

Feinstein, B. A., Goldfried, M. R., & Davila, J. (2012). The relationship between experiences of discrimination and mental health among lesbians and gay men: An examination of internalized homonegativity and rejection sensitivity as potential mechanisms. *Journal of Consulting and Clinical Psychology*, *80*(5), 917–927. DOI: 10.1037/a0029425 PMID: 22823860

Ferbežar, N., Kopinič, A., & Gavriloski Tretjak, M. (2024). Elements of Minority Stress and Resilience in LGBTQ+ Students' Experience of Education. *Journal of Homosexuality*, *72*(3), 520–543. DOI: 10.1080/00918369.2024.2326473 PMID: 38470515

Gaur, P. S., Saha, S., Goel, A., Ovseiko, P., Aggarwal, S., Agarwal, V., Haq, A. U., Danda, D., Hartle, A., Sandhu, N. K., & Gupta, L. (2023). Mental healthcare for young and adolescent LGBTQ+ individuals in the Indian subcontinent. *Frontiers in Psychology*, *14*, 1060543. DOI: 10.3389/fpsyg.2023.1060543 PMID: 36743255

Ghabrial, M. A. (2025). Stressed and oppressed: Insider perspectives on stress induction research with LGBTQA+ People of Color. *Psychoneuroendocrinology*, *174*, 107390. DOI: 10.1016/j.psyneuen.2025.107390 PMID: 39978213

Goldberg, S. B., Riordan, K. M., Sun, S., & Davidson, R. J. (2021). The Empirical Status of Mindfulness-Based Interventions: A Systematic Review of 44 Meta-Analyses of Randomized Controlled Trials. *Perspectives on Psychological Science*, *17*(1), 174569162096877. DOI: 10.1177/1745691620968771 PMID: 33593124

Goldberg, S. B., Tucker, R. P., Greene, P. A., Davidson, R. J., Wampold, B. E., Kearney, D. J., & Simpson, T. L. (2018). Mindfulness-based interventions for psychiatric disorders: A systematic review and meta-analysis. *Clinical Psychology Review*, *59*(59), 52–60. DOI: 10.1016/j.cpr.2017.10.011 PMID: 29126747

Grigoreva, D., & Szaszkó, B. (2024). Minority stress and psychological well-being in queer populations. *Scientific Reports*, *14*(1), 27084. DOI: 10.1038/s41598-024-78545-6 PMID: 39511355

Halli, S. S., Isac, S., Bhattacharjee, P., Dutta, S., Ramesh, B. M., Lorway, R., & Blanchard, J. (2021). Suicidality among gender minorities in Karnataka, South India. *BMC Psychiatry*, *21*(1), 25. DOI: 10.1186/s12888-021-03043-2 PMID: 33430838

Harrison, P. (2007). "How Shall I Say it …? " Relating the Nonrelational. *Environment & Planning A*, *39*(3), 590–608. DOI: 10.1068/a3825

Hatzenbuehler, M. L., Keyes, K. M., & Hasin, D. S. (2009). State-Level Policies and Psychiatric Morbidity In Lesbian, Gay, and Bisexual Populations. *American Journal of Public Health*, *99*(12), 2275–2281. DOI: 10.2105/AJPH.2008.153510 PMID: 19833997

Herek, G. M., & Garnets, L. D. (2007). Sexual Orientation and Mental Health. *Annual Review of Clinical Psychology, 3*(1), 353–375. DOI: 10.1146/annurev.clinpsy.3.022806.091510 PMID: 17716060

Iacono, G., Craig, S. L., Crowder, R., Brennan, D. J., & Loveland, E. K. (2022). A qualitative study of the LGBTQ+ youth affirmative mindfulness program for sexual and gender minority youth. *Mindfulness, 13*(1), 222–237. DOI: 10.1007/s12671-021-01787-2

Joshi, N., Vinu, V., Jois, S. N., Begum, F., & Salagame, K. K. (2022). The Need, Feasibility and Willingness to Explore "Meditation on Twin Hearts" as a Self-administered Tool for Mental Health Management among Transgender Women: An Exploratory Survey. *Community Mental Health Journal, 58*(4), 666–672. DOI: 10.1007/s10597-021-00869-8 PMID: 34255215

Juvonen, J., & Graham, S. (2014). Bullying in Schools: The Power of Bullies and the Plight of Victims. *Annual Review of Psychology, 65*(1), 159–185. DOI: 10.1146/annurev-psych-010213-115030 PMID: 23937767

Kattari, S. K., Walls, N. E., Speer, S. R., & Kattari, L. (2016). Exploring the relationship between transgender-inclusive providers and mental health outcomes among transgender/gender variant people. *Social Work in Health Care, 55*(8), 635–650. DOI: 10.1080/00981389.2016.1193099 PMID: 27351890

Khapre, M., Sahoo, K., Saxena, V., Sinha, S., Luthra, G., & Joshi, A. (2024). Exploring the utilization of targeted intervention services by transgender individuals in Uttarakhand, India: A qualitative study. *Frontiers in Public Health, 12*, 1476938. DOI: 10.3389/fpubh.2024.1476938 PMID: 39697287

Kidd, S. A., Howison, M., Pilling, M., Ross, L. E., & McKenzie, K. (2016). Severe Mental Illness in LGBT Populations: A Scoping Review. *Psychiatric Services (Washington, D.C.), 67*(7), 779–783. DOI: 10.1176/appi.ps.201500209 PMID: 26927576

Klimo, K. D., Wilson, J. W., Farewell, C., Grose, R. G., Puma, J. E., Brittain, D., Shomaker, L. B., & Quirk, K. (2024). A Pilot and Feasibility Study on a Mindfulness-Based Intervention Adapted for LGBTQ+ Adolescents. *International Journal of Environmental Research and Public Health, 21*(10), 1364. DOI: 10.3390/ijerph21101364 PMID: 39457337

Kosciw, J. G., Greytak, E. A., Giga, N. M., Villenas, C., & Danischewski, D. J. (2018). The 2017 national school climate survey. GLSEN. *The 2017 National School Climate Survey*, 2019-10.

Kurumaji, A. (2013). [The trends of mood disorders in ICD-11: Bipolar and depressive disorders]. *Seishin Shinkeigaku Zasshi = Psychiatria et Neurologia Japonica, 115*(1), 60–68. https://pubmed.ncbi.nlm.nih.gov/23691796/

Kuyken, W., Hayes, R., Barrett, B., Byng, R., Dalgleish, T., Kessler, D., Lewis, G., Watkins, E., Brejcha, C., Cardy, J., Causley, A., Cowderoy, S., Evans, A., Gradinger, F., Kaur, S., Lanham, P., Morant, N., Richards, J., Shah, P., & Byford, S. (2015). Effectiveness and cost-effectiveness of mindfulness-based cognitive therapy compared with maintenance antidepressant treatment in the prevention of depressive relapse or recurrence (PREVENT): A randomised controlled trial. *Lancet, 386*(9988), 63–73. DOI: 10.1016/S0140-6736(14)62222-4 PMID: 25907157

Kwon, P. (2013). Resilience in Lesbian, Gay, and Bisexual Individuals. *Personality and Social Psychology Review, 17*(4), 371–383. DOI: 10.1177/1088868313490248 PMID: 23904452

Lindahl, J. R., Fisher, N. E., Cooper, D. J., Rosen, R. K., & Britton, W. B. (2017). The varieties of contemplative experience: A mixed-methods study of meditation-related challenges in Western Buddhists. *PLoS One, 12*(5), e0176239. DOI: 10.1371/journal.pone.0176239 PMID: 28542181

Mamede, A., Merkelbach, I., Noordzij, G., & Denktas, S. (2022). Mindfulness as a protective factor against depression, anxiety and psychological distress during the COVID-19 pandemic: Emotion regulation and insomnia symptoms as mediators. *Frontiers in Psychology, 13*, 820959. Advance online publication. DOI: 10.3389/fpsyg.2022.820959 PMID: 35432084

Marshal, M. P., Dietz, L. J., Friedman, M. S., Stall, R., Smith, H. A., McGinley, J., Thoma, B. C., Murray, P. J., D'Augelli, A. R., & Brent, D. A. (2011). Suicidality and depression disparities between sexual minority and heterosexual youth: A meta-analytic review. *The Journal of Adolescent Health*, *49*(2), 115–123. DOI: 10.1016/j.jadohealth.2011.02.005 PMID: 21783042

Matsuzaka, S., Romanelli, M., & Hudson, K. D. (2021). "Render a service worthy of me": A qualitative study of factors influencing access to LGBTQ-specific health services. *SSM. Qualitative Research in Health*, *1*, 100019. DOI: 10.1016/j.ssmqr.2021.100019

Matthews, A. K., Hughes, T. L., Johnson, T., Razzano, L. A., & Cassidy, R. (2002). Prediction of Depressive Distress in a Community Sample of Women: The Role of Sexual Orientation. *American Journal of Public Health*, *92*(7), 1131–1139. DOI: 10.2105/AJPH.92.7.1131 PMID: 12084697

McConnell, E. A., Janulis, P., Phillips, G.II, Truong, R., & Birkett, M. (2018). Multiple Minority Stress and LGBT Community Resilience among Sexual Minority Men. *Psychology of Sexual Orientation and Gender Diversity*, *5*(1), 1–12. DOI: 10.1037/sgd0000265 PMID: 29546228

Mereish, E. H., & Bradford, J. B. (2014). Intersecting identities and substance use problems: Sexual orientation, gender, race, and lifetime substance use problems. *Journal of Studies on Alcohol and Drugs*, *75*(1), 179–188. DOI: 10.15288/jsad.2014.75.179 PMID: 24411810

Meyer, I. H. (2003). Prejudice, social stress, and mental health in lesbian, gay, and bisexual populations: Conceptual issues and research evidence. *Psychological Bulletin*, *129*(5), 674–697. DOI: 10.1037/0033-2909.129.5.674 PMID: 12956539

Meyer, I. H. (2013). Prejudice, social stress, and mental health in lesbian, gay, and bisexual populations: Conceptual issues and research evidence. *Psychology of Sexual Orientation and Gender Diversity*, *1*(S), 3–26. DOI: 10.1037/2329-0382.1.S.3

Meyer, I. H. (2015). Resilience in the study of minority stress and health of sexual and gender minorities. *Psychology of Sexual Orientation and Gender Diversity, 2*(3), 209–213. DOI: 10.1037/sgd0000132

Mishra, S. (2022). A Psychological Exploration Research on LGBT Community. *International Journal of Indian Psychology, 10*(2). Advance online publication. DOI: 10.25215/1002.068

Morris, B. J. (2023). A brief history of lesbian, gay, bisexual, and transgender social movements. *American psychological association, Psychology topics, Sexual orientation and gender diversity. Preuzeto s:* https://www.apa.org/topics/lgbtq/history

Mustanski, B., Andrews, R., & Puckett, J. A. (2016). The effects of cumulative victimization on mental health among lesbian, gay, bisexual, and transgender adolescents and young adults. *American Journal of Public Health, 106*(3), 527–533. DOI: 10.2105/AJPH.2015.302976 PMID: 26794175

Nishina, A., Juvonen, J., & Witkow, M. R. (2005). Sticks and Stones May Break My Bones, but Names Will Make Me Feel Sick: The Psychosocial, Somatic, and Scholastic Consequences of Peer Harassment. *Journal of Clinical Child and Adolescent Psychology, 34*(1), 37–48. DOI: 10.1207/s15374424jccp3401_4 PMID: 15677279

Pachankis, J. E. (2007). The psychological implications of concealing a stigma: A cognitive-affective-behavioral model. *Psychological Bulletin, 133*(2), 328–345. DOI: 10.1037/0033-2909.133.2.328 PMID: 17338603

Pachankis, J. E., Rendina, H. J., Restar, A., Ventuneac, A., Grov, C., & Parsons, J. T. (2015). A minority stress—Emotion regulation model of sexual compulsivity among highly sexually active gay and bisexual men. *Health Psychology, 34*(8), 829–840. DOI: 10.1037/hea0000180 PMID: 25528179

Plöderl, M., & Tremblay, P. (2015). Mental health of sexual minorities. A systematic review. *International Review of Psychiatry (Abingdon, England), 27*(5), 367–385. DOI: 10.3109/09540261.2015.1083949 PMID: 26552495

Pruessner, L., Timm, C., Kalmar, J., Bents, H., Barnow, S., & Mander, J. (2024). Sven Barnow, & Mander, J. (2024). Emotion Regulation as a Mechanism of Mindfulness in Individual Cognitive-Behavioral Therapy for Depression and Anxiety Disorders. *Depression and Anxiety*, *2024*(1), 1–16. DOI: 10.1155/2024/9081139 PMID: 40226724

Pullen Sansfaçon, A., Medico, D., Suerich-Gulick, F., & Temple Newhook, J. (2020). "I knew that I wasn't cis, I knew that, but I didn't know exactly": Gender identity development, expression and affirmation in youth who access gender affirming medical care. *International Journal of Transgender Health*, *21*(3), 307–320. DOI: 10.1080/26895269.2020.1756551 PMID: 34993511

Raj, P., & Dubey, A. (2024). Comprehending Health of the Transgender Population in India Through Bibliometric Analysis. *International Journal of Public Health*, *69*, 1606598. DOI: 10.3389/ijph.2024.1606598 PMID: 38665638

Ranade, K., Shankarappa, M. R., Kumar, N., & Somaiya, A. (2025). In quest of an authentic identity - an exploratory study of mental health assessment of gender incongruence in urban India. *BMC Psychiatry*, *25*(1), 387. DOI: 10.1186/s12888-025-06740-4 PMID: 40240909

Remes, O., Brayne, C., van der Linde, R., & Lafortune, L. (2016). A systematic review of reviews on the prevalence of anxiety disorders in adult populations. *Brain and Behavior*, *6*(7), e00497. Advance online publication. DOI: 10.1002/brb3.497 PMID: 27458547

Roselli, C. E. (2018). Neurobiology of gender identity and sexual orientation. *Journal of Neuroendocrinology*, *30*(7), e12562. DOI: 10.1111/jne.12562 PMID: 29211317

Russell, S. T., & Fish, J. N. (2016). Mental health in lesbian, gay, bisexual, and transgender (LGBT) youth. *Annual Review of Clinical Psychology*, *12*(1), 465–487. DOI: 10.1146/annurev-clinpsy-021815-093153 PMID: 26772206

Ryan, C., Russell, S. T., Huebner, D., Diaz, R., & Sanchez, J. (2010). Family acceptance in adolescence and the health of LGBT young adults. *Journal of Child and Adolescent Psychiatric Nursing, 23*(4), 205–213. DOI: 10.1111/j.1744-6171.2010.00246.x PMID: 21073595

Saewyc E. M. (2011). RESEARCH ON ADOLESCENT SEXUAL ORIENTATION: DEVELOPMENT, HEALTH DISPARITIES, STIGMA AND RESILIENCE. *Journal of research on adolescence: the official journal of the Society for Research on Adolescence, 21*(1), 256–272. DOI: 10.1111/j.1532-7795.2010.00727.x

Saha, S., Lim, C. C. W., Cannon, D. L., Burton, L., Bremner, M., Cosgrove, P., Huo, Y., & McGrath, J. (2020). Co-morbidity between mood and anxiety disorders: A systematic review and meta-analysis. *Depression and Anxiety, 38*(3), 286–306. DOI: 10.1002/da.23113 PMID: 33225514

Sandfort, T. G. M., de Graaf, R., ten Have, M., Ransome, Y., & Schnabel, P. (2014). Same-Sex Sexuality and Psychiatric Disorders in the Second Netherlands Mental Health Survey and Incidence Study (NEMESIS-2). *LGBT Health, 1*(4), 292–301. DOI: 10.1089/lgbt.2014.0031 PMID: 26609539

Savafi, S., Bazzazian, S., & Sirtori, C. R. (2024). The effectiveness of mindfulness training on social adjustment, self-esteem, and hope among transgender individuals in Tehran. *Journal of Neurology & Neuroscience Disorders, 10*(1), 1–8. DOI: 10.17352/jnnsd.000057

Schnabel, L. (2018). Sexual Orientation and Social Attitudes. *Socius: Sociological Research for a Dynamic World, 4*, 2378023118769550. Advance online publication. DOI: 10.1177/2378023118769550

Sekhon, S., & Gupta, V. (2023). *Mood Disorder*. PubMed; StatPearls Publishing. https://www.ncbi.nlm.nih.gov/books/NBK558911/

Selye, H. (1956). Stress and psychiatry. *The American Journal of Psychiatry, 113*(5), 423–427. DOI: 10.1176/ajp.113.5.423 PMID: 13362640

Semlyen, J., King, M., Varney, J., & Hagger-Johnson, G. (2016). Sexual orientation and symptoms of common mental disorder or low wellbeing: Combined meta-analysis of 12 UK population health surveys. *BMC Psychiatry, 16*(1), 67. Advance online publication. DOI: 10.1186/s12888-016-0767-z PMID: 27009565

Shaikh, A., Kamble, P., Daulatabad, V., Singhal, A., Madhusudhan, U., & John, N. A. (2024). Mental health challenges within the LGBTQ community: A societal imperative. *Journal of Family Medicine and Primary Care, 13*(9), 3529–3535. DOI: 10.4103/jfmpc.jfmpc_321_24 PMID: 39464965

Sharma, R. (2021). Rights of LGBTQ in India and the Struggle for Societal Acceptance. *Issue 3 Int'l JL Mgmt. & Human., 4*, 18, http://doi.one/10.1732/IJLMH.26695

Smith, B., Metzker, K., Waite, R., & Gerrity, P. (2015). Short-Form Mindfulness-Based Stress Reduction Reduces Anxiety and Improves Health-Related Quality of Life in an Inner-City Population. *Holistic Nursing Practice, 29*(2), 70–77. DOI: 10.1097/HNP.0000000000000075 PMID: 25658929

Snapp, S. D., Watson, R. J., Russell, S. T., Diaz, R. M., & Ryan, C. (2015). Social support networks for LGBT young adults: Low cost strategies for positive adjustment. *Family Relations, 64*(3), 420–430. DOI: 10.1111/fare.12124

Spijker, J., & Claes, S. (2014). [Mood disorders in the DSM-5]. *Tijdschrift voor Psychiatrie, 56*(3), 173–176. https://pubmed.ncbi.nlm.nih.gov/24643826/ PMID: 24643826

Srinivasan, S. P., & Chandrasekaran, S. (2020). Care of transgender individuals in India: A clinical perspective. *Indian Journal of Social Psychiatry, 36*(4), 284–288. DOI: 10.4103/ijsp.ijsp_88_20

Srinivasan, S. P., & Chandrasekaran, S. (2025). Mental Health Status and Its Psychosocial Correlates Among Help-Seeking Transgender Individuals: Experiences from a Clinic in South India. *Transgender Health, 10*(2), 201–209. DOI: 10.1089/trgh.2022.0150 PMID: 40309069

Steele, L. S., Ross, L. E., Dobinson, C., Veldhuizen, S., & Tinmouth, J. M. (2009). Women's Sexual Orientation and Health: Results from a Canadian Population-Based Survey. *Women & Health*, *49*(5), 353–367. DOI: 10.1080/03630240903238685 PMID: 19851942

Subhash, M., Jithesh, M., Rahmath, P. K., & Anjali, A. (2024). Integrated management with Ayurveda, yoga and counselling in gender dysphoria with conduct disorder. *Ayushdhara*, *10*(6), 158–164. DOI: 10.47070/ayushdhara.v10i6.1448

Toomey, R. B., & Russell, S. T. (2013). The Role of Sexual Orientation in School-Based Victimization: A Meta-Analysis. *Youth & Society*, *48*(2), 176–201. DOI: 10.1177/0044118X13483778 PMID: 26997680

Van Dam, N. T., van Vugt, M. K., Vago, D. R., Schmalzl, L., Saron, C. D., Olendzki, A., Meissner, T., Lazar, S. W., Kerr, C. E., Gorchov, J., Fox, K. C. R., Field, B. A., Britton, W. B., Brefczynski-Lewis, J. A., & Meyer, D. E. (2018). Mind the Hype: A Critical Evaluation and Prescriptive Agenda for Research on Mindfulness and Meditation. *Perspectives on Psychological Science: A Journal of the Association for Psychological Science, 13*(1), 36–61. DOI: 10.1177/1745691617709589

Wandrekar, J. R., & Nigudkar, A. S. (2020). What do we know about LGBTQIA+ mental health in India? A review of research from 2009 to 2019. *Journal of Psychosexual Health*, *2*(1), 26–36. DOI: 10.1177/2631831820918129

Wei, D., Wang, X., You, X., Luo, X., Hao, C., Gu, J., Peng, S., Yang, X., Hao, Y., Silenzio, V. M. B., Li, J., & Hou, F. (2020). Prevalence of depression, anxiety and suicide among men who have sex with men in China: A systematic review and meta-analysis. *Epidemiology and Psychiatric Sciences*, *29*, e136. Advance online publication. DOI: 10.1017/S2045796020000487 PMID: 32536353

Wittgens, C., Fischer, M. M., Buspavanich, P., Theobald, S., Schweizer, K., & Trautmann, S. (2022). Mental health in people with minority sexual orientations: A meta-analysis of population-based studies. *Acta Psychiatrica Scandinavica*, *145*(4), 357–372. DOI: 10.1111/acps.13405 PMID: 35090051

Wong, S. Y., Mak, W. W., Cheung, E. Y., Ling, C. Y., Lui, W. W., Tang, W., Wong, R. L., Lo, H. H., Mercer, S., & Ma, H. S. (2011). A randomized, controlled clinical trial: the effect of mindfulness-based cognitive therapy on generalized anxiety disorder among Chinese community patients: protocol for a randomized trial. *BMC Psychiatry*, *11*(1), 187. Advance online publication. DOI: 10.1186/1471-244X-11-187 PMID: 22126115

Yarns, B. C., Abrams, J. M., Meeks, T. W., & Sewell, D. D. (2016). The Mental Health of Older LGBT Adults. *Current Psychiatry Reports*, *18*(6), 60. Advance online publication. DOI: 10.1007/s11920-016-0697-y PMID: 27142205

Chapter 7
The Paradox of Emotional Intelligence:
Mindfulness-Based Interventions for Reducing Manipulative and Maladaptive Behaviors in Adolescents

Divya Dubey
http://orcid.org/0000-0002-3003-301X
Jindal Institute of Behavioural Sciences, O.P. Jindal Global University, Sonipat, India

Soni Kewalramani
http://orcid.org/0000-0002-8294-3314
Amity University, Lucknow, India

ABSTRACT

This chapter offers a critical examination of Emotional Intelligence (EI) in adolescence, challenging its uncritical celebration by highlighting its paradoxical nature. Drawing on theoretical frameworks and empirical findings from Indian adolescents, it reveals that emotionally competent youth particularly girls may also show elevated levels of neuroticism, psychoticism, and criminal propensity, suggesting that EI may mask internal distress or serve manipulative functions. In collectivist contexts,

DOI: 10.4018/979-8-2600-1202-4.ch007

emotional suppression driven by gendered norms may further distort emotional development. To address these dynamics, the chapter proposes a mindfulness-based EI framework incorporating ethical reflection, breathwork, meditation, and Positive Life Orientation (PLO), promoting resilience and emotional authenticity. It calls for ethically grounded, culturally responsive EI education that moves beyond skill acquisition to foster emotional maturity, integrity, and social responsibility. Practical recommendations for educators, psychologists, and policymakers are also presented.

INTRODUCTION

Adolescence is a critical period for emotional and social development, during which Emotional Intelligence (EI) exerts a profound influence. While high EI can promote resilience, adaptive decision-making, and interpersonal competence, it also carries the potential for ethical missteps, including manipulation, deception, and relational aggression. This paradox underscores the need for interventions that not only enhance emotional skills but also guide their ethical application. Mindfulness-based practices, by cultivating attention, self-reflection, and empathy, provide a promising framework to channel adolescent EI toward constructive outcomes. This chapter explores the dual nature of EI in adolescence and presents mindfulness-based interventions as a strategic, ethical corrective.

Emotional Intelligence, rooted in the foundational work of Salovey and Mayer (1990) and popularized by Goleman (1995), refers to the ability to perceive, understand, regulate, and use emotions constructively. For adolescents navigating peer pressure, identity conflicts, and future anxieties, EI has often been considered a protective factor. Research supports the notion that adolescents with higher EI show better stress management, lower rates of depression and anxiety, and improved interpersonal relationships (Mavroveli, Petrides, Rieffe, & Bakker, 2007).

However, new research suggests a more complex picture. As Kilduff, Chiaburu, and Menges (2010) argue, EI functions as a double-edged sword: while it can promote empathy and cooperation, it may also enable manipulation, impression management, and exploitation. This paradox is particularly significant in adolescence, where emotionally skilled youth may deploy EI not only for resilience and empathy but also for social advantage or concealment of distress. Without ethical grounding, EI may even contribute to antisocial behavior, relational aggression, or Machiavellian tendencies.

Empirical evidence illustrates this tension. For example, female adolescents often display high levels of emotional regulation while simultaneously showing elevated vulnerability to neuroticism and maladaptive behaviors a paradox discussed in greater detail later in this chapter. Such findings highlight why EI must be understood as context-dependent, shaped by developmental, social, and cultural forces.

In light of this, the present chapter proposes an integrative framework that reorients EI toward ethical self-regulation through mindfulness-based practices. Techniques such as meditation, breathwork, and yoga are considered not merely stress-reduction tools but methods that cultivate present-moment awareness, emotional responsibility, and compassionate action. The chapter also integrates Positive Life Orientation (PLO) as a complementary buffer against maladaptive outcomes, reinforcing resilience, optimism, and prosocial values.

Overall, this chapter critically examines the paradox of EI in adolescence and presents mindfulness-based interventions as a strategic corrective. The discussion proceeds by exploring the structural components of EI, its behavioral correlates, gendered patterns, and empirical findings, before turning to mindfulness-based interventions, practical frameworks, and policy implications.

EMOTIONAL INTELLIGENCE AND ADOLESCENT BEHAVIOR

Emotional Intelligence (EI), as defined by Salovey and Mayer (1990), refers to the ability to perceive, access, and generate emotions to assist thought, to understand emotions and emotional knowledge, and to regulate emotions to promote emotional and intellectual growth. Daniel Goleman (1995) expanded this concept for broader application in social and educational contexts, emphasizing five key components: self-awareness, self-regulation, motivation, empathy, and social skills. While these dimensions contribute to well-being, their behavioral implications during adolescence are multifaceted and complex.

Adolescence is a time of identity formation, peer affiliation, emotional volatility, and increased cognitive capacity for abstract thinking. During this phase, EI becomes not only a personal asset but also a social tool. Adolescents with well-developed emotional competencies tend to navigate peer relationships more effectively, manage academic stress more constructively, and avoid maladaptive coping strategies such as substance use or aggression (Brackett, Rivers, & Salovey, 2011).

Research has shown that higher emotional intelligence is positively correlated with adaptive coping strategies, increased self-esteem, and lower levels of externalizing behaviors such as delinquency and bullying (Mavroveli, Petrides, Rieffe, & Bakker, 2007). For instance, students with elevated EI scores demonstrate fewer symptoms of depression and anxiety, and are more likely to engage in prosocial behaviors like helping peers, volunteering, and conflict resolution (Extremera & Fernández-Berrocal, 2006).

However, recent literature has also pointed to the dual-edged nature of EI during adolescence. High EI, when not ethically grounded, can be utilized to manipulate peers, mask emotional distress, or engage in relational aggression (Austin, Farrelly, Black, & Moore, 2007). Adolescents who are emotionally intelligent may use their skills for impression management or to exert social control in peer groups. This paradox reveals the importance of integrating EI with ethical reasoning, mindfulness, and values education.

From a theoretical perspective, Bandura's Social Learning Theory (1977) helps explain how adolescents acquire emotional habits by observing parental, peer, and media models. Similarly, Erikson's (1968) theory of psychosocial development highlights adolescence as the stage of identity versus role confusion, during which EI plays a pivotal role in identity formation and self-concept.

More recent frameworks, such as Roeser and Eccles' (2015) contemplative education model, emphasize the integration of mindfulness with

EI, advocating for school-based interventions that foster self-awareness, compassion, and prosocial motivation. This approach resonates with CASEL's (Collaborative for Academic, Social, and Emotional Learning) five core competencies—self-awareness, self-management, social awareness, relationship skills, and responsible decision-making which align closely with Goleman's EI model.

Despite the growing body of evidence supporting the role of EI in adolescent behavior, most research focuses on general populations. There is a need for studies examining EI in at-risk youth, culturally diverse contexts, and among neurodivergent adolescents. Also, many current EI interventions lack longitudinal evaluation. Do benefits persist over time, particularly into adulthood? The ethical application of EI remains an understudied area. Future research must explore how values, cultural norms, and moral development mediate the behavioral expression of EI.

Emotional Intelligence significantly shapes adolescent behavior across academic, social, and psychological domains. Yet, to fully harness its potential, educators and practitioners must move beyond skill-building to embed EI within ethical, developmental, and cultural frameworks. This integrative approach will not only support adolescent well-being but also contribute to the formation of socially responsible, emotionally grounded adults.

EMOTIONAL INTELLIGENCE AND PROSOCIAL BEHAVIOR

Numerous studies have linked high Emotional Intelligence (EI) with prosocial outcomes, including empathy, cooperation, altruism, and ethical decision-making. Adolescents with high EI exhibit superior conflict resolution skills, lower levels of aggression, and enhanced interpersonal functioning (Mestre, Guil, Lopes, Salovey, & Gil-Olarte, 2006). These competencies translate into more supportive peer relationships, increased resistance to negative peer pressure, and healthier social affiliations.

Empirical evidence suggests that emotionally intelligent adolescents are more likely to engage in peer support, demonstrate empathic concern, and maintain long-term friendships characterized by trust and mutual respect (Eisenberg, Spinrad, & Morris, 2013). The cultivation of self-awareness and emotional regulation has also been shown to reduce bullying behaviors and promote greater inclusion and social acceptance (Ciarrochi, Heaven, & Davies, 2007).

Moreover, EI contributes significantly to psychological resilience. Adolescents with higher emotional competencies report lower levels of anxiety, depression, and stress (Extremera & Fernández-Berrocal, 2006). By accurately interpreting emotional cues, they respond more sensitively to others' needs, thus enhancing group cohesion and fostering interpersonal trust. This dynamic not only supports individual well-being but also strengthens the overall school climate.

School-based interventions grounded in Social-Emotional Learning (SEL) have demonstrated positive outcomes in both academic and behavioral domains. Durlak et al. (2011), in a meta-analysis of 213 SEL programs, found that participants showed improved academic performance, increased prosocial behavior, and decreased conduct problems and emotional distress. These findings are supported by CASEL's core framework, which emphasizes self-awareness, self-management, social awareness, relationship skills, and responsible decision-making.

From a theoretical standpoint, empathy development theories (Hoffman, 2001) and moral development frameworks (Kohlberg, 1984) highlight the centrality of emotional understanding in prosocial behavior. Emotional competencies enable adolescents to take the perspective of others, engage in moral reasoning, and align their actions with ethical principles. Also, Attachment Theory (Bowlby, 1969) suggests that emotionally secure adolescents are more likely to develop trusting, caring relationships and respond compassionately to others' distress.

However, some scholars caution against overgeneralizing the prosocial impact of EI. For example, Petrides et al. (2016) argue that trait EI may also be used for strategic self-presentation or emotional manipulation, particularly in competitive or high-stress environments. This ambivalence calls for a nuanced understanding of how context, personality, and ethical grounding mediate the prosocial potential of EI.

Much of the literature focuses on general populations in Western contexts. There is a need to investigate prosocial behavior and EI across diverse cultures, particularly in collectivist societies. Research should also explore how digital socialization (e.g., social media, online gaming) influences the development and expression of EI and prosociality. The role of gender and neurodiversity in shaping prosocial behaviors linked to EI warrants deeper exploration.

EMOTIONAL INTELLIGENCE AND ANTISOCIAL TENDENCIES: THE DARK SIDE

Contrary to the dominant narrative of Emotional Intelligence (EI) as inherently prosocial and psychologically beneficial, a growing body of literature emphasizes the darker potential of EI protecting against some externalizing behaviors, yet also equipping adolescents with tools for covert manipulation or emotional exploitation.

Austin, Farrelly, Black, and Moore (2007) observed significant correlations between high EI and "dark triad" traits, Machiavellianism, narcissism, and psychopathy. These individuals exhibit high levels of strategic emotional regulation, enabling them to deceive or exploit others while maintaining a socially acceptable façade. Hyde, Grieve, and Roberts (2018) further demonstrated that adolescents with high EI but low moral reasoning are more likely to engage in relational aggression, such as gossip, exclusion, or emotional manipulation.

Côté and Miners (2006) introduced the concept of strategic EI, noting that individuals may use emotional regulation not to promote well-being, but to manipulate social outcomes for personal gain. Similarly, Kilduff, Chiaburu, and Menges (2010) argue that high EI can serve as a "social weapon," enabling individuals to manage impressions and influence group dynamics subtly, often without detection.

These concerns are particularly salient during adolescence a developmental period marked by experimentation with power, identity, and peer hierarchies. Adolescents who are praised for their emotional awareness but not taught ethical decision-making may internalize the belief that emotional control is a tool for self-promotion rather than social cohesion.

The Social Information Processing (SIP) model (Crick & Dodge, 1994) helps explain how adolescents with high EI may interpret emotional cues through biased schemas, especially if shaped by aggressive environments. Such adolescents are adept at reading social situations but may choose aggressive or coercive responses if their internal moral scripts or environmental cues reward such behavior.

In a school context, these patterns can manifest as relational bullying, emotional blackmail, or subtle peer manipulation behaviors that are often difficult for educators to detect due to the socially skilled nature of the perpetrators. This underscores the importance of integrating EI education with ethical frameworks, mindfulness, and character development.

Much of the literature on the dark side of EI is cross-sectional and lacks longitudinal insight into how manipulative use of EI evolves over time. There is limited research on how cultural norms, peer group dynamics, and family environments influence the ethical or unethical deployment of emotional competencies. More empirical work is needed on the neurobiological underpinnings of manipulative EI, especially concerning impulse control, empathy deficits, and reward sensitivity.

Educators and mental health professionals must move beyond promoting emotional awareness alone and instead focus on intentional, value-based emotional practices. EI interventions should include scenarios involving ethical dilemmas and teach adolescents to weigh the social consequences of emotionally manipulative behavior. There is a need to develop assessment tools that differentiate between constructive and destructive applications of EI, potentially through peer ratings, teacher observations, and narrative interviews.

While EI holds tremendous promise for adolescent development, it is not an ethical safeguard in itself. Without moral orientation, emotional intelligence can become a mechanism of control rather than connection, a means of manipulation rather than mutual understanding. Recognizing this dark side is essential for designing responsible and transformative EI curricula.

EMPIRICAL FINDINGS FROM ADOLESCENT POPULATIONS

Empirical studies on Emotional Intelligence (EI) in adolescent populations, especially within diverse cultural contexts like India, reveal complex and sometimes contradictory patterns. In the current study on Indian adolescents, it was observed that emotionally competent individuals particularly female adolescents reported high scores on emotional regulation, yet simultaneously displayed elevated levels of neuroticism and psychoticism. This duality suggests that emotional control, while adaptive in external settings, may also serve to mask internal distress or be strategically deployed for managing interpersonal relationships.

These findings are consistent with prior studies indicating that emotionally literate adolescents, especially girls, may internalize societal expectations of emotional poise, resulting in emotional suppression and increased vulnerability to anxiety or psychosomatic complaints (Nolen-Hoeksema & Girgus, 1994; Zahn-Waxler, Shirtcliff, & Marceau, 2008). Such adolescents might meet external demands for emotional appropriateness while neglecting internal emotional authenticity, creating a dissonance between outer composure and inner turmoil.

Moreover, high criminal propensity scores among emotionally adept adolescents underscore a critical dimension: Emotional Intelligence, in the absence of ethical grounding, can enable morally ambiguous behavior. This aligns with findings by Cauffman, Steinberg, and Piquero (2005), who reported that youth with advanced emotional understanding sometimes engaged in calculated delinquent acts when it served their personal goals. The dual application of EI either to build empathetic connections or manipulate outcomes highlights the pressing need for moral and contemplative frameworks in emotional training programs.

Another significant finding involved adolescents from urban, academically competitive environments. These individuals often demonstrated high social desirability scores, maintaining appearances of emotional competence while concealing behavioral or psychological difficulties. This phenomenon aligns with research on impression management in adolescents (Paulhus & Reid, 1991) and suggests that EI may sometimes be internalized as a performative tool rather than a sincere emotional skill. Adolescents in high-pressure contexts may learn to use EI to fulfill academic or social expectations, while bypassing emotional integration or ethical reflection.

These empirical patterns call for a paradigm shift in how Emotional Intelligence is conceptualized and taught. Current findings bolster the argument for embedding EI development within:

- Mindfulness-based interventions (Zoogman et al., 2015) that enhance present-moment awareness and emotional authenticity.
- Ethical frameworks that encourage adolescents to reflect on the intention and consequences behind emotional expression (Goleman, 1995).
- Trauma-informed pedagogy, especially for female adolescents who may be using emotional control as a survival strategy (Jennings et al., 2011)

Emotional Intelligence remains a critical developmental asset, its impact on adolescent behavior must be contextualized within gender, ethics, culture, and psychological well-being. Emotionally intelligent adolescents may thrive or struggle, depending on whether their emotional skills are accompanied by ethical reflection, internal alignment, and systemic support.

While these findings shed light on the paradoxical role of EI in adolescence, it is important to recognize that most empirical studies rely on short-term assessments. There is a lack of longitudinal evidence examining whether such patterns both beneficial and maladaptive are sustained across developmental transitions. Future research should track adolescents over time to determine whether mindfulness-based EI training can alter these trajectories in lasting ways.

GENDERED EMOTIONAL INTELLIGENCE

The Shadow Side of Female Emotional Intelligence

When Emotional Intelligence (EI) is cultivated in contexts emphasizing compliance, likability, and emotional labor, girls may develop externally adaptive but internally costly emotional control. This aligns with Hochschild's (1983) concept of *emotion work*, which involves managing one's own and others' emotions to meet social expectations. Girls, often rewarded for being nurturing and agreeable, may mask authentic emotions, suppress anger, or prioritize others' needs, leading to stress, low self-esteem, and emotional exhaustion—a form of internal dissonance explained by Festinger's (1957) Cognitive Dissonance Theory.

High EI can also be misused. The ability to read and influence emotions may fuel relational aggression—covert harm through exclusion, gossip, or manipulation (Crick & Grotpeter, 1995). Austin et al. (2007) note that instrumental empathy can facilitate emotional manipulation, and when combined with high psychoticism (as observed in doctoral research), EI can mask antisocial tendencies. Impression Management Theory (Leary & Kowalski, 1990) further explains how girls may strategically manage social perceptions rather than authentically express emotions.

This shadow side of female EI underscores the need for interventions that go beyond skill promotion, integrating ethics, mindfulness, and emotional authenticity to support well-being, integrity, and genuine emotional competence rather than mere social approval.

Male Emotional Intelligence: A Repressed Potential

Boys' Emotional Intelligence (EI) is often hidden or underdeveloped due to cultural norms equating masculinity with emotional stoicism. From a young age, boys are socialized to view vulnerability as weakness and emotional detachment as strength, reinforced by caregivers, peers, media, and schools. Hegemonic masculinity (Connell, 1995) explains this suppression, as societal emphasis on dominance and self-reliance encourages boys to mask emotions like sadness or fear, sometimes expressing discomfort through aggression or risk-taking (Pollack, 1998).

Gender role conflict (Mahalik et al., 2003) further highlights the tension boys experience when their emotional needs clash with traditional male norms, potentially leading to emotional dysregulation, withdrawal, or mental health issues. Yet, research shows that boys can develop EI when nurtured in psychologically safe environments. Mindfulness programs and Social-Emotional Learning (SEL) interventions improve emotional awareness, reduce aggression, and enhance overall well-being (Schonert-Reichl & Lawlor, 2010; Greenberg et al., 2003). Secure attachment relationships (Bowlby, 1969) also foster emotional openness and regulation.

Traditional EI assessments often overlook boys' competencies, favoring verbal and relational expressions over action-oriented or protective forms of empathy. Positive masculinity frameworks (Kiselica & Englar-Carlson, 2010) promote integrating strength with sensitivity and leadership with compassion, encouraging boys to develop EI without compromising identity or social standing.

Supporting boys' EI requires emotionally safe spaces, inclusive assessments, positive role models, and family and community engagement to challenge stereotypes. Male EI is not absent—it is often unseen or culturally suppressed. With targeted support, boys can cultivate emotional skills that enhance well-being, relationships, and societal contributions.

Toward a Non-Binary Understanding of Emotional Intelligence

While gender-based analysis helps understand Emotional Intelligence (EI) in adolescence, it is crucial to move beyond binary frameworks. Non-binary, transgender, and gender-fluid adolescents face unique emotional challenges, including societal stigma, misgendering, identity invalidation, limited access to affirming environments, and heightened discrimination, all of which affect emotional development and self-regulation.

Kosciw et al. (2020) report that LGBTQ+ students, particularly gender-diverse youth, experience elevated emotional distress—anxiety, depression, and isolation—often worsened in unsupportive school environments. Fear of rejection or violence may lead these adolescents to suppress authentic emotional expression, hindering healthy EI development. Minority Stress Theory (Meyer, 2003) explains how chronic prejudice, discrimination, and internalized stigma uniquely impact mental health and emotional functioning, highlighting the need for EI interventions that are both emotionally supportive and identity-affirming.

An intersectional lens (Crenshaw, 1989) further clarifies that emotional experiences are shaped not only by gender identity but also by race, class, disability, and culture. For example, a non-binary adolescent of color navigating economic hardship faces distinct emotional challenges compared to a white, middle-class cisgender peer. Emotional education must therefore address both gender diversity and social inequalities.

Queer-affirming pedagogy (Airton, 2013; Robinson & Ferfolja, 2008) emphasizes creating learning environments that resist heteronormative and binary assumptions—using inclusive language, validating non-binary emotional expression, and facilitating identity-conscious discussions. Neurodivergent, gender-diverse adolescents may require trauma-informed and neuroaffirming approaches, as standard EI programs often fail to capture subtle communication or regulation styles. Protective factors such as family support, affirming peer relationships, and access to gender-affirming care enhance emotional regulation and psychological health (Singh et al., 2014).

Mindful self-compassion practices (Neff, 2003) can be particularly powerful, helping gender-diverse adolescents counter internalized stigma and body image distress, and fostering emotional healing and self-worth beyond societal judgment.

ROLE OF CULTURAL AND CONTEXTUAL FACTORS

The expression of Emotional Intelligence (EI) is deeply shaped by sociocultural norms, values, and expectations. In collectivist societies like India, adolescents are often socialized to suppress or moderate emotions to maintain group harmony and familial honor (Markus & Kitayama,

1991; Mesquita, 2001). Emotional regulation may prioritize compliance over authenticity, balancing social expectations against personal feelings.

Research shows that Indian adolescents frequently suppress distress to avoid disrupting family or peer group stability (Saraswathi & Larson, 2002). Gopalan & Nelson (2019) found that emotional suppression supports academic self-presentation but undermines psychological well-being, reflecting a tension between success and self-expression. Gender norms compound this effect: girls are expected to display empathy, patience, and self-sacrifice, while boys are socialized toward stoicism and emotional restraint (Pollack, 1998; Chaplin & Aldao, 2013). Girls often internalize emotional burdens silently, whereas boys may externalize distress through aggression or risk-taking.

This can blur the line between authentic empathy and socially conditioned performance. Adolescents may mimic culturally and gender-appropriate emotional displays without reflecting internal states—a phenomenon termed "emotional conformity" (Matsumoto et al., 2008). In collectivist families, adolescents also navigate intergenerational expectations, managing both their own emotions and those of parents or elders, adding further emotional labor, particularly for girls (Chadda & Deb, 2013).

Integrating Cultural Intelligence (CQ) with EI provides a framework for understanding how adolescents navigate emotional expression within relational hierarchies, gender norms, and cultural codes (Earley & Ang, 2003).

Policy and Practice Implications

- EI curricula should incorporate cultural humility and gender sensitivity, reflecting traditions, family dynamics, and social norms.
- Schools must provide safe spaces for adolescents to process and express emotions without fear of social or familial repercussions.
- Mindfulness-based programs, framed within cultural ethics and indigenous practices, can help adolescents balance inner authenticity with social harmony.

By considering cultural and gendered contexts, EI development can be understood not just as a personal skill but as a socially embedded competence, guiding interventions that are inclusive, ethical, and effective.

THE NEED FOR ETHICAL GROUNDING

The dual nature of Emotional Intelligence (EI) as both a facilitator of prosocial behavior and a potential enabler of manipulation highlights the urgent need for ethical grounding in emotional education. Emotional skills should not be taught as value-neutral competencies, but must be embedded within frameworks that nurture compassion, integrity, accountability, and social justice.

Research indicates that EI, when detached from moral grounding, can be diverted toward manipulative or self-serving purposes. Joseph and Newman (2010) and Brackett and Mayer (2003) emphasize that adolescents with high emotional awareness but limited ethical orientation may exploit their skills to deceive or dominate others, particularly in competitive or hierarchical contexts. Hyde et al. (2020) similarly note that such "strategic EI" may manifest as relational aggression, emotional coercion, or peer exclusion, undermining the empathetic values EI is often assumed to promote.

This calls for a paradigm shift toward what Narvaez (2010) terms *"ethical skill development"*, in which emotional awareness and regulation are taught alongside virtue ethics such as empathy, humility, fairness, and respect. Narvaez's Integrative Ethical Education (IEE) model demonstrates how moral sensitivity, judgment, motivation, and action can be systematically cultivated in tandem with cognitive and emotional competencies. In adolescence, a developmental stage where identity and morality are still forming, this integration becomes particularly crucial.

Goleman's (1995) mixed model of EI originally included empathy and social skills, yet critics argue it underemphasized the ethical orientation of these competencies. More recent work in emotional education stresses the need for intentionality, relational ethics, and emotional justice, concepts that ensure EI is used to strengthen human connection rather than manipulate it.

Mindfulness-based interventions (MBIs) provide a promising pathway for embedding ethical awareness into EI. Practices such as loving-kindness meditation, compassion training, and yogic principles of *ahimsa* (non-harm) and *satya* (truthfulness) cultivate reflection not only on *what* adolescents feel, but also on *why* they feel it and *how* they choose to act. Studies by Roeser (2014) and Greenberg & Harris (2012) demonstrate that MBIs enhance perspective-taking, moral reasoning, and emotional responsibility, strengthening both psychological resilience and ethical engagement.

However, significant gaps remain. Few EI programs have standardized ethical benchmarks or curricula that explicitly measure whether emotional competencies translate into ethical conduct. Longitudinal studies are scarce, leaving questions about whether EI training sustains moral outcomes into adulthood. Research on how adolescents interpret the ethical implications of their emotional skills is also limited, signaling a critical area for future research.

To ensure Emotional Intelligence (EI) education and Mindfulness-Based Interventions (MBIs) are used responsibly in adolescent contexts, the following ethical guidelines are recommended:

1. **Embed Ethics Explicitly** – Integrate moral reasoning exercises, ethical dilemmas, and reflective dialogues into EI curricula.
2. **Adopt Trauma-Informed Practices** – Ensure mindfulness activities are safe, avoid retraumatization, and provide adequate psychological support.
3. **Respect Autonomy and Agency** – Give adolescents choice and voice in emotional education, avoiding coercive compliance.
4. **Ensure Cultural and Gender Sensitivity** – Adapt interventions to local traditions, family dynamics, and gender norms.
5. **Safeguard Against Instrumentalization** – Frame EI as a pathway to empathy, justice, and well-being, not merely as a tool for academic or career advantage.

6. **Evaluate Holistically** – Use mixed-methods assessment that captures not only skills but also ethical orientation, relational outcomes, and adolescent voices.

MINDFULLNESS AND INTERVENTIONS

Mindfulness-Based Interventions for Ethical and Self-Regulated Emotional Intelligence

Adolescence is a stage marked by impulsivity, heightened emotions, and vulnerability to social pressures. Emotional Intelligence (EI), while valuable, risks being used manipulatively without ethical grounding. Mindfulness, defined as non-judgmental present-moment awareness, provides a corrective pathway by enhancing self-regulation, emotional clarity, empathy, and compassion.

Mindfulness-Based Emotional Regulation Theory (Garland et al., 2015) explains how mindfulness interrupts automatic thought–emotion cycles, allowing adolescents to respond rather than react. Similarly, Gross's Process Model of Emotion Regulation (1998) aligns with mindfulness by showing how early awareness enables healthier regulation strategies, reducing the need for suppression or aggression. This is particularly crucial in adolescence, when the prefrontal cortex is still maturing (Steinberg, 2005).

Research demonstrates that mindfulness strengthens EI while reducing maladaptive behaviors. School-based mindfulness programs improve classroom climate, prosocial behavior, and attention regulation (Schonert-Reichl & Lawlor, 2010; Flook et al., 2010). A meta-analysis by Zoogman et al. (2015) found that mindfulness interventions led to reductions in anxiety, depression, and stress, while Tan (2016) reported improvements in executive function and emotional regulation. More recently, Noorollahi, Shahabizadeh, and Nasri (2024) compared mindfulness-based therapy with paradoxical treatment and found that both approaches significantly improved distress tolerance in adolescents with social anxiety symptoms. This highlights the contemporary relevance of mindfulness in addressing adolescent emotional vulnerabilities. Neuroscientific studies further show that mindfulness increases prefrontal cortex activation (executive control) and decreases amygdala reactivity (fear/emotional overdrive) (Hölzel et al., 2011), thereby enhancing impulse control.

Mindfulness-Based Stress Reduction (MBSR) and Mindfulness-Based Cognitive Therapy (MBCT) have proven effective for adolescent anxiety, depression, and trauma (Biegel et al., 2009; Sibinga et al., 2016). In classrooms, mindfulness cultivates calm attention and improves peer relationships, aligning with India's National Education Policy (NEP 2020), which emphasizes socio-emotional learning, yoga, and ethical values. Emerging digital tools such as *Headspace* and *Calm* also show promise for youth engagement (Dunning et al., 2019).

Beyond enhancing resilience and well-being, mindfulness plays a corrective role in addressing the manipulative potential of Emotional Intelligence. Adolescents with high EI may sometimes deploy emotional skills strategically to gain social advantage, manage impressions, or conceal inner distress. Mindfulness interrupts these tendencies by cultivating non-judgmental awareness and compassion. Practices such as loving-kindness meditation (Neff, 2003) and mindful self-compassion (Jennings, 2015) shift the focus from performance and impression management toward authentic emotional processing. In this way, mindfulness reduces emotional masking, challenges the use of EI as a tool of manipulation, and reorients emotional competence toward empathy, integrity, and ethical connection.

Most studies on adolescent mindfulness interventions assess only short-term outcomes such as reduced anxiety, improved attention, and increased prosocial behavior. There is limited longitudinal evidence to show whether these benefits persist across critical developmental transitions, such as the shift from adolescence to emerging adulthood. This highlights the need for follow-up studies that evaluate the durability of mindful EI training over time.

Breathwork and Embodied Awareness

One of the most accessible and effective forms of mindfulness practice is breathwork, which engages both physiological and psychological mechanisms for emotional regulation. Focusing attention on the breath not only anchors the mind and reduces cognitive distractions but also calms physiological arousal by modulating autonomic nervous system activity. For adolescents experiencing emotional turbulence, impulsivity, or anxiety, breathwork offers a portable, cost-effective, and immediate intervention for emotional grounding.

The Polyvagal Theory (Porges, 2007) provides a compelling framework for understanding the connection between breath and emotional states. This theory highlights how slow, deep breathing activates the vagal nerve and shifts the body from a sympathetic "fight or flight" mode into a parasympathetic "rest and digest" state. By facilitating this shift, breathwork helps adolescents regulate emotional responses, increase heart rate variability (HRV), and return to a state of physiological calm.

Breathing techniques such as diaphragmatic breathing, box breathing, coherent breathing, and alternate-nostril breathing (Nadi Shodhana) have been empirically validated. For instance, Brown & Gerbarg (2005) found that yogic breathing techniques improved mood and cognitive flexibility while reducing symptoms of anxiety and PTSD. Similarly, Zaccaro et al. (2018) conducted a systematic review and found that slow-paced breathing techniques significantly improved emotional well-being and stress resilience across various populations, including adolescents.

Furthermore, embodied awareness an awareness of bodily sensations and their emotional correlates enhances self-understanding and emotional intelligence. Adolescents who learn to recognize the physical cues of emotional states (e.g., tightening of the chest in anxiety or shallow breathing in stress) are better equipped to intervene early and regulate their emotions effectively. This aligns with Interoceptive Awareness Theory (Craig, 2002), which posits that increased awareness of internal bodily states is linked to improved emotional clarity and regulation.

School-based interventions that incorporate breathwork into daily routines such as the "MindUP" curriculum or India's "Fit India Movement" and AYUSH protocols demonstrate how culturally adapted breath practices can be scaled for broader impact. In these settings, adolescents have reported greater attention, fewer disciplinary incidents, and improved emotional balance (Schonert-Reichl et al., 2015). Public health policies are increasingly recognizing the value of breathwork. India's National Education Policy (NEP) 2020 encourages the integration of yogic and contemplative practices into education to enhance students' holistic well-being. Similarly, global organizations such as WHO and UNICEF advocate for mind-body interventions to support adolescent mental health in school environments, especially in post-COVID recovery frameworks.

Despite its advantages, breathwork remains understudied in clinical psychology and educational neuroscience, especially with respect to long-term efficacy and variations in individual responsiveness. Concerns also exist about accessibility and cultural sensitivity, particularly in communities where breath practices may be unfamiliar or stigmatized. More intersectional research is needed to explore how breathwork affects adolescents across diverse cultural, neurodiverse, and gender-diverse populations.

Innovative trends involve combining breathwork with biofeedback technology, allowing adolescents to visualize physiological changes in real time. Early-stage studies (Lehrer et al., 2020) suggest that biofeedback-enhanced breath training significantly improves self-regulation and emotional resilience. These tools can bridge the gap between abstract mindfulness concepts and tangible experiences, making emotional regulation more accessible to tech-savvy youth.

Meditation and Emotional Clarity

Meditative practices especially those emphasizing loving-kindness (metta), self-compassion, open monitoring, and body scan techniques play a crucial role in helping adolescents develop emotional awareness, acceptance, and clarity. These practices cultivate a non-reactive and non-judgmental stance toward emotional experiences, allowing individuals to observe their feelings without being immediately overtaken by them. This fosters a sense of psychological distance that enhances reflection, emotional integration, and ethical decision-making.

Cognitive-Behavioral Theories and Mindfulness-Based Cognitive Therapy (MBCT) (Segal, Williams, & Teasdale, 2012) provide a robust theoretical framework for meditation's impact on emotional processing. These theories emphasize the importance of decentering from thoughts and emotional narratives a process that meditation strengthens. Through repeated exposure to internal states during meditation, adolescents can learn to disidentify from distressing emotions, reducing rumination and emotional reactivity.

Research has consistently shown that Loving-Kindness Meditation (LKM) improves emotional well-being by increasing positive affect and social connectedness. Fredrickson et al. (2008) found that LKM practices led to upward spirals of positive emotion, which in turn enhanced psychological resilience, life satisfaction, and empathy. Similarly, Neff and Germer (2013) demonstrated that self-compassion training through meditation significantly reduced anxiety, self-criticism, and emotional suppression in adolescents and young adults.

Meditative practices also enhance emotional clarity, a subdomain of Emotional Intelligence that involves identifying and labeling emotions accurately. Through techniques such as body scans and open monitoring, adolescents learn to recognize subtle physical sensations and thought-emotion connections, which improves interoceptive awareness (Mehling et al., 2009). Enhanced emotional clarity contributes to better self-regulation, reduced impulsivity, and more thoughtful responses in interpersonal situations.

Contemplative Neuroscience offers additional validation, showing that regular meditation alters neural activity in regions such as the anterior cingulate cortex, insula, and prefrontal cortex, which are linked to emotion regulation, empathy, and attention (Tang, Hölzel, & Posner, 2015). Adolescents who meditate regularly may therefore develop more adaptive neurocognitive pathways for managing stress and emotional conflict.

Policy frameworks are increasingly acknowledging the value of meditation. In India, the National Education Policy (NEP) 2020 advocates integrating yogic and meditative practices into the curriculum to promote mental health and holistic development. Internationally, programs like Inner Explorer, Calm Classroom, and Mindfulness in Schools Project (UK) provide scalable meditation modules that support students' emotional clarity, resilience, and ethical awareness.

Despite these strengths, gaps remain. Meditation is often introduced in schools without sufficient cultural adaptation, developmental tailoring, or trauma-informed safeguards. Adolescents with unresolved trauma or high anxiety may initially struggle with meditative silence or body-based awareness. Research by Treleaven (2018) emphasizes the need for trauma-sensitive mindfulness that accommodates different emotional thresholds and offers options for grounding.

Furthermore, most studies on meditation and emotional clarity are short-term and conducted on small, non-diverse samples. There is a need for longitudinal, intersectional, and culturally diverse studies that assess meditation's impact across race, gender identity, neurodiversity, and socio-economic contexts.

To strengthen the role of meditation in Emotional Intelligence development, the following recommendations are proposed:

- Integrate age-appropriate, trauma-sensitive meditative practices into school curricula with trained facilitators
- Combine meditation with emotion labeling exercises and reflective writing for enhanced clarity
- Include family and community engagement to destigmatize contemplative practices
- Offer digital tools for guided meditation tailored to adolescent needs and cultural backgrounds

Yoga as a Holistic Mind-Body Practice

Yoga, an ancient practice with roots in Indian philosophy, combines physical movement (asana), breath control (pranayama), and meditative awareness (dhyana) offering a comprehensive modality for enhancing Emotional Intelligence (EI). This triadic integration supports the development of self-regulation, emotional clarity, and embodied awareness, which are especially beneficial during adolescence a period characterized by neurobiological change, identity exploration, and emotional volatility.

The Neurovisceral Integration Model (Thayer & Lane, 2000) provides a useful framework to understand how yoga supports emotion regulation. This model posits that bodily states, particularly those regulated through the vagus nerve, influence cognitive and emotional processes. Yoga's emphasis on breath and postural alignment stimulates parasympathetic activity, enhances heart rate variability (HRV), and fosters a calm, emotionally balanced state.

Empirical research supports yoga's benefits for adolescent emotional health. In a randomized controlled trial, Khalsa et al. (2012) found that high school students participating in a yoga program reported reduced anger, depression, and fatigue compared to a control group. Similarly, Sahaja yoga meditation has been associated with increased emotional resilience and reduced stress responses among adolescents (Manocha et al., 2011).

Yoga also facilitates emotional embodiment, the process of recognizing, processing, and integrating emotional experiences through physical sensations. As adolescents engage in yoga postures, they learn to notice how emotions manifest in the body (e.g., tightness in the chest with anxiety or restlessness in the limbs with agitation), which contributes to interoceptive awareness and emotional literacy (Price & Hooven, 2018).

From a policy standpoint, yoga is gaining traction as a mental health strategy. India's National Education Policy (NEP) 2020 explicitly promotes yoga as part of holistic education. The Ministry of AYUSH has developed school-based yoga curricula, and programs like "Fit India Movement" include yoga for cultivating emotional and physical well-being. Internationally, organizations such as UNESCO and WHO have acknowledged yoga as an effective strategy for psychosocial support, especially in post-pandemic mental health recovery.

Despite these advances, several gaps and challenges remain. Research on yoga's effects often suffers from small sample sizes, lack of active control groups, and variability in intervention protocols. Cultural attitudes toward yoga especially in non-Indian or secular contexts can also influence participation and outcomes. Moreover, few studies have investigated how yoga affects different subgroups of adolescents, such as LGBTQ+ youth, trauma survivors, or those with learning disabilities.

Innovative practices are now emerging to make yoga more inclusive and trauma-informed. Trauma-Sensitive Yoga (TSY) (Emerson & Hopper, 2011) emphasizes choice, consent, and body autonomy, ensuring that yoga does not inadvertently retraumatize individuals. In educational settings, school-based yoga programs like "Yoga Ed" and "Little Flower

Yoga" integrate SEL frameworks with age-appropriate asanas, creating structured pathways to emotional intelligence development.

ETHICAL AND SPIRITUAL DIMENSIONS OF MINDFUL PRACTICE

While mindfulness is often presented as a secular technique in contemporary educational and clinical settings, its origins lie deeply embedded in spiritual and philosophical traditions, particularly those of Buddhism, Hinduism, and Jainism. These traditions emphasize ethical living, compassion, and interconnectedness, which are integral when applying mindfulness to Emotional Intelligence (EI). Without this ethical grounding, EI risks becoming a set of instrumental skills focused on personal or social advantage rather than a transformative approach to living with integrity, empathy, and wisdom.

Theoretical frameworks such as Ethical Mindfulness (Monteiro, Musten, & Compson, 2015) argue for a reintegration of mindfulness with its moral roots. This perspective critiques the Western adaptation of mindfulness that often strips it of its ethical underpinnings. When mindfulness is taught without moral context, emotional awareness may be sharpened, but not necessarily directed toward prosocial outcomes. Emotional manipulation, relational aggression, or self-centered control may result if mindfulness and EI are not aligned with compassion and moral reasoning.

Integrating spiritual concepts such as ahimsa (non-violence), satya (truthfulness), karuna (compassion), and aparigraha (non-possessiveness) drawn from Indian philosophical systems—reinforces the moral context of emotional practice. These values invite adolescents to consider the intentions behind their emotional behaviors and to reflect on how emotions affect others, thus grounding Emotional Intelligence in social ethics and emotional justice.

Empirical studies support the value of ethical mindfulness. Roeser et al. (2014) demonstrated that mindfulness training in educators increased not only self-regulation but also ethical sensitivity and compassionate response toward students. Similarly, Van Gordon et al. (2017) found that spiritually framed mindfulness interventions, such as Meditation Awareness Training (MAT), improved not only emotional regulation but also altruistic behavior, humility, and life purpose in adolescents and young adults.

Spiritual dimensions of mindfulness are also supported by eudaimonic well-being theory (Ryan & Deci, 2001), which emphasizes flourishing through meaning, virtue, and self-realization. Adolescents who view mindfulness as a path to self-knowledge and service are more likely to develop an emotionally intelligent identity that is resilient, socially engaged, and ethically anchored.

Policy frameworks increasingly recognize the importance of value-based education. India's National Curriculum Framework (NCF) 2023 and NEP 2020 advocate for character development, moral reasoning, and contemplative practices as part of holistic education. Globally, UNESCO's Education for Sustainable Development (ESD) includes socio-emotional and ethical competencies as vital for peacebuilding and global citizenship.

However, there are notable gaps and controversies. Critics argue that integrating spiritual content into public education may blur the line between secularism and religious instruction. Moreover, adolescents from non-religious or differing faith backgrounds may find spiritually inflected practices alienating if not presented with cultural sensitivity and inclusivity. This underscores the need for pluralistic, choice-based mindfulness programs that accommodate diverse belief systems while upholding core ethical principles.

Novel practices are emerging to bridge these divides. Programs like Ethics-Based Mindfulness (EBM) and Compassionate Systems Framework blend mindfulness with global ethics, social justice, and systems thinking. These approaches situate Emotional Intelligence within broader conversations on equity, sustainability, and collective well-being.

PRACTICAL FRAMEWORK FOR SCHOOLS AND PRACTITIONERS

To translate the theoretical insights and empirical findings into actionable strategies, this section outlines a comprehensive framework for integrating mindful, ethical Emotional Intelligence (EI) into school curricula and youth development settings. Grounded in developmental psychology, contemplative pedagogy, and whole-child education models, this framework aims to support educators, counselors, and program designers in cultivating emotionally intelligent, ethically aware, and resilient adolescents.

Foundational Principles

This framework is built upon the following key principles:

Developmental appropriateness: Aligning content with the cognitive and emotional capacities of different age groups (Piaget, 1972; Erikson, 1968)

Cultural responsiveness: Incorporating diverse values, narratives, and modes of expression (Gay, 2000; Ladson-Billings, 1995)

Ethical anchoring: Embedding practices in values such as compassion, non-harm, and integrity (Noddings, 2005)

Experiential learning: Utilizing reflective, embodied, and dialogical approaches for deeper integration (Kolb, 2014)

Systems alignment: Connecting classroom practices with institutional policies and community goals (Fullan, 2006)

Main Components

The following components operationalize the framework:

1. **Curricular Integration Mindful EI should be woven into existing subjects (e.g., language, social studies, health) through:**
    - Emotion-focused learning activities
    - Literature and media analysis through an emotional lens
    - Group projects requiring collaboration, empathy, and conflict resolution Research by CASEL (2020) and Jones & Kahn (2017) supports the integration of SEL and mindfulness across academic domains to enhance both socio-emotional and cognitive outcomes.

2. **Dedicated Mindful EI Sessions Weekly or bi-weekly sessions can include:**
    - Guided meditations (e.g., body scan, loving-kindness)
    - Group dialogues on emotions and ethical dilemmas
    - Breathing and grounding exercises
    - Role plays and storytelling Programs like MindUP, Learning to BREATHE, and India's "Happiness Curriculum" offer replicable models.
3. **Teacher and Staff Development Teachers are the emotional climate setters of the classroom. Ongoing professional development should include:**
    - Mindfulness practice and emotional literacy for teachers
    - Trauma-informed pedagogy
    - Reflective supervision and peer coaching Studies by Jennings & Greenberg (2009) and Roeser et al. (2012) show that teacher well-being and mindful presence significantly influence student outcomes.
4. **Family and Community Engagement Sustainable EI development requires alignment between home and school. Strategies include:**
    - Family mindfulness nights
    - Emotional literacy newsletters
    - Parent workshops on adolescent development and communication
5. **Policy and Administrative Support School leadership plays a pivotal role in systematizing mindful EI. Key actions:**
    - Embedding EI in the mission and vision of the school
    - Allocating time and resources
    - Creating emotionally safe disciplinary practices Policies like NEP 2020, NCF 2023, and UNESCO's Happy Schools Framework advocate for emotional well-being as a central pillar of education.

Recommendations

- Co-create programs with adolescents for contextual relevance
- Invest in teacher capacity building and well-being

- Use mixed-method evaluation to capture affective and behavioral outcomes
- Anchor programs in ethics and justice, not only performance
- Build alliances with local mental health organizations and contemplative communities

A practical framework for mindful, ethical EI must be multi-layered, culturally grounded, and ethically guided. It must go beyond reducing adolescent distress and aim to nurture emotionally intelligent changemakers capable of shaping compassionate, inclusive, and resilient societies.

Core Modules and Sample Activities

1. **Self-Awareness**
    - Activity: Emotion identification cards
    - Journaling prompt: "When I feel angry, I usually…"
    - Practice: Body scan meditation
2. **Self-Regulation**
    - Activity: "STOP" technique (Stop, Take a breath, Observe, Proceed)
    - Practice: Alternate-nostril breathing
    - Reflection: Triggers and emotional patterns
3. **Motivation and Goal-Setting**
    - Activity: Vision board creation
    - Discussion: Short-term vs. long-term gratification
    - Practice: Visualization meditation
4. **Empathy and Compassion**
    - Activity: "Walk in Their Shoes" role-play
    - Practice: Loving-kindness meditation
    - Discussion: Boundaries vs. enmeshment
5. **Social Skills and Ethical Behavior**
    - Activity: Conflict resolution wheel
    - Practice: Deep listening in pairs
    - Reflection: Acts of kindness journal
6. **Integration with PLO (Positive Life Orientation)**
    - Activity: Life purpose statement writing

- Discussion: Optimism in the face of failure
- Practice: Gratitude meditation

Assessment Tools

Assessment should be ongoing and multidimensional, capturing both quantitative and qualitative outcomes:

- **Pre- and Post-Intervention Surveys**
  - Emotional Quotient Inventory: Youth Version (EQ-i:YV)
  - Rosenberg Self-Esteem Scale
  - Positive Life Orientation Scale
- **Behavioral Observations**
  - Teacher and counselor logs of behavioral incidents, peer interaction quality, and participation
- **Reflective Journals and Portfolios**
  - Review student journals for emotional insight, ethical reasoning, and personal growth

Family and Community Engagement

The impact of a mindful EI program is amplified when families and communities are involved:

- **Workshops for Parents**
  - Help parents understand and reinforce EI strategies at home
  - Teach co-regulation and mindful parenting skills
- **Community Projects**
  - Engage students in service-learning to practice compassion in action
  - Foster a sense of contribution and interconnectedness

Adapting for Diverse Contexts

Schools and programs operate in varied contexts. Adaptation is key:

- Urban schools may emphasize stress management and peer dynamics
- Rural schools may integrate indigenous wisdom and local practices
- Under-resourced settings can use no-cost, body-based practices
- Inclusive schools may adapt for neurodiverse learners using visual supports and routine-based instruction

Case Example: Urban High School Implementation

At a metropolitan public school in Delhi, a pilot 10-week mindful EI program was implemented with 60 ninth-grade students. The sessions integrated breathing practices, emotion mapping, role-plays, and journaling. Results included:

- 25% reduction in reported interpersonal conflicts
- 30% increase in emotional vocabulary usage
- Qualitative feedback from students indicated greater emotional clarity and peer empathy

Teachers observed improved classroom climate and more respectful communication. The school subsequently integrated mindfulness practices into morning assemblies and launched a peer mentorship program.

CHALLENGES AND CONSIDERATIONS

Despite their demonstrated benefits, mindfulness-based interventions (MBIs) for adolescents are not without significant challenges. These complexities must be acknowledged to ensure ethical, effective, and inclusive practice.

Firstly, adolescent receptivity to mindfulness varies. Some adolescents may resist introspective practices due to discomfort with silence, emotional vulnerability, or perceived irrelevance. Cultural norms and religious beliefs may also affect acceptance particularly in communities where contemplative practices are viewed as spiritual or incompatible with dominant faith systems. According to Greenberg and Harris (2012), adolescent skepticism can be mitigated through peer modeling, relevance-based framing, and gradual integration of mindfulness activities.

Secondly, MBIs can inadvertently trigger distress or anxiety, especially for trauma-exposed adolescents. Practices that encourage stillness and inward attention may resurface unresolved trauma, grief, or suppressed emotions. This underscores the need for trauma-informed adaptations, such as options for movement-based mindfulness, grounding exercises, and safe exit strategies. Treleaven (2018) emphasizes that mindfulness must be delivered with safety, choice, and relational trust to avoid retraumatization.

Another critical consideration is the authenticity and integrity of mindfulness delivery. In some educational contexts, mindfulness is commodified packaged as a stress-reduction technique devoid of its ethical and contemplative roots. This can reduce mindfulness to a performance metric or behavioral control tool, rather than a practice of self-awareness and ethical clarity. Monteiro, Musten, and Compson (2015) warn that decontextualized mindfulness may inadvertently reinforce conformity, compliance, or emotional suppression.

The "McMindfulness" critique (Purser, 2019) further highlights the risk of using mindfulness as a corporate or institutional strategy to manage distress without addressing systemic inequities. This critique is particularly relevant in under-resourced school settings, where mindfulness may be introduced without concurrent efforts to address teacher burnout, bullying, or socio-economic stressors affecting students.

Moreover, evaluation of MBIs should include not only behavioral and cognitive outcomes but also measures of emotional authenticity, relational quality, and ethical growth. Participatory action research, narrative assessments, and feedback loops can enrich the evaluation process.

IMPLICATIONS FOR POLICY AND PRACTICE

The findings and framework of this chapter carry significant implications for educational policy, curriculum design, mental health support, and practitioner training. A system-wide integration of ethically grounded Emotional Intelligence (EI) and mindfulness practices requires strategic, culturally sensitive, and evidence-informed approaches. Below are key recommendations supported by theory and research:

Policy Integration: Educational frameworks should mandate the inclusion of social-emotional learning (SEL) and mindfulness-based ethical development as core curricular components, not optional supplements. As recommended by UNESCO's *Happy Schools Framework* and India's *National Education Policy (NEP) 2020*, education must be holistic and values-based, embedding emotional, ethical, and civic learning from early grades (UNESCO, 2016; MHRD, 2020). Alongside NEP 2020, the *National Curriculum Framework (NCF 2023)* reinforces socio-emotional learning, mindfulness, and life skills as central to adolescent development. At the international level, CASEL's five SEL competencies—self-awareness, self-management, social awareness, relationship skills, and responsible decision-making align with UNESCO's emphasis on holistic and values-driven education. Together, these frameworks establish Mindful EI as both a national and global priority.

Teacher Preparation and Support: Pre-service and in-service teacher education programs should include training in trauma-informed care, contemplative pedagogy (Roeser, 2006), and ethical classroom leadership. Teachers must be empowered to cultivate their own Emotional Intelligence and mindfulness capacities, which research suggests has a cascading positive effect on classroom climate and student outcomes (Jennings & Greenberg, 2009).

Mental Health and EI Synergy: School psychologists, counselors, and SEL facilitators should work collaboratively to ensure that Emotional Intelligence programs align with broader mental health goals. This includes using early screening tools to detect emotional distress masked by high EI and ensuring access to trauma-responsive care (Substance Abuse and Mental Health Services Administration [SAMHSA], 2014).

Cultural Responsiveness and Inclusion: Emotional learning programs must avoid Western-centric, one-size-fits-all models. Instead, they should incorporate local cultural practices, community ethics, and indigenous contemplative wisdom (e.g., yoga, Sufi zikr, tribal rituals). Theoretical models such as Culturally Responsive Teaching (Gay, 2018) and Intersectionality Theory (Crenshaw, 1991) can guide the development of inclusive frameworks.

Evaluation and Continuous Feedback: Programs should be rigorously evaluated using mixed-methods designs that combine quantitative measures (e.g., self-reports, behavior scales) with qualitative tools like narrative interviews, journaling, and participatory reflection. This ensures responsiveness to students' lived experiences and supports iterative program development (Patton, 2015).

Community and Family Involvement: Emotionally intelligent development does not occur in isolation. Schools should actively engage families, caregivers, and community leaders to co-create emotionally nurturing ecosystems. Parenting workshops, community mindfulness circles, and intergenerational dialogue sessions can extend the impact of school-based programs (Elias et al., 2003).

Ethical Safeguards and Accountability: As Emotional Intelligence tools become more embedded in educational and therapeutic spaces, there is a need for ethical oversight. Clear frameworks must guide the use of EI assessments, prevent misuse (e.g., labeling or emotional manipulation), and uphold student dignity and autonomy (Zeidner, Matthews, & Roberts, 2009).

Digital and Hybrid Innovations: With the rise of EdTech, emotionally intelligent digital tools must be designed with data privacy, accessibility, and inclusivity in mind. Platforms offering mindfulness and SEL content should align with ethical standards and avoid the commodification of emotional practices (Zhao et al., 2021).

By consolidating insights from India's NEP 2020 and NCF 2023 with international frameworks such as CASEL and UNESCO, educational systems can ensure that EI interventions are scalable, culturally legitimate, and ethically grounded. Such integration supports not only individual well-being but also prepares adolescents to participate as ethical, compassionate global citizens. Embedding Mindful EI into policy and practice thus demands an integrated, ethics-centered, and systemic approach. When education becomes not just about performance but about presence, purpose, and people, we empower adolescents to flourish in emotionally intelligent, ethically anchored, and socially engaged ways.

DIRECTIONS FOR FUTURE RESEARCH

While Emotional Intelligence (EI) has been extensively studied in various domains, its ethical dimensions, particularly during adolescence, remain under-explored and theoretically underdeveloped. The following directions outline key areas for future inquiry, grounded in emerging research, theoretical innovation, and sociocultural realities:

- **Longitudinal Impacts of Mindful EI Programs**: Existing studies have established short-term benefits of mindfulness-based EI interventions in reducing stress and improving self-regulation (Zoogman et al., 2015; Felver & Jennings, 2016). However, longitudinal research is needed to evaluate lasting effects on adolescent behavior, identity formation, mental health, and life satisfaction. Do these programs foster sustained emotional resilience and ethical decision-making into adulthood?
- **Gender-Diverse and Neurodiverse Experiences**: The majority of EI research still relies on gender-binary frameworks and neurotypical assumptions. Future studies must explore how non-binary, transgender, and neurodivergent adolescents experience, express, and internalize EI. Integrating neurodiversity paradigms (Armstrong, 2010) and gender-expansive theories (Gilligan, 1982) can lead to more inclusive, affirming EI practices.
- **Intersectional and Cultural Dimensions**: There is a critical need to explore intersectionality in emotional development how factors like socioeconomic status, caste, race, language, and religion shape emotional expression and ethical empathy (Crenshaw, 1991; hooks, 2000). Research should also examine indigenous and collectivist emotional frameworks, contrasting them with dominant Western models of EI.
- **Secular vs. Spiritually-Informed Mindfulness Models**: Comparative studies should assess whether spiritual mindfulness traditions (e.g., Buddhist metta, Christian centering prayer, Sufi dhikr) promote greater ethical attunement and emotional depth than secular protocols like MBSR or Learning to BREATHE. Spiritual traditions often embed EI in moral and communal contexts, a poten-

tial advantage over utility-based secular models (Roeser & Eccles, 2015).

- **Digital Tools and Technological Influence**: The digital ecosystem increasingly mediates adolescents' emotional lives. Studies must examine the efficacy and risks of AI-driven emotional assessments, emotional literacy apps, and gamified mindfulness platforms. While tech-based solutions may increase access, they also pose risks of emotional commodification, privacy breaches, and reduced face-to-face empathy (Zhao et al., 2021).
- **Development of Ethical EI Assessments**: Current EI tools such as MSCEIT or EQ-i focus heavily on cognitive accuracy or behavioral frequency. Future tools should assess ethical intentionality, relational consequences, and values alignment. Qualitative instruments and narrative-based tools could complement self-report metrics to better capture moral reasoning and emotional impact (Zeidner et al., 2009).

POLICY RECOMMENDATIONS FOR FUTURE RESEARCH

- Fund interdisciplinary, international collaborations to study EI in diverse cultural and educational contexts
- Mandate gender and neurodiversity representation in adolescent EI studies
- Develop open-access ethical EI assessment tools for schools and practitioners
- Encourage youth participatory action research (YPAR) to co-create emotionally intelligent and just spaces

In conclusion, future research must move beyond the optimization of emotional skills to a critical, culturally embedded, and ethically grounded inquiry. Only then can we nurture adolescents who are not just emotionally competent but also conscious, compassionate, and committed to collective well-being.

CONCLUSION

While this chapter emphasizes the paradoxical and sometimes darker aspects of EI, it is important to note that the majority of research continues to demonstrate its benefits for resilience, social connection, and academic achievement. Future studies should balance these perspectives to avoid overgeneralization.

This chapter also underscores the paradox of Emotional Intelligence in adolescence: a capacity that can promote resilience and empathy, yet also fuel manipulation, emotional masking, and maladaptive behaviors. Empirical findings reveal that emotionally competent adolescents, particularly girls, may simultaneously display heightened psychological vulnerability and antisocial tendencies. Left ungrounded, EI risks functioning as a tool for control rather than connection.

In a world increasingly shaped by emotional disconnection, performative empathy, and algorithm-driven behavior, the cultivation of ethical Emotional Intelligence (EI) through mindfulness-based practices is not just beneficial, it is imperative. Social media, political polarization, economic precarity, and competitive educational environments often normalize emotional manipulation, suppression, or commodification. Within this turbulent context, adolescents stand at a developmental crossroads. The emotional patterns they internalize today will influence their relationships, mental health, civic engagement, and ethical orientation for years to come.

Equipping adolescents with mindful, ethically grounded EI means empowering them to:

- Pause before reacting, making space for reflection and self-awareness
- Act with compassion, even in moments of personal or social conflict
- Establish healthy emotional boundaries, rooted in self-respect and mutual dignity
- Contribute to peacebuilding, empathy, and justice in their schools and communities

Mindfulness-based interventions provide a crucial corrective to this paradox. By embedding emotional skills in compassion, authenticity, and ethical orientation, mindfulness interrupts manipulative patterns and reduces emotional masking. It reorients Emotional Intelligence away from self-serving strategies and toward prosocial development, ensuring that emotional competence supports integrity, empathy, and social responsibility.

While this chapter critically interrogates the widespread, sometimes uncritical embrace of EI as a panacea for psychological or academic success, it ultimately reaffirms its transformative potential when embedded within ethics, mindfulness, and social consciousness. The call is not to abandon EI but to reimagine it as a framework for human flourishing rather than strategic self-optimization.

To this end, researcher urge:

- Educators to integrate contemplative, trauma-informed, and justice-oriented SEL frameworks
- Psychologists and counselors to detect the shadow sides of EI and promote emotional authenticity
- Parents and caregivers to model vulnerability, active listening, and mindful presence
- Policymakers to embed ethical EI and mindfulness education in national curricula and adolescent mental health programs

Emotional Intelligence, when cultivated not just for performance but for purpose, can support adolescents in becoming not merely emotionally competent but also ethically courageous, emotionally resilient, and socially transformative. In this way, EI becomes more than a skill it becomes a moral compass, guiding the next generation toward lives of inner peace, relational harmony, and global compassion.

REFERENCES

Airton, L. (2013). Leave "those kids" alone: On the conflation of school homophobia and suffering queers. *Curriculum Inquiry*, *43*(5), 532–562. DOI: 10.1111/curi.12031

Armstrong, M. (2010). *Armstrong's essential human resource management practice: A guide to people management*. Kogan Page Publishers.

Austin, E. J., Farrelly, D., Black, C., & Moore, H. (2007). Emotional intelligence, Machiavellianism and emotional manipulation: Does EI have a dark side? *Personality and Individual Differences*, *43*(1), 179–189. DOI: 10.1016/j.paid.2006.11.019

Bandura, A., & Walters, R. H. (1977). *Social learning theory* (Vol. 1). Prentice hall.

Biegel, G. M., Brown, K. W., Shapiro, S. L., & Schubert, C. M. (2009). Mindfulness-based stress reduction for the treatment of adolescent psychiatric outpatients: A randomized clinical trial. *Journal of Consulting and Clinical Psychology*, *77*(5), 855–866. DOI: 10.1037/a0016241 PMID: 19803566

Brackett, M. A., & Mayer, J. D. (2003). Convergent, discriminant, and incremental validity of competing measures of emotional intelligence. *Personality and Social Psychology Bulletin*, *29*(9), 1147–1158. DOI: 10.1177/0146167203254596 PMID: 15189610

Brackett, M. A., Rivers, S. E., & Salovey, P. (2011). Emotional intelligence: Implications for personal, social, academic, and workplace success. *Social and Personality Psychology Compass*, *5*(1), 88–103. DOI: 10.1111/j.1751-9004.2010.00334.x

Brown, R. P., & Gerbarg, P. L. (2005). Sudarshan Kriya yogic breathing in the treatment of stress, anxiety, and depression: Part I—neurophysiologic model. *Journal of Alternative and Complementary Medicine (New York, N.Y.)*, *11*(1), 189–201. DOI: 10.1089/acm.2005.11.189 PMID: 15750381

Cauffman, E., Steinberg, L., & Piquero, A. R. (2005). Psychological, neuropsychological and physiological correlates of serious antisocial behavior in adolescence: The role of self-control. *Criminology*, *43*(1), 133–176. DOI: 10.1111/j.0011-1348.2005.00005.x

Chadda, R. K., & Deb, K. S. (2013). Indian family systems, collectivistic society and psychotherapy. *Indian Journal of Psychiatry*, *55*(6, Suppl 2), S299–S309. DOI: 10.4103/0019-5545.105555 PMID: 23858272

Chaplin, T. M., & Aldao, A. (2013). Gender differences in emotion expression in children: A meta-analytic review. *Psychological Bulletin*, *139*(4), 735–765. DOI: 10.1037/a0030737 PMID: 23231534

Ciarrochi, J., Heaven, P. C., & Davies, F. (2007). The impact of hope, self-esteem, and attributional style on adolescents' school grades and emotional well-being: A longitudinal study. *Journal of Research in Personality*, *41*(6), 1161–1178. DOI: 10.1016/j.jrp.2007.02.001

Connell, R. W. (1995). *Masculinities*. Polity.

Côté, S., & Miners, C. T. (2006). Emotional intelligence, cognitive intelligence, and job performance. *Administrative Science Quarterly*, *51*(1), 1–28. DOI: 10.2189/asqu.51.1.1

Craig, A. D. (2002). How do you feel? Interoception: The sense of the physiological condition of the body. *Nature Reviews. Neuroscience*, *3*(8), 655–666. DOI: 10.1038/nrn894 PMID: 12154366

Crenshaw, K. (1989) "Demarginalizing the Intersection of Race and Sex: A Black Feminist Critique of Antidiscrimination Doctrine, Feminist Theory and Antiracist Politics," *University of Chicago Legal Forum*: Vol. 1989, Article 8.

Crenshaw, K. (1991). Race, gender, and sexual harassment. s. *California Law Review*, *65*, 1467.

Crick, N. R., & Dodge, K. A. (1994). A review and reformulation of social information-processing mechanisms in children's social adjustment. *Psychological Bulletin*, *115*(1), 74–101. DOI: 10.1037/0033-2909.115.1.74

Crick, N. R., & Grotpeter, J. K. (1995). Relational aggression, gender, and social-psychological adjustment. *Child Development, 66*(3), 710–722. DOI: 10.2307/1131945 PMID: 7789197

Dunning, D. L., Griffiths, K., Kuyken, W., Crane, C., Foulkes, L., Parker, J., & Dalgleish, T. (2019). Research Review: The effects of mindfulness-based interventions on cognition and mental health in children and adolescents–a meta-analysis of randomized controlled trials. *Journal of Child Psychology and Psychiatry, and Allied Disciplines, 60*(3), 244–258. DOI: 10.1111/jcpp.12980 PMID: 30345511

Durlak, J. A., Weissberg, R. P., Dymnicki, A. B., Taylor, R. D., & Schellinger, K. B. (2011). The impact of enhancing students' social and emotional learning: A meta-analysis of school-based universal interventions. *Child Development, 82*(1), 405–432. DOI: 10.1111/j.1467-8624.2010.01564.x PMID: 21291449

. Earley, P. C., & Ang, S. (2003). Cultural intelligence: Individual interactions across cultures.

Eisenberg, N., Spinrad, T. L., & Morris, A. S. (2013). 13 Prosocial Development. The Oxford handbook of developmental psychology, Vol. 2: Self and other, 2, 300.

Elias, M. J., Zins, J. E., Graczyk, P. A., & Weissberg, R. P. (2003). Implementation, sustainability, and scaling up of social-emotional and academic innovations in public schools. *School Psychology Review, 32*(3), 303–319. DOI: 10.1080/02796015.2003.12086200

Emerson, D., & Hopper, E. (2011). *Overcoming trauma through yoga: Reclaiming your body*. North Atlantic Books.

Erikson, E. H. (1968). On the nature of psycho-historical evidence: In search of Gandhi. *Daedalus*, •••, 695–730.

Extremera, N., & Fernández-Berrocal, P. (2006). Emotional intelligence as predictor of mental, social, and physical health in university students. *The Spanish Journal of Psychology, 9*(1), 45–51. DOI: 10.1017/S1138741600005965 PMID: 16673622

Felver, J. C., & Jennings, P. A. (2016). Applications of mindfulness-based interventions in school settings: An introduction. *Mindfulness*, *7*(1), 1–4. DOI: 10.1007/s12671-015-0478-4

Flook, L., Smalley, S. L., Kitil, M. J., Galla, B. M., Kaiser-Greenland, S., Locke, J., Ishijima, E., & Kasari, C. (2010). Effects of mindful awareness practices on executive functions in elementary school children. *Journal of Applied School Psychology*, *26*(1), 70–95. DOI: 10.1080/15377900903379125

Fredrickson, B. L., Cohn, M. A., Coffey, K. A., Pek, J., & Finkel, S. M. (2008). Open hearts build lives: Positive emotions, induced through loving-kindness meditation, build consequential personal resources. *Journal of Personality and Social Psychology*, *95*(5), 1045–1062. DOI: 10.1037/a0013262 PMID: 18954193

Fullan, M. (2006). The future of educational change: System thinkers in action. *Journal of Educational Change*, *7*(3), 113–122. DOI: 10.1007/s10833-006-9003-9

Garland, E. L., Farb, N. A. R., Goldin, P., & Fredrickson, B. L. (2015). Mindfulness broadens awareness and builds eudaimonic meaning: A process model of mindful positive emotion regulation. *Psychological Inquiry*, *26*(4), 293–314. DOI: 10.1080/1047840X.2015.1064294 PMID: 27087765

. Gay, G. (2000). Culturally responsive teaching: Theory, research, and practice. teachers college press.

. Gay, G. (2018). Culturally responsive teaching: Theory, research, and practice. teachers college press.

. Gilligan, C. (1982). The contribution of women's thought to developmental theory: The elimination of sex bias in moral development research and education.

Goleman, D. (1995). *Emotional intelligence: Why it can matter more than IQ*. Bantam Books.

Gopalan, M., & Nelson, A. A. (2019). Understanding the racial discipline gap in schools. *AERA Open*, *5*(2), 2332858419844613. DOI: 10.1177/2332858419844613

Greenberg, M. T., & Harris, A. R. (2012). Nurturing mindfulness in children and youth: Current state of research. *Child Development Perspectives*, *6*(2), 161–166. DOI: 10.1111/j.1750-8606.2011.00215.x

Greenberg, M. T., Weissberg, R. P., O'Brien, M. U., Zins, J. E., Fredericks, L., Resnik, H., & Elias, M. J. (2003). Enhancing school-based prevention and youth development through coordinated social, emotional, and academic learning. *The American Psychologist*, *58*(6-7), 466–474. DOI: 10.1037/0003-066X.58.6-7.466 PMID: 12971193

Gross, J. J. (1998). The emerging field of emotion regulation: An integrative review. *Review of General Psychology*, *2*(3), 271–299. DOI: 10.1037/1089-2680.2.3.271

Hochschild, A. R. (1983). *The managed heart: Commercialization of human feeling*. University of California Press.

. Hoffman, M. L. (2001). Toward a comprehensive empathy-based theory of prosocial moral development.

Hölzel, B. K., Carmody, J., Vangel, M., Congleton, C., Yerramsetti, S. M., Gard, T., & Lazar, S. W. (2011). Mindfulness practice leads to increases in regional brain gray matter density. *Psychiatry Research: Neuroimaging*, *191*(1), 36–43. DOI: 10.1016/j.pscychresns.2010.08.006 PMID: 21071182

Hooks, B. (2000). *Feminist theory: From margin to center*. Pluto press.

Hyde, J., Grieve, R., Norris, K., & Kemp, N. (2020). The dark side of emotional intelligence: The role of gender and the Dark Triad in emotional manipulation at work. *Australian Journal of Psychology*, *72*(4), 307–317. DOI: 10.1111/ajpy.12294

Jennings, P. A. (2015). Early childhood teachers' well-being, mindfulness, and self-compassion in relation to classroom quality and attitudes towards challenging students. *Mindfulness*, *6*(4), 732–743. DOI: 10.1007/s12671-014-0312-4

Jennings, P. A., & Greenberg, M. T. (2009). The prosocial classroom: Teacher social and emotional competence in relation to student and classroom outcomes. *Review of Educational Research*, *79*(1), 491–525. DOI: 10.3102/0034654308325693

Jennings, P. A., Snowberg, K. E., Coccia, M. A., & Greenberg, M. T. (2011). Improving classroom learning environments by cultivating awareness and resilience in education (CARE): Results of two pilot studies. *Journal of Classroom Interaction*, •••, 37–48.

Jones, S. M., & Kahn, J. (2017). *The Evidence Base for How We Learn: Supporting Students' Social, Emotional, and Academic Development. Consensus Statements of Evidence from the Council of Distinguished Scientists*. Aspen Institute.

Joseph, D. L., & Newman, D. A. (2010). Emotional intelligence: An integrative meta-analysis and cascading model. *The Journal of Applied Psychology*, *95*(1), 54–78. DOI: 10.1037/a0017286 PMID: 20085406

Khalsa, S. B. S., Hickey-Schultz, L., Cohen, D., Steiner, N., & Cope, S. (2012). Evaluation of the mental health benefits of yoga in a secondary school: A preliminary randomized controlled trial. *The Journal of Behavioral Health Services & Research*, *39*(1), 80–90. DOI: 10.1007/s11414-011-9249-8 PMID: 21647811

Kilduff, M., Chiaburu, D. S., & Menges, J. I. (2010). Strategic use of emotional intelligence in organizational settings: Exploring the dark side. *Research in Organizational Behavior*, *30*, 129–152. DOI: 10.1016/j.riob.2010.10.002

Kiselica, M. S., & Englar-Carlson, M. (2010). Identifying, affirming, and building upon male strengths: The positive psychology/positive masculinity model of psychotherapy with boys and men. *Psychotherapy (Chicago, Ill.)*, *47*(3), 276–287. DOI: 10.1037/a0021159 PMID: 22402085

Kohlberg, L., Ricks, D., & Snarey, J. (1984). Childhood development as a predictor of adaptation in adulthood. *Genetic Psychology Monographs*.

. Kolb, D. A. (2014). Experiential learning: Experience as the source of learning and development. FT press.

Kosciw, J. G., Clark, C. M., Truong, N. L., & Zongrone, A. D. (2020). The 2019 National School Climate Survey: The Experiences of Lesbian, Gay, Bisexual, Transgender, and Queer Youth in Our Nation's Schools. A Report from GLSEN. Gay, Lesbian and Straight Education Network (GLSEN). 121 West 27th Street Suite 804, New York, NY 10001.

Ladson-Billings, G. (1995). Toward a theory of culturally relevant pedagogy. *American Educational Research Journal*, *32*(3), 465–491. DOI: 10.3102/00028312032003465

Leary, M. R., & Kowalski, R. M. (1990). Impression management: A literature review and two-component model. *Psychological Bulletin*, *107*(1), 34–47. DOI: 10.1037/0033-2909.107.1.34

Lehrer, P., Kaur, K., Sharma, A., Shah, K., Huseby, R., Bhavsar, J., Sgobba, P., & Zhang, Y. (2020, September). Heart Rate Variability Biofeedback Improves Emotional and Physical Health and Performance: A Systematic Review and Meta Analysis. [Erratum in: Appl Psychophysiol Biofeedback. 2021 Dec;46] [4] [:389. doi: 10.1007/s10484-021-09526-y. PMID: 32385728]. *Applied Psychophysiology and Biofeedback*, *45*(3), 109–129. DOI: 10.1007/s10484-020-09466-z PMID: 32385728

Mahalik, J. R., Locke, B., Ludlow, L., Diemer, M., Scott, R. P. J., Gottfried, M., & Freitas, G. (2003). Development of the Conformity to Masculine Norms Inventory. *Psychology of Men & Masculinity*, *4*(1), 3–25. DOI: 10.1037/1524-9220.4.1.3

Manocha, R., Black, D., Sarris, J., & Stough, C. (2011). A randomized, controlled trial of meditation for work stress, anxiety and depressed mood in full-time workers. *Evidence-Based Complementary and Alternative Medicine : eCAM*, *2011*(1), 960583. DOI: 10.1155/2011/960583 PMID: 21716708

Markus, H. R., & Kitayama, S. (1991). Cultural variation in the self-concept. In *The self: Interdisciplinary approaches* (pp. 18–48). Springer New York. DOI: 10.1007/978-1-4684-8264-5_2

Matsumoto, D., Yoo, S. H., & Nakagawa, S. (2008). Culture, emotion regulation, and adjustment. *Journal of Personality and Social Psychology*, *94*(6), 925–937. DOI: 10.1037/0022-3514.94.6.925 PMID: 18505309

Mavroveli, S., Petrides, K. V., Rieffe, C., & Bakker, F. (2007). Trait emotional intelligence, psychological well-being and peer-rated social competence in adolescence. *British Journal of Developmental Psychology, 25*(2), 263–275. DOI: 10.1348/026151006X118577

Mehling, W. E., Gopisetty, V., Daubenmier, J., Price, C. J., Hecht, F. M., & Stewart, A. (2009). Body awareness: Construct and self-report measures. *PLoS One, 4*(5), e5614. DOI: 10.1371/journal.pone.0005614 PMID: 19440300

Mesquita, B. (2001). Emotions in collectivist and individualist contexts. *Journal of Personality and Social Psychology, 80*(1), 68–74. DOI: 10.1037/0022-3514.80.1.68 PMID: 11195892

Mestre, J. M., Guil, R., Lopes, P. N., Salovey, P., & Gil-Olarte, P. (2006). Emotional intelligence and social and academic adaptation to school. *Psicothema, 18*(suppl), 112–117. PMID: 17295967

Monteiro, L. M., Musten, R. F., & Compson, J. (2015). Traditional and contemporary mindfulness: Finding the middle path in the tangle of concerns. *Mindfulness, 6*(1), 1–13. DOI: 10.1007/s12671-014-0301-7

Narvaez, D. (2010). Building a sustaining classroom climate for purposeful ethical citizenship. In *International research handbook on values education and student wellbeing* (pp. 659–673). Springer Netherlands. DOI: 10.1007/978-90-481-8675-4_38

Neff, K. (2003). Self-compassion: An alternative conceptualization of a healthy attitude toward oneself. *Self and Identity, 2*(2), 85–101. DOI: 10.1080/15298860309032

Neff, K. D., & Germer, C. K. (2013). A pilot study and randomized controlled trial of the mindful self-compassion program. *Journal of Clinical Psychology, 69*(1), 28–44. DOI: 10.1002/jclp.21923 PMID: 23070875

Noddings, N. (2005). Identifying and responding to needs in education. *Cambridge Journal of Education, 35*(2), 147–159. DOI: 10.1080/03057640500146757

Nolen-Hoeksema, S., & Girgus, J. S. (1994). The emergence of gender differences in depression during adolescence. *Psychological Bulletin, 115*(3), 424–443. DOI: 10.1037/0033-2909.115.3.424 PMID: 8016286

Noorollahi, A., Shahabizadeh, F., & Nasri, M. (2024). Comparing The Effectiveness of Mindfulness-Based Therapy and Paradoxical Treatment on Distress Tolerance in Adolescents with Social Anxiety Symptoms. *International Journal of Education and Cognitive Sciences*, *5*(3), 157–168. DOI: 10.61838/kman.ijecs.5.3.18

. Patton, M. Q. 2015. Qualitative research & evaluation methods: integrating theory and practice.

Paulhus, D. L., & Reid, D. B. (1991). Enhancement and denial in socially desirable responding. *Journal of Personality and Social Psychology*, *60*(2), 307–317. DOI: 10.1037/0022-3514.60.2.307

Petrides, K. V., Mikolajczak, M., Mavroveli, S., Sanchez-Ruiz, M. J., Furnham, A., & Pérez-González, J. C. (2016). Developments in trait emotional intelligence research. *Emotion Review*, *8*(4), 335–341. DOI: 10.1177/1754073916650493

. Piaget, J. (1972). Development and learning. Reading in child behavior and development, 38-46.

Pollack, W. S. (1998). *Real boys: Rescuing our sons from the myths of boyhood.* Henry Holt and Company.

Porges, S. W. (2007). The polyvagal perspective. *Biological Psychology*, *74*(2), 116–143. DOI: 10.1016/j.biopsycho.2006.06.009 PMID: 17049418

Price, C. J., & Hooven, C. (2018). Interoceptive awareness skills for emotion regulation: Theory and approach of mindful awareness in body-oriented therapy (MABT). *Frontiers in Psychology*, *9*, 798. DOI: 10.3389/fpsyg.2018.00798 PMID: 29892247

Purser, R. (2019). *McMindfulness: How mindfulness became the new capitalist spirituality*. Repeater.

Robinson, K. H., & Ferfolja, T. (2008). Playing it up, playing it down, playing it safe: Queering teacher education. *Teaching and Teacher Education, 24*(4), 846–858. DOI: 10.1016/j.tate.2007.11.004

Roeser, R. W. (2014). The emergence of mindfulness-based interventions in educational settings. In *Motivational interventions* (Vol. 18, pp. 379–419). Emerald Group Publishing Limited. DOI: 10.1108/S0749-742320140000018010

Roeser, R. W., & Eccles, J. S. (2015). Mindfulness and compassion in human development: Introduction to the special section. *Developmental Psychology, 51*(1), 1–6. DOI: 10.1037/a0038453 PMID: 25546594

Roeser, R. W., Skinner, E., Beers, J., & Jennings, P. A. (2012). Mindfulness training and teachers' professional development: An emerging area of research and practice. *Child Development Perspectives, 6*(2), 167–173. DOI: 10.1111/j.1750-8606.2012.00238.x

Roeser, S. (2006). The role of emotions in judging the moral acceptability of risks. *Safety Science, 44*(8), 689–700. DOI: 10.1016/j.ssci.2006.02.001

Ryan, R. M., & Deci, E. L. (2001). On happiness and human potentials: A review of research on hedonic and eudaimonic well-being. *Annual Review of Psychology, 52*(1), 141–166. DOI: 10.1146/annurev.psych.52.1.141 PMID: 11148302

Salovey, P., & Mayer, J. D. (1990). Emotional intelligence. *Imagination, Cognition and Personality, 9*(3), 185–211. DOI: 10.2190/DUGG-P24E-52WK-6CDG

. Saraswathi, T. S., & Larson, R. W. (2002). Adolescence in Global Perspective. The world's youth: Adolescence in eight regions of the globe, 344.

Schonert-Reichl, K. A., & Lawlor, M. S. (2010). The effects of a mindfulness-based education program on pre-and early adolescents' well-being and social and emotional competence. *Mindfulness, 1*(3), 137–151. DOI: 10.1007/s12671-010-0011-8

Schonert-Reichl, K. A., Oberle, E., Lawlor, M. S., Abbott, D., Thomson, K., Oberlander, T. F., & Diamond, A. (2015). Enhancing cognitive and social–emotional development through a simple-to-administer mindfulness-based school program for elementary school children: A randomized controlled trial. *Developmental Psychology*, *51*(1), 52–66. DOI: 10.1037/a0038454 PMID: 25546595

Segal, Z., Williams, M., & Teasdale, J. (2012). *Mindfulness-based cognitive therapy for depression*. Guilford press.

Sibinga, E., Webb, L., Ghazarian, S. R., & Ellen, J. M. (2016). School-based mindfulness instruction: An RCT. *Pediatrics*, *137*(1), e20152532. DOI: 10.1542/peds.2015-2532 PMID: 26684478

Singh, A. A., Meng, S. E., & Hansen, A. W. (2014). "I am my own gender": Resilience strategies of trans youth. *Journal of Counseling and Development*, *92*(2), 208–218. DOI: 10.1002/j.1556-6676.2014.00150.x

Steinberg, L. (2005). Cognitive and affective development in adolescence. *Trends in Cognitive Sciences*, *9*(2), 69–74. DOI: 10.1016/j.tics.2004.12.005 PMID: 15668099

Tang, Y. Y., Hölzel, B. K., & Posner, M. I. (2015). The neuroscience of mindfulness meditation. *Nature Reviews. Neuroscience*, *16*(4), 213–225. DOI: 10.1038/nrn3916 PMID: 25783612

Thayer, J. F., & Lane, R. D. (2000). A model of neurovisceral integration in emotion regulation and dysregulation. *Journal of Affective Disorders*, *61*(3), 201–216. DOI: 10.1016/S0165-0327(00)00338-4 PMID: 11163422

Treleaven, D. A. (2018). *Trauma-sensitive mindfulness: Practices for safe and transformative healing*. WW Norton & Company.

Van Gordon, W., Shonin, E., Dunn, T., Garcia-Campayo, J., & Griffiths, M. (2017). Van Gordon, W., Shonin, E., Dunn, T., Garcia-Campayo, J., & Griffiths, MD (2017). Meditation Awareness Training for the treatment of fibromyalgia: A randomised controlled trial. *British Journal of Health Psychology*, *22*, 186–206. DOI: 10.1111/bjhp.12224 PMID: 27885763

Zaccaro, A., Piarulli, A., Laurino, M., Garbella, E., Menicucci, D., Neri, B., & Gemignani, A. (2018). How breath-control can change your life: A systematic review on psycho-physiological correlates of slow breathing. *Frontiers in Human Neuroscience, 12*, 409421. DOI: 10.3389/fnhum.2018.00353 PMID: 30245619

Zahn-Waxler, C., Shirtcliff, E. A., & Marceau, K. (2008). Disorders of childhood and adolescence: Gender and psychopathology. *Annual Review of Clinical Psychology, 4*(1), 275–303. DOI: 10.1146/annurev.clinpsy.3.022806.091358 PMID: 18370618

Zeidner, M., Matthews, G., & Roberts, R. D. (2009). *What we know about emotional intelligence: How it affects learning, work, relationships, and our mental health.* Boston Review., DOI: 10.7551/mitpress/7404.001.0001

Zhao, Y., Llorente, A. M. P., & Gómez, M. C. S. (2021). Digital competence in higher education research: A systematic literature review. *Computers & Education, 168*, 104212. DOI: 10.1016/j.compedu.2021.104212 PMID: 36568577

Zoogman, S., Goldberg, S. B., Hoyt, W. T., & Miller, L. (2015). Mindfulness interventions with youth: A meta-analysis. *Mindfulness, 6*(2), 290–302. DOI: 10.1007/s12671-013-0260-4

Compilation of References

Ahammed, S. (2019). Caste-based Oppression, Trauma and Collective Victimhood in Erstwhile South India: The Collective Therapeutic Potential of Theyyam. *Psychology and Developing Societies*, *31*(1), 88–105. DOI: 10.1177/0971333618825051

Airton, L. (2013). Leave "those kids" alone: On the conflation of school homophobia and suffering queers. *Curriculum Inquiry*, *43*(5), 532–562. DOI: 10.1111/curi.12031

Alam, A. (2022). Contemplative pedagogy: An experiment with school students for demystifying the philosophy of contemplative education. *Resilience and Transformation in Global Restructuring*, *1*, 289–300.

Alamer, A., & Almulhim, F. (2021). The interrelation between language anxiety and self-determined motivation; a mixed methods approach. *Frontiers in Education*, *6*, 618655. DOI: 10.3389/feduc.2021.618655

Alejandria, M. C. P., Casimiro, K. M. D., Gibe, J. A. L., Fernandez, N. S. F., Tumaneng, D. C., Sandoval, E. C. A., Hernandez, P. J. S., Quan-Nalus, M. A., Alipao, F. A., & Alejandria, M. A. C. P. (2023). Attaining well-being beyond the home: A socio-cultural framing of mental health among university students in the Philippines. *Health Education Journal*, *82*(2), 143–155. DOI: 10.1177/00178969221141547

Álvarez-Pérez, Y., Rivero-Santana, A., Perestelo-Pérez, L., Duarte-Díaz, A., Ramos-García, V., Toledo-Chávarri, A., Torres-Castaño, A., León-Salas, B., Infante-Ventura, D., González-Hernández, N., Rodríguez-Rodríguez, L., & Serrano-Aguilar, P. (2022). Effectiveness of Mantra-Based Meditation on Mental Health: A Systematic Review and Meta-Analysis. *International Journal of Environmental Research and Public Health, 19*(6), 3380. DOI: 10.3390/ijerph19063380

Alvear, D., Soler, J., & Cebolla, A. (2022). A. Meditators' Non-academic Definition of Mindfulness. *Mindfulness, 13*(6), 1544–1554. DOI: 10.1007/s12671-022-01899-3 PMID: 35634214

American Psychiatric Association. (2022). *DSM-5 TM guidebook the essential companion to the diagnostic and statistical manual of mental disorders* (5th ed.). Dc American Psychiatric Publishing.

American Psychological Association. (2018). Community. *APA Dictionary of Psychology.* APA website. https://dictionary.apa.org/community

American Psychological Association. (2018). Trauma. *APA dictionary of psychology*. APA website. https://dictionary.apa.org/trauma

Andres, F. (2025). The Role of Emotional Intelligence in Self-Awareness and Well-Being. In *Development of Self-Awareness and Wellbeing: Global Learning Challenges in a Shifting Society* (pp. 1-46). IGI Global Scientific Publishing. DOI: 10.4018/979-8-3373-0360-4.ch001

Antony, S., & Neelakantan, M. S. (2025). Exploring the effectiveness of mindfulness-based intervention among college students in India. *Current Psychology (New Brunswick, N.J.), 44*(10), 8232–8244. DOI: 10.1007/s12144-024-07148-1

Armstrong, M. (2010). *Armstrong's essential human resource management practice: A guide to people management*. Kogan Page Publishers.

Arvind, A., Pandya, A., Amin, L., Aggarwal, M., Agrawal, D., Tiwari, K., Singh, S., Nemkul, M., & Agarwal, P. (2021). Social strain, distress, and gender dysphoria among transgender women and Hijra in Vadodara, India. *International Journal of Transgender Health, 23*(1-2), 149–163. DOI: 10.1080/26895269.2020.1845273 PMID: 35403111

Ashkanasy, N., & Kay, A. (2023). Mindfulness and emotion: A five-level analysis. *Journal of Management & Organization, 29*(3), 406–424. DOI: 10.1017/jmo.2023.22

Austin, E. J., Farrelly, D., Black, C., & Moore, H. (2007). Emotional intelligence, Machiavellianism and emotional manipulation: Does EI have a dark side? *Personality and Individual Differences, 43*(1), 179–189. DOI: 10.1016/j.paid.2006.11.019

Azadmarzabadi, E. (2013). The effectiveness of mindfulness training on psychological symptoms in veterans with post-traumatic stress disorder. *International Journal of Behavioral Sciences, 7*(1), 67–74.

Baams, L., & Kaufman, T. M. L. (2023). Sexual Orientation and Gender Identity/Expression in Adolescent Research: Two Decades in Review. *Journal of Sex Research, 60*(7), 1004–1019. DOI: 10.1080/00224499.2023.2219245 PMID: 37307300

Baer, R., Crane, C., Miller, E., & Kuyken, W. (2019). Doing no harm in mindfulness-based programs: Conceptual issues and empirical findings. *Clinical Psychology Review, 71*(1), 101–114. DOI: 10.1016/j.cpr.2019.01.001 PMID: 30638824

Bakker, A. B., & Demerouti, E. (2007). The job demands-resources model: State of the art. *Journal of Managerial Psychology, 22*(3), 309–328. DOI: 10.1108/02683940710733115

Bak, T. (2025). Exploring the contemplative: A meditative self-inquiry of Individual Consultations practice. *Journal of Academic Language and Learning, 19*(1), 102–122.

Ballaret, J. R. (2024). Navigating the New Normal: An in-Depth Study of Adaptation and Change in Filipino Family Structures Postpandemic. *The Family Journal (Alexandria, Va.)*, •••, 10664807231225209. DOI: 10.1177/10664807231225209

Balsam, K. F., Molina, Y., Beadnell, B., Simoni, J., & Walters, K. (2011). Measuring multiple minority stress: The LGBT People of Color Microaggressions Scale. *Cultural Diversity & Ethnic Minority Psychology*, *17*(2), 163–174. DOI: 10.1037/a0023244 PMID: 21604840

Bandura, A., & Walters, R. H. (1977). *Social learning theory* (Vol. 1). Prentice hall.

Banwari, A. (2019). Re-imaginations of Yoga in the 21st Century: A Journey of Healing and Community- Building. *University of Cape Town.* https://www.researchgate.net/publication/354076309

Bartels, A., Peterson, S., & Reina, C. (2019). Understanding well-being at work: Development and validation of the eudaimonic workplace well-being scale. *PLoS One*, *14*(4), e0215957. DOI: 10.1371/journal.pone.0215957 PMID: 31022285

Barudin, J. (2024). Weaving threads of collective liberation: Intercultural wisdom among indigenous and south asian women in the indigenous yoga collective. *Race and Yoga*, *8*(1). Advance online publication. DOI: 10.5070/R38163528

Basavaraddi, I. (2015). Yoga: Its Origin, History and Development. https://doi.org/https://www.redtwigyoga.com/uploads/1/2/1/9/12195443/yoga__its_origin_history_and_development.pdf

Batrakoulis, A. (2022). Psychophysiological Adaptations to Yoga Practice in Overweight and Obese Individuals: A Topical Review. *Diseases (Basel, Switzerland)*, *10*(4), 107. DOI: 10.3390/diseases10040107

Baumeister, R. F., & Vohs, K. D. (2004). Self-regulation. *Character strengths and virtues: A handbook and classification*, 499-516.

Bazzano, A. N., Anderson, C. E., Hylton, C., & Gustat, J. (2018). Effect of mindfulness and yoga on quality of life for elementary school students and teachers: Results of a randomized controlled school-based study. *Psychology Research and Behavior Management, 11*, 81–89. DOI: 10.2147/PRBM.S157503 PMID: 29695937

Bazzano, A. N., Sun, Y., Chavez-Gray, V., Akintimehin, T., Gustat, J., Barrera, D., & Roi, C. (2022). Effect of Yoga and Mindfulness Intervention on Symptoms of Anxiety and Depression in Young Adolescents Attending Middle School: A Pragmatic Community-Based Cluster Randomized Controlled Trial in a Racially Diverse Urban Setting. *International Journal of Environmental Research and Public Health, 19*(19), 12076. DOI: 10.3390/ijerph191912076 PMID: 36231378

Bazzano, A. N., Sun, Y., Zu, Y., Fleckman, J. M., Blackson, E. A., Patel, T., Shorty-Belisle, A., Liederman, K. H., & Roi, C. (2023). Yoga and mindfulness for social-emotional development and resilience in 3–5 year-old children: Non-randomized, controlled intervention. *Psychology Research and Behavior Management, 16*, 109–118. DOI: 10.2147/PRBM.S385413 PMID: 36660255

Bennett, L. M., & Starnino, V. R. (2022). The experience of yoga for persons with complex interpersonal trauma: A phenomenological approach. *Complementary Therapies in Clinical Practice, 49*, 101674. DOI: 10.1016/j.ctcp.2022.101674

Bergen-Cico, D., Possemato, K., & Pigeon, W. (2014). Reductions in cortisol associated with primary care brief mindfulness program for veterans with PTSD. *Medical Care, 52*(Supplement 5), S25–S31. DOI: 10.1097/MLR.0000000000000224 PMID: 25397819

BeyondBlue. (2019). *BeyondBlue national mental health and wellbeing study of police and emergency services: Phase 3A—Knowledge translation guide and workbook* (Unpublished report).

Biegel, G. M., Brown, K. W., Shapiro, S. L., & Schubert, C. M. (2009). Mindfulness-based stress reduction for the treatment of adolescent psychiatric outpatients: A randomized clinical trial. *Journal of Consulting and Clinical Psychology, 77*(5), 855–866. DOI: 10.1037/a0016241 PMID: 19803566

Bigelow, L. B. (2023). Mindfulness Meditation Programs Informed by Transgender Youth. *Mindfulness, 14*(1), 128–140. DOI: 10.1007/s12671-022-02048-6 PMID: 36590761

Bishop, S. R., Lau, M., Shapiro, S., Carlson, L., Anderson, N. D., Carmody, J., Segal, Z. V., Abbey, S., Speca, M., Velting, D., & Devins, G. (2004). Mindfulness: A proposed operational definition. *Clinical Psychology : a Publication of the Division of Clinical Psychology of the American Psychological Association, 11*(3), 230–241. DOI: 10.1093/clipsy.bph077

Black, D. S. (2011). *A brief definition of mindfulness*. Mindfulness Research Guide.

Black, D. S., & Fernando, R. (2014). Mindfulness training and classroom behavior among lower-income and ethnic minority elementary school children. *Journal of Child and Family Studies, 23*(7), 1242–1246. DOI: 10.1007/s10826-013-9784-4 PMID: 25624749

Blair, C. (2010). Stress and the development of self-regulation in context. *Child Development Perspectives, 4*(3), 181–188. DOI: 10.1111/j.1750-8606.2010.00145.x PMID: 21779305

Blair, C., & Ku, S. (2022). A hierarchical integrated model of self-regulation. *Frontiers in Psychology, 13*, 725828. DOI: 10.3389/fpsyg.2022.725828 PMID: 35317011

Bloom, D. E., Cafiero, E. T., Jané-Llopis, E., Abrahams-Gessel, S., Bloom, L. R., Fathima, S., Feigl, A. B., Gaziano, T., Mowafi, M., Pandya, A., ... (2011). *The global economic burden of noncommunicable diseases*. World Economic Forum.

Bock, B. C., Dunsiger, S. I., Rosen, R. K., Thind, H., Jennings, E., Fava, J. L., Becker, B. M., Carmody, J., & Marcus, B. H. (2019). Yoga as a Complementary Therapy for Smoking Cessation: Results From BreathEasy, a Randomized Clinical Trial. *Nicotine & Tobacco Research: Official Journal of the Society for Research on Nicotine and Tobacco, 21*(11), 1517–1523. DOI: 10.1093/ntr/nty212

Bogaert, A. F., & Skorska, M. N. (2020). A short review of biological research on the development of sexual orientation. *Hormones and Behavior, 119*, 104659. DOI: 10.1016/j.yhbeh.2019.104659 PMID: 31911036

Boss, P., Beaulieu, L., Wieling, E., Turner, W., & LaCruz, S. (2003). Healing loss, ambiguity, and trauma: A community-based intervention with families of union workers missing after the 9/11 attack in New York City. *Journal of Marital and Family Therapy, 29*(4), 455–467. DOI: 10.1111/j

Bostock, S., Crosswell, A. D., Prather, A. A., & Steptoe, A. (2019). Mindfulness on-the-go: Effects of a mindfulness meditation app on work stress and well-being. *Journal of Occupational Health Psychology, 24*(1), 127–138. DOI: 10.1037/ocp0000118 PMID: 29723001

Bowlby, J. (1969). Attachment and Loss: Vol. 1. *Attachment. Attachment and Loss*. Basic Books.

Brackett, M. A., & Mayer, J. D. (2003). Convergent, discriminant, and incremental validity of competing measures of emotional intelligence. *Personality and Social Psychology Bulletin, 29*(9), 1147–1158. DOI: 10.1177/0146167203254596 PMID: 15189610

Brackett, M. A., Rivers, S. E., & Salovey, P. (2011). Emotional intelligence: Implications for personal, social, academic, and workplace success. *Social and Personality Psychology Compass, 5*(1), 88–103. DOI: 10.1111/j.1751-9004.2010.00334.x

Braun, V., & Clarke, V. (2023). Toward good practice in thematic analysis: Avoiding common problems and be (com) ing a knowing researcher. *International Journal of Transgender Health, 24*(1), 1–6. DOI: 10.1080/26895269.2022.2129597 PMID: 36713144

Breedvelt, J. J., Amanvermez, Y., Harrer, M., Karyotaki, E., Gilbody, S., Bockting, C. L., Cuijpers, P., & Ebert, D. D. (2019). The effects of meditation, yoga, and mindfulness on depression, anxiety, and stress in tertiary education students: A meta-analysis. *Frontiers in Psychiatry, 10*, 193. DOI: 10.3389/fpsyt.2019.00193 PMID: 31068842

Broderick, P. C. (2013). *Learning to Breathe: A Mindfulness Curriculum for Adolescents to Cultivate Emotion Regulation, Attention, and Performance*. New Harbinger Publications.

Brooks, A. W., Schroeder, J., Risen, J. L., Gino, F., Galinsky, A. D., Norton, M. I., & Schweitzer, M. E. (2016). RETRACTED: Don't stop believing: Rituals improve performance by decreasing anxiety. *Organizational Behavior and Human Decision Processes, 137*, 71–85. DOI: 10.1016/j.obhdp.2016.07.004

Brown, L. A. (2025). Narrative Inquiry as Contemplative Methodology. *Journal of Contemplative and Holistic Education, 3*(1), 6. DOI: 10.25035/jche.03.01.06

Brown, R. P., & Gerbarg, P. L. (2005). Sudarshan Kriya yogic breathing in the treatment of stress, anxiety, and depression: Part I—neurophysiologic model. *Journal of Alternative and Complementary Medicine (New York, N.Y.), 11*(1), 189–201. DOI: 10.1089/acm.2005.11.189 PMID: 15750381

Bruce, M. A., Skrine Jeffers, K., King Robinson, J., & Norris, K. C. (2018). Contemplative Practices: A Strategy to Improve Health and Reduce Disparities. *International Journal of Environmental Research and Public Health, 15*(10), 2253. DOI: 10.3390/ijerph15102253

Bruce-Martin, M. (2022). *Higher education lecturers' experiences of contemplative practices and mindful learning: a self-determination theory perspective*. University of Northumbria at Newcastle.

Bryant, E. F., Khanna, M., Bronkhorst, J., Myrvold, K., Shaw, S., Samuel, G., & Holen, A. (2016). *Asian traditions of meditation*. University of Hawaii Press.

Buckner, R. (2020). Zen in distress: Theorizing gender dysphoria and traumatic remembrance within Sōtō Zen meditation. *Religions, 11*(11), 582. DOI: 10.3390/rel11110582

Cahill, S., & Makadon, H. (2014). Sexual orientation and gender identity data collection in clinical settings and in electronic health records: A key to ending LGBT health disparities. *LGBT Health, 1*(1), 34–41. DOI: 10.1089/lgbt.2013.0001 PMID: 26789508

Calafato, R. (2023). Charting the motivation, self-efficacy beliefs, language learning strategies, and achievement of multilingual university students learning Arabic as a foreign language. *Asian-Pacific Journal of Second and Foreign Language Education, 8*(1), 20. DOI: 10.1186/s40862-023-00194-5

Can, A., Poyrazl, S., & Pillay, Y. (2021). Eleven Types of Adjustment Problems and Psychological Well-Being among International Students. *Eurasian Journal of Educational Research, 91*(91), 1–20. DOI: 10.14689/ejer.2021.91.1

Cao, X., Hangeldiyeva, N., Ali, A., & Pitafi, A. H. (2025). A social comparison perspective to investigating the influence of social media on employee creativity. *International Journal of Human-Computer Interaction, 41*(13), 8481–8494. DOI: 10.1080/10447318.2024.2410533

Carrière, K., Khoury, B., Günak, M. M., & Knäuper, B. (2018). Mindfulness-based interventions for weight loss: A systematic review and meta-analysis. *Obesity Reviews, 19*(2), 164–177. DOI: 10.1111/obr.12623

Carroll, A., Hepburn, S. J., & Bower, J. (2022, August). Mindful practice for teachers: Relieving stress and enhancing positive mindsets. []). Frontiers Media SA.]. *Frontiers in Education, 7*, 954098. DOI: 10.3389/feduc.2022.954098

Casey, B. J., Jones, R. M., & Hare, T. A. (2008). The adolescent brain. *Annals of the New York Academy of Sciences, 1124*(1), 111–126. DOI: 10.1196/annals.1440.010 PMID: 18400927

Casey, L. S., Reisner, S. L., Findling, M. G., Blendon, R. J., Benson, J. M., Sayde, J. M., & Miller, C. (2019). Discrimination in the United States: Experiences of lesbian, gay, bisexual, transgender, and queer Americans. *Health Services Research, 54*(S2), 1454–1466. DOI: 10.1111/1475-6773.13229 PMID: 31659745

Cauffman, E., Steinberg, L., & Piquero, A. R. (2005). Psychological, neuropsychological and physiological correlates of serious antisocial behavior in adolescence: The role of self-control. *Criminology, 43*(1), 133–176. DOI: 10.1111/j.0011-1348.2005.00005.x

Chadda, R. K., & Deb, K. S. (2013). Indian family systems, collectivistic society and psychotherapy. *Indian Journal of Psychiatry, 55*(6, Suppl 2), S299–S309. DOI: 10.4103/0019-5545.105555 PMID: 23858272

Chand, S. P., & Marwaha, R. (2023). *Anxiety*. National Library of Medicine; StatPearls Publishing. https://www.ncbi.nlm.nih.gov/books/NBK470361/

Chaplin, T. M., & Aldao, A. (2013). Gender differences in emotion expression in children: A meta-analytic review. *Psychological Bulletin, 139*(4), 735–765. DOI: 10.1037/a0030737 PMID: 23231534

Chauhan, V., & Saxena, M. T. (2024). Yoga and mindfulness in educational settings: Impact on student well-being and performance. *The Journal of Research Administration, 6*(1).

Chenowith, N. H. (2014). Cultural and linguistic obstacles for ELLs. *Beyond Words, 2*(2), 91-120. https://doi.org/DOI: 10.33508/bw.v2i2.594

Chiesa, A., & Serretti, A. (2009). Mindfulness-based stress reduction for stress management in healthy people: A review and meta-analysis. *Journal of Alternative and Complementary Medicine (New York, N.Y.), 15*(5), 593–600. DOI: 10.1089/acm.2008.0495 PMID: 19432513

Chioneso, N. A., Hunter, C. D., Gobin, R. L., McNeil Smith, S., Mendenhall, R., & Neville, H. A. (2020). Community Healing and Resistance Through Storytelling: A Framework to Address Racial Trauma in Africana Communities. *The Journal of Black Psychology, 46*(2-3), 95–121. DOI: 10.1177/0095798420929468

Choi, S. K., Divsalar, S., Flórez-Donado, J., Kittle, K., Lin, A., Meyer, I. H., & Torres-Salazar, P. (2020). Stress, health, and well-being of LGBT people in Colombia.

Chrisinger, B. W., & Rich, T. (2020). Contemplation by Design: Leveraging the "Power of the Pause" on a Large University Campus Through Built and Social Environments. *Frontiers in Public Health*, *8*, 31. DOI: 10.3389/fpubh.2020.00031

Chugh-Gupta, N., Baldassarre, F. G., & Vrkljan, B. H. (2013). Canadian Journal of Occupational. *Canadian Journal of Occupational Therapy*, *80*(3), 150–170. DOI: 10.1177/0008417413500930 PMID: 24224228

Ciarrochi, J., Heaven, P. C., & Davies, F. (2007). The impact of hope, self-esteem, and attributional style on adolescents' school grades and emotional well-being: A longitudinal study. *Journal of Research in Personality*, *41*(6), 1161–1178. DOI: 10.1016/j.jrp.2007.02.001

Cillessen, L., Johannsen, M., Speckens, A. E. M., & Zachariae, R. (2019). Mindfulness-based interventions for psychological and physical health outcomes in cancer patients and survivors: A systematic review and meta-analysis of randomized controlled trials. *Psycho-Oncology*, *28*(12), 2257–2269. DOI: 10.1002/pon.5214

Colzato, L. S., Ozturk, A., & Hommel, B. (2012). Meditate to create: The impact of focused-attention and open-monitoring training on convergent and divergent thinking. *Frontiers in Psychology*, *3*, 116. DOI: 10.3389/fpsyg.2012.00116 PMID: 22529832

Conboy, L. A., Noggle, J. J., Frey, J. L., Kudesia, R. S., & Khalsa, S. B. S. (2013). Qualitative evaluation of a high school yoga program: Feasibility and perceived benefits. *Explore (New York, N.Y.)*, *9*(3), 171–180. DOI: 10.1016/j.explore.2013.02.001 PMID: 23643372

Condon, P., Desbordes, G., Miller, W. B., & DeSteno, D. (2013). Meditation Increases Compassionate Responses to Suffering. *Psychological Science*, *24*(10), 2125–2127. DOI: 10.1177/0956797613485603

Connell, R. W. (1995). *Masculinities*. Polity.

Connell, R. W. (2015). Pride and prejudice and professionalism: The right to be out—Sexual orientation and gender identity in America's public schools. *Contexts, 12*(4), 371–391. DOI: 10.1177/1536504215611898

Conway, S. M. (2022). The role of meditation in the fight for social justice. *Mindworks Meditation & Buddhist Path*. https://mindworks.org/blog/role-meditation-social-justice/

Cook, C. C. H. (2020). The causes of human sexual orientation. *Theology and Sexuality, 27*(1), 1–19. DOI: 10.1080/13558358.2020.1818541

Cook-Cottone, C. P. (2015). *Mindfulness and yoga for self-regulation: A primer for mental health professionals*. Springer Publishing Company. DOI: 10.1891/9780826198631

Cook-Cottone, C., & Douglass, L. (2017). Yoga communities and eating disorders: Creating safe space for positive embodiment. *International Journal of Yoga Therapy, 27*(1), 87–93. DOI: 10.17761/1531-2054-27.1.87 PMID: 29131729

Copeland, W. E., Shanahan, L., Hinesley, J., Chan, R. F., Aberg, K. A., Fairbank, J. A., van den Oord, E. J. C. G., & Costello, E. J. (2018). Association of childhood trauma exposure with adult psychiatric disorders and functional outcomes. *JAMA Network Open, 1*(7), e184493. DOI: 10.1001/jamanetworkopen.2018.4493 PMID: 30646356

Čopelj, E. (2022). Mindfulness and attention: Towards a phenomenology of mindfulness as the feeling of being tuned in. *Asian Philosophy, 32*(2), 126–151. DOI: 10.1080/09552367.2022.2031015

Corrigan, L., Moran, P., McGrath, N., Eustace-Cook, J., & Daly, D. (2022). The characteristics and effectiveness of pregnancy yoga interventions: A systematic review and meta-analysis. *BMC Pregnancy and Childbirth, 22*(1), 250. DOI: 10.1186/s12884-022-04474-9

Cosker-Rowland, R. (2023). Recent work on gender identity and gender. *Analysis, 83*(4), 801–820. DOI: 10.1093/analys/anad027

Côté, S., & Miners, C. T. (2006). Emotional intelligence, cognitive intelligence, and job performance. *Administrative Science Quarterly, 51*(1), 1–28. DOI: 10.2189/asqu.51.1.1

Cott, C. A., Finch, E., Gasner, D., Yoshida, K., Thomas, S. G., & Verrier, M. C. (2004). The movement continuum theory of physical therapy. *Physiotherapy Canada. Physiotherapie Canada, 56*(4), 179–187. DOI: 10.3138/ptc.56.4.179

Craig, A. D. (2002). How do you feel? Interoception: The sense of the physiological condition of the body. *Nature Reviews. Neuroscience, 3*(8), 655–666. DOI: 10.1038/nrn894 PMID: 12154366

Craney, R. S., Watson, L. B., Brownfield, J., & Flores, M. J. (2018). Bisexual women's discriminatory experiences and psychological distress: Exploring the roles of coping and LGBTQ community connectedness. *Psychology of Sexual Orientation and Gender Diversity, 5*(3), 324–337. DOI: 10.1037/sgd0000276

Crasta, A., & Dmello, L. (2024). Empowering Women: An Analysis of Needs and Preferences for Self-Discovery, Self-Esteem, and Positive Attitude Development Training. [PIJTRCS]. *Poornaprajna International Journal of Teaching & Research Case Studies, 1*(1), 308–325. DOI: 10.64818/PIJTRCS.3107.8494.0012

Crenshaw, K. (1989) "Demarginalizing the Intersection of Race and Sex: A Black Feminist Critique of Antidiscrimination Doctrine, Feminist Theory and Antiracist Politics," *University of Chicago Legal Forum*: Vol. 1989, Article 8.

Crenshaw, K. (1991). Race, gender, and sexual harassment. s. *California Law Review, 65*, 1467.

Crick, N. R., & Dodge, K. A. (1994). A review and reformulation of social information-processing mechanisms in children's social adjustment. *Psychological Bulletin, 115*(1), 74–101. DOI: 10.1037/0033-2909.115.1.74

Crick, N. R., & Grotpeter, J. K. (1995). Relational aggression, gender, and social-psychological adjustment. *Child Development, 66*(3), 710–722. DOI: 10.2307/1131945 PMID: 7789197

Csala, B., Springinsfeld, C. M., & Köteles, F. (2021). The relationship between yoga and spirituality: A systematic review of empirical research. *Frontiers in Psychology, 12*, 695939. DOI: 10.3389/fpsyg.2021.695939 PMID: 34408712

D'augelli, A. R. (2002). Mental health problems among lesbian, gay, and bisexual youths ages 14 to 21. *Journal of Technological Advancements, 7*(3), 433–456. DOI: 10.1177/1359104502007003039

Dahl, R. E., Allen, N. B., Wilbrecht, L., & Suleiman, A. B. (2018). Importance of investing in adolescence from a developmental science perspective. *Nature, 554*(7693), 441–450. DOI: 10.1038/nature25770 PMID: 29469094

Daly, M., & Robinson, E. (2022). Depression and anxiety during COVID-19. *Lancet, 399*(10324), 518. DOI: 10.1016/S0140-6736(22)00187-8 PMID: 35123689

Das, H. K., & Govindappa, L. (2023). Anxiety, depression and social support of LGBTIQ during COVID-19 in Kerala, India. *The International Journal of Social Psychiatry, 69*(8), 1971–1978. DOI: 10.1177/00207640231183913 PMID: 37353961

Dash, B. (2024). Yama and niyama in modern leadership. *JIER, 4*(3). Advance online publication. DOI: 10.52783/jier.v4i3.1878

Datta, S., & Mukherjee, T. (2017). A clinical case study using acceptance and commitment therapy. *Indian Journal of Clinical Psychology, 44*(1), 68–74.

Davidson, R. J., & Dahl, C. J. (2016). Varieties of Contemplative Practice. *JAMA Psychiatry*. Advance online publication. DOI: 10.1001/jamapsychiatry.2016.3469

De', A. (2024). Approaches to eliminate mental health stigma, sexism, and racism in the workplace. *Journal of Women's Health Care and Management, 5*(1). Advance online publication. DOI: 10.47275/2692-0948-154

DeLuca, S. M., Kelman, A. R., & Waelde, L. C. (2018). A systematic review of ethnoracial representation and cultural adaptation of mindfulness-and meditation-based interventions. *Psychological Studies, 63*(2), 117–129. DOI: 10.1007/s12646-018-0452-z

Demerouti, E., Bakker, A. B., Nachreiner, F., & Schaufeli, W. B. (2001). The job demands-resources model of burnout. *The Journal of Applied Psychology, 86*(3), 499–512. DOI: 10.1037/0021-9010.86.3.499 PMID: 11419809

Derks, D., & Bakker, A. B. (2014). Smartphone use, work-home interference, and burnout: A diary study on the role of recovery. *Applied Psychology, 63*(3), 411–440. DOI: 10.1111/j.1464-0597.2012.00530.x

Di Marco, D., Hoel, H., & Lewis, D. (2021). Discrimination and Exclusion on Grounds of Sexual and Gender Identity: Are LGBT People's Voices Heard at the Workplace? *The Spanish Journal of Psychology, 24*, e18. Advance online publication. DOI: 10.1017/SJP.2021.16 PMID: 33745498

Dimitropoulos, G., Cullen, E., Cullen, O., Pawluk, C., McLuckie, A., Patten, S., Bulloch, A., Wilcox, G., & Arnold, P. D. (2022). "Teachers often see the red flags first": Perceptions of school staff regarding their roles in supporting students with mental health concerns. *School Mental Health, 14*(2), 402–415. DOI: 10.1007/s12310-021-09475-1

Donnelly, K. Z., Goldberg, S., & Fournier, D. (2020). A qualitative study of LoveYourBrain Yoga: A group-based yoga with psychoeducation intervention to facilitate community integration for people with traumatic brain injury and their caregivers. *Disability and Rehabilitation, 42*(17), 2482–2491. DOI: 10.1080/09638288.2018.1563638

Draper-Clarke, J. L., & Green, C. (2023). Cultivating well-being, community cohesion and sense of purpose through African contemplative practices. *University of the Witwatersrand.* https://doi.org/DOI: 10.21203/rs.3.rs-3119401/v1

Dunning, D. L., Griffiths, K., Kuyken, W., Crane, C., Foulkes, L., Parker, J., & Dalgleish, T. (2019). Research Review: The effects of mindfulness-based interventions on cognition and mental health in children and adolescents–a meta-analysis of randomized controlled trials. *Journal of Child Psychology and Psychiatry, and Allied Disciplines*, *60*(3), 244–258. DOI: 10.1111/jcpp.12980 PMID: 30345511

Durlak, J. A., Weissberg, R. P., Dymnicki, A. B., Taylor, R. D., & Schellinger, K. B. (2011). The impact of enhancing students' social and emotional learning: A meta-analysis of school-based universal interventions. *Child Development*, *82*(1), 405–432. DOI: 10.1111/j.1467-8624.2010.01564.x PMID: 21291449

Dutta, G., & Vimal, K. (2025). Educating the Whole Child: The Power of Contemplative Practices. In *Handbook of Positive Psychology and Indian Thought Systems: Transforming Education for Well-being and Happiness* (pp. 127–149). Springer Nature Singapore. DOI: 10.1007/978-981-96-4210-6_9

Earnshaw, V. A., Reisner, S. L., Juvonen, J., Hatzenbuehler, M. L., Perrotti, J., & Schuster, M. A. (2017). LGBTQ Bullying: Translating Research to Action in Pediatrics. *Pediatrics*, *140*(4), e20170432. DOI: 10.1542/peds.2017-0432 PMID: 28947607

Edyburn, K. L., & Meek, S. (2021). Seeking safety and humanity in the harshest immigration climate in a generation: A review of the literature on the effects of separation and detention on migrant and asylum-seeking children and families in the United States during the Trump administration. *Social Policy Report*, *34*(1), 1–46.

Einarsen, S., Hoel, H., Zapf, D., & Cooper, C. L. (2011). *Bullying and harassment in the workplace: Developments in theory, research, and practice* (2nd ed.). CRC Press.

Eisenberg, N., Spinrad, T. L., & Morris, A. S. (2013). 13 Prosocial Development. The Oxford handbook of developmental psychology, Vol. 2: Self and other, 2, 300.

Elias, M. J., Zins, J. E., Graczyk, P. A., & Weissberg, R. P. (2003). Implementation, sustainability, and scaling up of social-emotional and academic innovations in public schools. *School Psychology Review*, *32*(3), 303–319. DOI: 10.1080/02796015.2003.12086200

ElKayal, M. M., & Metwaly, S. M. (2022). Effectiveness of mindfulness-based intervention on post-traumatic stress symptoms among emergency nursing students. *Middle East Curr Psychiatry*, *29*, 40. DOI: 10.1186/s43045-022-00208-x

Elwy, A., Groessl, E., Eisen, S., Riley, K., Maiya, M., Lee, J., & Park, C. (2014). A systematic scoping review of yoga intervention components and study quality. *American Journal of Preventive Medicine*, *47*(2), 220–232. DOI: 10.1016/j.amepre.2014.03.012 PMID: 24996759

Emerson, D., & Hopper, E. (2011). *Overcoming trauma through yoga: Reclaiming your body*. North Atlantic Books.

Emerson, D., & Hopper, E. (2011). *Overcoming Trauma through Yoga: Reclaiming Your Body*. North Atlantic Books.

Engert, V., Klimecki, O., & Kanske, P. (2023). Spreading positive change: Societal benefits of men. *Frontiers in Psychiatry*, *14*. Advance online publication. DOI: 10.3389/fpsyt.2023.1038051

English, A., McKibben, E., Sivaramakrishnan, D., Hart, N., Richards, J., & Kelly, P. (2022). A Rapid Review Exploring the Role of Yoga in Healing Psychological Trauma. *International Journal of Environmental Research and Public Health*, *19*(23), 16180. DOI: 10.3390/ijerph192316180

Erikson, E. H. (1968). On the nature of psycho-historical evidence: In search of Gandhi. *Daedalus*, •••, 695–730.

Erikson, K. (1976). *Everything In its Path*. Simon and Schuster.

Erikson, K. (1991). Notes on Trauma and Community. *The American Imago*, *48*(4), 455–472. http://www.jstor.org/stable/26303923

Extremera, N., & Fernández-Berrocal, P. (2006). Emotional intelligence as predictor of mental, social, and physical health in university students. *The Spanish Journal of Psychology*, *9*(1), 45–51. DOI: 10.1017/S1138741600005965 PMID: 16673622

Eyerman, R., Alexander, J. C., Giesen, B., Smelser, N. J., & Sztompka, P. (2004). *Cultural Trauma and Collective Identity*. University of California Press.

Fanahei, R. (2024). Community-based social healing, community healing, and the role of "healing leader.". *Grail of Science*, *36*, 501–510. DOI: 10.36074/grail-of-science.16.02.2024.088

Farb, N. A. S., Anderson, A. K., & Segal, Z. V. (2012). The Mindful Brain and Emotion Regulation in Mood Disorders. *Canadian Journal of Psychiatry*, *57*(2), 70–77. DOI: 10.1177/070674371205700203 PMID: 22340146

Farrell, S. J., Aubry, T., & Coulombe, D. (2003). Neighborhoods and neighbors: Do they contribute to personal well-being? *Journal of Community Psychology*, *32*(1), 9–25. DOI: 10.1002/jcop.10082

Fedewa, A. L., Ahn, S., & Aspiranti, K. B. (2022). Mindfulness in Elementary School Teachers: Effects on Teacher Stress, Mental Health, and Mindfulness in the Classroom. Int. J. School. *Health*, *9*(2), 73–82. DOI: 10.30476/INTJSH.2022.92252.1169

Feinstein, B. A., Goldfried, M. R., & Davila, J. (2012). The relationship between experiences of discrimination and mental health among lesbians and gay men: An examination of internalized homonegativity and rejection sensitivity as potential mechanisms. *Journal of Consulting and Clinical Psychology*, *80*(5), 917–927. DOI: 10.1037/a0029425 PMID: 22823860

Felver, J. C., Butzer, B., Olson, K. J., Smith, I. M., & Khalsa, S. B. S. (2015). Yoga in public school improves adolescent mood and affect. *Contemporary School Psychology*, *19*(4), 184–192. DOI: 10.1007/s40688-014-0031-9 PMID: 26478825

Felver, J. C., & Jennings, P. A. (2016). Applications of mindfulness-based interventions in school settings: An introduction. *Mindfulness*, *7*(1), 1–4. DOI: 10.1007/s12671-015-0478-4

Ferbežar, N., Kopinič, A., & Gavriloski Tretjak, M. (2024). Elements of Minority Stress and Resilience in LGBTQ+ Students' Experience of Education. *Journal of Homosexuality*, *72*(3), 520–543. DOI: 10.1080/00918369.2024.2326473 PMID: 38470515

Fisher, V., Li, W. W., & Malabu, U. (2023). The effectiveness of mindfulness-based stress reduction (MBSR) on the mental health, HbA1C, and mindfulness of diabetes patients: A systematic review and meta-analysis of randomised controlled trials. *Applied Psychology. Health and Well-Being*, *15*(4), 1733–1749. DOI: 10.1111/aphw.12441 PMID: 36855248

Fiske E, Martin S, Luetkemeyer J. (2020). Building Nurses 'Resilience to Trauma through Contemplative Practices. *Creative Nursing*. 26(4):090-096. doi:DOI: 10.1891/CRNR-D-20-00054

Flanagan, B., & Clough, K. (Eds.). (2024). *The Routledge handbook of research methods in spirituality and contemplative studies*. Taylor & Francis. DOI: 10.4324/9781003341598

Flook, L., Smalley, S. L., Kitil, M. J., Galla, B. M., Kaiser-Greenland, S., Locke, J., Ishijima, E., & Kasari, C. (2010). Effects of mindful awareness practices on executive functions in elementary school children. *Journal of Applied School Psychology*, *26*(1), 70–95. DOI: 10.1080/15377900903379125

Follette, V. Palm, K.M. & Pearson, A.N. (2006). Mindfulness and trauma: implications for treatment. *J Rat-Emo Cognitive-Behav Ther 24*, 45–61/. https://doi.org/DOI: 10.1007/s10942-006-0025-2

Francis, S. E., Shawyer, F., Cayoun, B. A., Grabovac, A., & Meadows, G. (2024). Differentiating mindfulness-integrated cognitive behavior therapy and mindfulness-based cognitive therapy clinically: The why, how, and what of evidence-based practice. *Frontiers in Psychology*, *15*, 1342592. DOI: 10.3389/fpsyg.2024.1342592 PMID: 38384351

Fredrickson, B. L., Cohn, M. A., Coffey, K. A., Pek, J., & Finkel, S. M. (2008). Open hearts build lives: Positive emotions, induced through loving-kindness meditation, build consequential personal resources. *Journal of Personality and Social Psychology*, *95*(5), 1045–1062. DOI: 10.1037/a0013262 PMID: 18954193

Fullan, M. (2006). The future of educational change: System thinkers in action. *Journal of Educational Change*, *7*(3), 113–122. DOI: 10.1007/s10833-006-9003-9

Fürstenberg, N., Alfes, K., & Kearney, E. (2021). How and when paradoxical leadership benefits work engagement: The role of goal clarity and work autonomy. *Journal of Occupational and Organizational Psychology*, *94*(3), 672–705. DOI: 10.1111/joop.12344

Gaiswinkler, L., & Unterrainer, H. F. (2016). The relationship between yoga involvement, mindfulness and psychological well-being. *Complementary Therapies in Medicine*, *26*, 123–127. DOI: 10.1016/j.ctim.2016.03.011 PMID: 27261992

Gardner, P. (2021). Contemplative pedagogy: Fostering transformative learning in a critical service learning course. *Journal of Experiential Education*, *44*(2), 152–166. DOI: 10.1177/1053825920952086

Garland, E. L., Farb, N. A. R., Goldin, P., & Fredrickson, B. L. (2015). Mindfulness broadens awareness and builds eudaimonic meaning: A process model of mindful positive emotion regulation. *Psychological Inquiry*, *26*(4), 293–314. DOI: 10.1080/1047840X.2015.1064294 PMID: 27087765

Garland, E., & Howard, M. (2018). Mindfulness-based treatment of addiction: Current state of the field and envisioning the next wave of research. *Addiction Science & Clinical Practice*, *13*(1), 14. Advance online publication. DOI: 10.1186/s13722-018-0115-3 PMID: 29669599

Garnett, B. (2010). Toward understanding the academic trajectories of ESL youth. *Canadian Modern Language Review*, *66*(5), 677–710. DOI: 10.3138/cmlr.66.5.677

Gaur, P. S., Saha, S., Goel, A., Ovseiko, P., Aggarwal, S., Agarwal, V., Haq, A. U., Danda, D., Hartle, A., Sandhu, N. K., & Gupta, L. (2023). Mental healthcare for young and adolescent LGBTQ+ individuals in the Indian subcontinent. *Frontiers in Psychology*, *14*, 1060543. DOI: 10.3389/fpsyg.2023.1060543 PMID: 36743255

Gey, J. W., Yap, C. K., Leow, K., & Lo, Y. Y. (2025). Resilience as a mediator between emotional intelligence (EI) and perceived stress among young adults in Malaysia. *Discover Mental Health*, *5*(1), 1–13. DOI: 10.1007/s44192-025-00166-w PMID: 40108032

Ghabrial, M. A. (2025). Stressed and oppressed: Insider perspectives on stress induction research with LGBTQA+ People of Color. *Psychoneuroendocrinology*, *174*, 107390. DOI: 10.1016/j.psyneuen.2025.107390 PMID: 39978213

Gilbert, P., & Van Gordon, W. (2023). Compassion as a skill: A comparison of contemplative and evolution-based approaches. *Mindfulness*, *14*(10), 2395–2416. DOI: 10.1007/s12671-023-02173-w

Ginwright, S. A. (2015). Radically Healing Black Lives: A Love Note to Justice. *New Directions for Student Leadership*, *2015*(148), 33–44. DOI: 10.1002/yd.20151

Goldberg, S. B., Riordan, K. M., Sun, S., & Davidson, R. J. (2021). The Empirical Status of Mindfulness-Based Interventions: A Systematic Review of 44 Meta-Analyses of Randomized Controlled Trials. *Perspectives on Psychological Science*, *17*(1), 174569162096877. DOI: 10.1177/1745691620968771 PMID: 33593124

Goldberg, S. B., Tucker, R. P., Greene, P. A., Davidson, R. J., Wampold, B. E., Kearney, D. J., & Simpson, T. L. (2018). Mindfulness-based interventions for psychiatric disorders: A systematic review and meta-analysis. *Clinical Psychology Review*, *59*(59), 52–60. DOI: 10.1016/j.cpr.2017.10.011 PMID: 29126747

Goleman, D. (1995). *Emotional intelligence: Why it can matter more than IQ*. Bantam Books.

Gomez, E. C. (2024, July 8). Impact of Values Education in Daily Lives of Students: A Qualitative Study. *Southeast Asian Journal of Multidisciplinary Studies.* https://research.cmc.edu.ph/index.php/journals/article/view/161

Gopalan, M., & Nelson, A. A. (2019). Understanding the racial discipline gap in schools. *AERA Open*, *5*(2), 2332858419844613. DOI: 10.1177/2332858419844613

Gordon, T. (2019). Contemplativ practices. In *Holistic healing: Theories, practice and social change*. Canadian Scholars.

Government of India. (n.d.). Community. *National portal of India.* Retrieved July 31, 2025, from https://www.india.gov.in/people-groups/community

Greenberg, M. T., & Harris, A. R. (2012). Nurturing mindfulness in children and youth: Current state of research. *Child Development Perspectives*, *6*(2), 161–166. DOI: 10.1111/j.1750-8606.2011.00215.x

Greenberg, M. T., Weissberg, R. P., O'Brien, M. U., Zins, J. E., Fredericks, L., Resnik, H., & Elias, M. J. (2003). Enhancing school-based prevention and youth development through coordinated social, emotional, and academic learning. *The American Psychologist*, *58*(6-7), 466–474. DOI: 10.1037/0003-066X.58.6-7.466 PMID: 12971193

Grigoreva, D., & Szaszkó, B. (2024). Minority stress and psychological well-being in queer populations. *Scientific Reports*, *14*(1), 27084. DOI: 10.1038/s41598-024-78545-6 PMID: 39511355

Groessl, E., Maiya, M., Elwy, A., Riley, K., Sarkin, A., Eisen, S., & Park, C. (2015). The essential properties of yoga questionnaire: Development and methods. *International Journal of Yoga Therapy*, *25*(1), 51–59. DOI: 10.17761/1531-2054-25.1.51 PMID: 26667289

Gross, J. J. (1998). The emerging field of emotion regulation: An integrative review. *Review of General Psychology*, *2*(3), 271–299. DOI: 10.1037/1089-2680.2.3.271

Grover, L. T. (2020). Surviving hell Summer: Baton Rouge, Louisiana, racial polarization, and implications for community healing. *Community Development (Columbus, Ohio)*, *51*(3), 283–296. 10.1080

Gunnlaugson, O., Cueto de Souza, R., Zhao, S., Yee, A., Scott, C., & Bai, H. (2022). Revisiting the Nature of Transformative Learning Experiences in Contemplative Higher Education. *Journal of Transformative Education, 21*(1), 84-101. https://doi.org/ (Original work published 2023)DOI: 10.1177/15413446211067285

Gururaj, G., Varghese, M., Benegal, V., Rao, G. N., Pathak, K., & Singh, L. K.NMHS collaborators group. (2016). *National Mental Health Survey of India, 2015–16: Summary*. NIMHANS Publication.

Hagins, M., & Rundle, A. (2016). Yoga improves academic performance in urban high school students compared to physical education: A randomized controlled trial. *Mind, Brain and Education : the Official Journal of the International Mind, Brain, and Education Society*, *10*(2), 105–116. DOI: 10.1111/mbe.12107

Haider, T., Dai, L., & Sharma, M. (2021). Efficacy of Meditation-Based Interventions on Post-Traumatic Stress Disorder (PTSD) Among Veterans: A Narrative Review. *Advances*, *35*(1).

Halbesleben, J. R. B. (2006). Sources of social support and burnout: A meta-analytic test of the conservation of resources model. *The Journal of Applied Psychology*, *91*(5), 1134–1145. DOI: 10.1037/0021-9010.91.5.1134 PMID: 16953774

Halli, S. S., Isac, S., Bhattacharjee, P., Dutta, S., Ramesh, B. M., Lorway, R., & Blanchard, J. (2021). Suicidality among gender minorities in Karnataka, South India. *BMC Psychiatry*, *21*(1), 25. DOI: 10.1186/s12888-021-03043-2 PMID: 33430838

Hamid, T. M. H. T. A., & Idrus, F. (2021). A correlational study of the English listening and speaking anxiety in rural areas. *English Language Teaching*, *14*(2), 9–19. DOI: 10.5539/elt.v14n2p9

Harker, R., Pidgeon, A. M., Klaassen, F., & King, S. (2016). Exploring resilience and mindfulness as preventative factors for psychological distress burnout and secondary traumatic stress among human service professionals. *Work (Reading, Mass.)*, *54*(3), 631–637. DOI: 10.3233/WOR-162311 PMID: 27286075

Harrison, P. (2007). "How Shall I Say it …? " Relating the Nonrelational. *Environment & Planning A*, *39*(3), 590–608. DOI: 10.1068/a3825

Harvey, M. R., Mondesir, A. V., & Aldrich, H. (2007). Fostering resilience in traumatized communities: A community empowerment model of intervention. *Journal of Aggression, Maltreatment & Trauma*, *14*(1–2), 265–285. DOI: 10.1300/J146v14n01_14

Ha, T., & Moon, K. (2023). Distributive justice, goal clarity, and organizational citizenship behavior: The moderating role of transactional and transformational leadership. *Sustainability (Basel)*, *15*(9), 7403. DOI: 10.3390/su15097403

Hatzenbuehler, M. L., Keyes, K. M., & Hasin, D. S. (2009). State-Level Policies and Psychiatric Morbidity In Lesbian, Gay, and Bisexual Populations. *American Journal of Public Health*, *99*(12), 2275–2281. DOI: 10.2105/AJPH.2008.153510 PMID: 19833997

Hayes, S. C., Strosahl, K. D., & Wilson, K. G. (2012). *Acceptance and Commitment Therapy: The Process and Practice of Mindful Change*. Guilford Press. DOI: 10.1037/17335-000

Healing foundation. (2019). A theory of change for healing. https://cdn.healingfoundation.org.au/app/uploads/2019/04/18122127/HF_Theory_of_Change_A4_Mar2019_WEB.pdf

He, H., Zhao, L., & Liu, B. (2025). Make or break? How positive and negative family experiences affect workplace creativity: The role of energy and mindfulness. *The Journal of Creative Behavior*, *59*(1), e70002. Advance online publication. DOI: 10.1002/jocb.70002

Herek, G. M., & Garnets, L. D. (2007). Sexual Orientation and Mental Health. *Annual Review of Clinical Psychology*, *3*(1), 353–375. DOI: 10.1146/annurev.clinpsy.3.022806.091510 PMID: 17716060

Hick, S. F., & Furlotte, C. R. (2009). Mindfulness and social justice-oriented approaches: Bridging the mind and society together in social work practice. *Canadian Association for Social Work Education, 26*(1), 5–24. https://www.researchgate.net/publication/321642093

Hilton, L., Maher, A. R., Colaiaco, B., Apaydin, E., Sorbero, M. E., Booth, M., Shanman, R. M., & Hempel, S. (2017). Meditation for posttraumatic stress: Systematic review and meta-analysis. *Psychological Trauma: Theory, Research, Practice, and Policy*, *9*(4), 453–460. DOI: 10.1037/tra0000180

Hirschberger, G. (2018). Collective Trauma and the Social Construction of Meaning. *Frontiers in Psychology*, *9*, 1441. DOI: 10.3389/fpsyg.2018.01441

Hochschild, A. R. (1983). *The managed heart: Commercialization of human feeling*. University of California Press.

Hölzel, B. K., Carmody, J., Vangel, M., Congleton, C., Yerramsetti, S. M., Gard, T., & Lazar, S. W. (2011). Mindfulness practice leads to increases in regional brain gray matter density. *Psychiatry Research: Neuroimaging*, *191*(1), 36–43. DOI: 10.1016/j.pscychresns.2010.08.006 PMID: 21071182

Hooks, B. (2000). *Feminist theory: From margin to center*. Pluto press.

Horwitz, E. (2001). Language anxiety and achievement. *Annual Review of Applied Linguistics*, *21*, 112–126. DOI: 10.1017/S0267190501000071

Hülsheger, U. R., Alberts, H. J., Feinholdt, A., & Lang, J. W. (2013). Benefits of mindfulness at work: The role of mindfulness in emotion regulation, emotional exhaustion, and job satisfaction. *The Journal of Applied Psychology*, *98*(2), 310–325. DOI: 10.1037/a0031313 PMID: 23276118

Hunt, J. (2017). The impact of immigration on the educational attainment of natives. *The Journal of Human Resources*, *52*(4), 1060–1118. DOI: 10.3368/jhr.52.4.0115-6913R1

Hunt, M., Al-Braiki, F., Dailey, S., Russell, R., & Simon, K. (2018). Mindfulness training, yoga, or both? Dismantling the active components of a mindfulness-based stress reduction intervention. *Mindfulness*, *9*(2), 512–520. DOI: 10.1007/s12671-017-0793-z

Hurst, S., Maiya, M., Casteel, D., Sarkin, A., Libretto, S., Elwy, A., Park, C. L., & Groessl, E. (2018). Yoga therapy for military personnel and veterans: Qualitative perspectives of yoga students and instructors. *Complementary Therapies in Medicine*, *40*, 222–229. DOI: 10.1016/j.ctim.2017.10.008 PMID: 30219455

Huseynova, G., & İslamoğlu, M. (2024). Mind over matter: Mindfulness as a buffer against workplace incivility. *Frontiers in Psychology*, *15*, 1409326. Advance online publication. DOI: 10.3389/fpsyg.2024.1409326 PMID: 39205969

Hussain, M. S., Salam, A., & Farid, A. (2020). Students' motivation in English language learning (ELL): An exploratory study of motivation-al factors for EFL and ESL adult learners. *International Journal of Applied Linguistics and English Literature*, *9*(4), 15–28. DOI: 10.7575/aiac.ijalel.v.9n.4p.15

Hyde, J., Grieve, R., Norris, K., & Kemp, N. (2020). The dark side of emotional intelligence: The role of gender and the Dark Triad in emotional manipulation at work. *Australian Journal of Psychology*, *72*(4), 307–317. DOI: 10.1111/ajpy.12294

Hytman, L., Amestoy, M. E., Ueberholz, R. Y., & Fiocco, A. J. (2025). Cultural adaptations of mindfulness-based interventions for psychosocial well-being in ethno-racial minority populations: A systematic narrative review. *Mindfulness*, *16*(1), 21–41. DOI: 10.1007/s12671-024-02501-8

Iacono, G., Craig, S. L., Crowder, R., Brennan, D. J., & Loveland, E. K. (2022). A qualitative study of the LGBTQ+ youth affirmative mindfulness program for sexual and gender minority youth. *Mindfulness*, *13*(1), 222–237. DOI: 10.1007/s12671-021-01787-2

Ijadi-Maghsoodi, R., Koushkaki, S. R., Klomhaus, A., Aralis, H., Venegas-Murillo, A., Marlotte, L., Siddiqi, S., Lee, K., De La Cruz, S. A., & Kataoka, S. (2025). Resilience and traumatic stress among Latinx English language learners: A cross-sectional study of students from an urban school district. *BMC Public Health, 25*(1), 2458. DOI: 10.1186/s12889-025-23105-4 PMID: 40665267

Iloka, P. C. (2025). Teaching Integrity: Strategies for Fostering Ethical Behavior in Students. *UNIZIK Journal of Educational Research and Policy Studies, 19*(1).

International Labor Organization. (n.d.). *The work stress conundrum.* https://www.ilo.org/safework/events/safeday/33thinkpieces/WCMS_681594/lang--en/index.htm

Ioannou, A. (2023). Mindfulness and technostress in the workplace: A qualitative approach. *Frontiers in Psychology, 14*, 1252187. Advance online publication. DOI: 10.3389/fpsyg.2023.1252187 PMID: 38022994

Iyer, S. S. (2025). Indian Community Development – A bottom-to-top Prospective. *Global Journal of Human Social Science, 4*(3), 23–59. https://doi.org/ https://doi.org/10.55640/gjhss/Volume04Issue03-03

James, A. C., James, G., Cowdrey, F. A., Soler, A., & Choke, A. (2015). Cognitive behavioural therapy for anxiety disorders in children and adolescents. *Cochrane Database of Systematic Reviews*, 2. PMID: 25692403

James-Palmer, A., Anderson, E. Z., Zucker, L., Kofman, Y., & Daneault, J. F. (2020). Yoga as an Intervention for the Reduction of Symptoms of Anxiety and Depression in Children and Adolescents: A Systematic Review. *Frontiers in Pediatrics, 8*, 78. DOI: 10.3389/fped.2020.00078

Jansen, S., Niyonzima, J. B., & Gerbarg, P. (2024). Evaluating effects of community-based social healing model on Ubuntu, mental health and psychosocial functioning in post-genocide Rwanda: Protocol for cluster randomized control trial. *Trials, 25*, 773. DOI: 10.1186/s13063-024-08632-6

Jennings, P. A. (2015). Early childhood teachers' well-being, mindfulness, and self-compassion in relation to classroom quality and attitudes towards challenging students. *Mindfulness, 6*(4), 732–743. DOI: 10.1007/s12671-014-0312-4

Jennings, P. A., & Greenberg, M. T. (2009). The prosocial classroom: Teacher social and emotional competence in relation to student and classroom outcomes. *Review of Educational Research, 79*(1), 491–525. DOI: 10.3102/0034654308325693

Jennings, P. A., Snowberg, K. E., Coccia, M. A., & Greenberg, M. T. (2011). Improving classroom learning environments by cultivating awareness and resilience in education (CARE): Results of two pilot studies. *Journal of Classroom Interaction*, •••, 37–48.

Jiwa, A., Kelly, L., & Pierre-Hansen, N. (2008). Healing the community to heal the individual: Literature review of aboriginal community-based alcohol and substance abuse programs. *Canadian Family Physician Médecin de Famille Canadien, 54*(7), 1000–1000.e7.

Jones, S. M., & Kahn, J. (2017). *The Evidence Base for How We Learn: Supporting Students' Social, Emotional, and Academic Development. Consensus Statements of Evidence from the Council of Distinguished Scientists.* Aspen Institute.

Joseph, D. L., & Newman, D. A. (2010). Emotional intelligence: An integrative meta-analysis and cascading model. *The Journal of Applied Psychology, 95*(1), 54–78. DOI: 10.1037/a0017286 PMID: 20085406

Joshi, N., Vinu, V., Jois, S. N., Begum, F., & Salagame, K. K. (2022). The Need, Feasibility and Willingness to Explore "Meditation on Twin Hearts" as a Self-administered Tool for Mental Health Management among Transgender Women: An Exploratory Survey. *Community Mental Health Journal, 58*(4), 666–672. DOI: 10.1007/s10597-021-00869-8 PMID: 34255215

Juvonen, J., & Graham, S. (2014). Bullying in Schools: The Power of Bullies and the Plight of Victims. *Annual Review of Psychology, 65*(1), 159–185. DOI: 10.1146/annurev-psych-010213-115030 PMID: 23937767

Kabat-Zinn, J. (1990). *Full Catastrophe Living: Using the Wisdom of Your Body and Mind to Face Stress, Pain, and Illness*. Delacorte Press.

Kabat-Zinn, J. (2003). Mindfulness-based interventions in context: Past, present, and future. *Clinical Psychology : a Publication of the Division of Clinical Psychology of the American Psychological Association, 10*(2), 144–156. DOI: 10.1093/clipsy.bpg016

Kalayjian, A. S. (1995). Disaster and mass trauma: Global perspectives on post disaster mental health management. Long Branch, NJ: Vista.

Kanchibhotla, D., Rao, M. V., & Reddy, P. (2021). The prevalence of musculoskeletal disorders among Indian IT professionals and their association with mental health. *Indian Journal of Occupational and Environmental Medicine, 25*(3), 125–131. DOI: 10.4103/ijoem.ijoem_179_21 PMID: 34759597

Kao, P. C. (2024). Exploring the roles of academic expectation stress, adaptive coping, and academic resilience on perceived English proficiency. *BMC Psychology, 12*(1), 158. DOI: 10.1186/s40359-024-01630-y PMID: 38493172

Karakurt, N., & Durmaz, H. (2025). The impact of mindfulness intervention on the subjective well-being of nursing students: An experimental study. *BMC Psychology, 13*(1), 955. DOI: 10.1186/s40359-025-03334-3 PMID: 40846982

Karasek, R., & Theorell, T. (1990). *Healthy work: Stress, productivity, and the reconstruction of working life*. Basic Books.

Karas, K. J. (2021). *Discovering the Contemplative Practices, Communication Techniques and Teaching Methods of Holistic Educators Demonstrating Presence with Students*. The University of Akron.

Kattari, S. K., Walls, N. E., Speer, S. R., & Kattari, L. (2016). Exploring the relationship between transgender-inclusive providers and mental health outcomes among transgender/gender variant people. *Social Work in Health Care, 55*(8), 635–650. DOI: 10.1080/00981389.2016.1193099 PMID: 27351890

Kazemipour, F., Amin, S., & Pourseidi, B. (2012). Relationship between workplace spirituality and organizational citizenship behavior among nurses through mediation of affective organizational commitment. *Journal of Nursing Scholarship*, *44*(3), 302–310. DOI: 10.1111/j.1547-5069.2012.01456.x PMID: 22804973

Kemeny, M. E., Foltz, C., Cavanagh, J. F., Cullen, M., Giese-Davis, J., Jennings, P., Rosenberg, E. L., Gillath, O., Shaver, P. R., Wallace, B. A., & Ekman, P. (2012). Contemplative/emotion training reduces negative emotional behavior and promotes prosocial responses. *Emotion (Washington, D.C.)*, *12*(2), 338–350. DOI: 10.1037/a0026118

Kendall, P. C., Safford, S., Flannery-Schroeder, E., & Webb, A. (2004). Child anxiety treatment: Outcomes in adolescence and impact on substance use and depression at 7.4-year follow-up. *Journal of Consulting and Clinical Psychology*, *72*(2), 276–287. DOI: 10.1037/0022-006X.72.2.276 PMID: 15065961

Keng, S. L., Smoski, M. J., & Robins, C. J. (2011). Effects of mindfulness on psychological health: A review of empirical studies. *Clinical Psychology Review*, *31*(6), 1041–1056. DOI: 10.1016/j.cpr.2011.04.006

Kessler, R. C., Avenevoli, S., & Merikangas, K. R. (2012). Mood disorders in children and adolescents: An epidemiologic perspective. *Biological Psychiatry*, *49*(12), 1002–1014. DOI: 10.1016/S0006-3223(01)01129-5 PMID: 11430842

Khalsa, S. B. S., & Butzer, B. (2016). Yoga in school settings: A research review. *Annals of the New York Academy of Sciences*, *1373*(1), 45–55. DOI: 10.1111/nyas.13025 PMID: 26919395

Khalsa, S. B. S., Hickey-Schultz, L., Cohen, D., Steiner, N., & Cope, S. (2012). Evaluation of the mental health benefits of yoga in a secondary school: A preliminary randomized controlled trial. *The Journal of Behavioral Health Services & Research*, *39*(1), 80–90. DOI: 10.1007/s11414-011-9249-8 PMID: 21647811

Khapre, M., Sahoo, K., Saxena, V., Sinha, S., Luthra, G., & Joshi, A. (2024). Exploring the utilization of targeted intervention services by transgender individuals in Uttarakhand, India: A qualitative study. *Frontiers in Public Health, 12*, 1476938. DOI: 10.3389/fpubh.2024.1476938 PMID: 39697287

Khezerlou, E. (2023). Iranian EFL Students' Perceptions of Foreign Language Writing Anxiety and Perfectionism in Essay Writing. *Journal of English Language Teaching and Linguistics, 8*(3), 277–295. DOI: 10.21462/jeltl.v8i3.1167

Khoury, B., Sharma, M., Rush, S. E., & Fournier, C. (2015). Mindfulness-based stress reduction for healthy individuals: A meta-analysis. *Journal of Psychosomatic Research, 78*(6), 519–528. DOI: 10.1016/j.jpsychores.2015.03.009 PMID: 25818837

Kidd, S. A., Howison, M., Pilling, M., Ross, L. E., & McKenzie, K. (2016). Severe Mental Illness in LGBT Populations: A Scoping Review. *Psychiatric Services (Washington, D.C.), 67*(7), 779–783. DOI: 10.1176/appi.ps.201500209 PMID: 26927576

Kilduff, M., Chiaburu, D. S., & Menges, J. I. (2010). Strategic use of emotional intelligence in organizational settings: Exploring the dark side. *Research in Organizational Behavior, 30*, 129–152. DOI: 10.1016/j.riob.2010.10.002

Kiselica, M. S., & Englar-Carlson, M. (2010). Identifying, affirming, and building upon male strengths: The positive psychology/positive masculinity model of psychotherapy with boys and men. *Psychotherapy (Chicago, Ill.), 47*(3), 276–287. DOI: 10.1037/a0021159 PMID: 22402085

Klimo, K. D., Wilson, J. W., Farewell, C., Grose, R. G., Puma, J. E., Brittain, D., Shomaker, L. B., & Quirk, K. (2024). A Pilot and Feasibility Study on a Mindfulness-Based Intervention Adapted for LGBTQ+ Adolescents. *International Journal of Environmental Research and Public Health, 21*(10), 1364. DOI: 10.3390/ijerph21101364 PMID: 39457337

Knell, S. M. (1993). *Cognitive-Behavioral Play Therapy*. Jason Aronson.

Kohlberg, L., Ricks, D., & Snarey, J. (1984). Childhood development as a predictor of adaptation in adulthood. *Genetic Psychology Monographs*.

Koileri, V. (2025). Healing The Psyche from Caste Violence: Addressing the Cumulative Psychological Trauma of Generations of Oppression and Deprivation Among the SC/ST Community in India. *International Journal of Indian Psychology, 13*(2). Advance online publication. DOI: 10.25215/1302.125

Kosciw, J. G., Clark, C. M., Truong, N. L., & Zongrone, A. D. (2020). The 2019 National School Climate Survey: The Experiences of Lesbian, Gay, Bisexual, Transgender, and Queer Youth in Our Nation's Schools. A Report from GLSEN. Gay, Lesbian and Straight Education Network (GLSEN). 121 West 27th Street Suite 804, New York, NY 10001.

Kosciw, J. G., Greytak, E. A., Giga, N. M., Villenas, C., & Danischewski, D. J. (2018). The 2017 national school climate survey. GLSEN. *The 2017 National School Climate Survey*, 2019-10.

Kumar, A., Chawla, K., Mishra, A., Singh, G., Pandey, A., & Rikhari, P. (2023). Are doctors feeling burnout? Multicenter cross-sectional study on burnout syndrome and its determinants during the ongoing pandemic. *Indian Journal of Psychiatry*, *65*(5), 541–549. DOI: 10.4103/indianjpsychiatry.indianjpsychiatry_726_22 PMID: 37397848

Kurumaji, A. (2013). [The trends of mood disorders in ICD-11: Bipolar and depressive disorders]. *Seishin Shinkeigaku Zasshi = Psychiatria et Neurologia Japonica, 115*(1), 60–68. https://pubmed.ncbi.nlm.nih.gov/23691796/

Kuyken, W., Hayes, R., Barrett, B., Byng, R., Dalgleish, T., Kessler, D., Lewis, G., Watkins, E., Brejcha, C., Cardy, J., Causley, A., Cowderoy, S., Evans, A., Gradinger, F., Kaur, S., Lanham, P., Morant, N., Richards, J., Shah, P., & Byford, S. (2015). Effectiveness and cost-effectiveness of mindfulness-based cognitive therapy compared with maintenance antidepressant treatment in the prevention of depressive relapse or recurrence (PREVENT): A randomised controlled trial. *Lancet*, *386*(9988), 63–73. DOI: 10.1016/S0140-6736(14)62222-4 PMID: 25907157

Kwon, P. (2013). Resilience in Lesbian, Gay, and Bisexual Individuals. *Personality and Social Psychology Review*, *17*(4), 371–383. DOI: 10.1177/1088868313490248 PMID: 23904452

Ladson-Billings, G. (1995). Toward a theory of culturally relevant pedagogy. *American Educational Research Journal*, *32*(3), 465–491. DOI: 10.3102/00028312032003465

Lambert, A. B., & Stapp, A. C. (2020). The Impact of Mindfulness-Based Yoga Interventions on Fifth-Grade Students Perceived Stress and Anxiety. *International Electronic Journal of Elementary Education*, *12*(5), 471–480. DOI: 10.26822/iejee.2020562137

LaMontagne, A. D., Martin, A., Page, K. M., Reavley, N. J., Noblet, A. J., Milner, A. J., Keegel, T., & Smith, P. M. (2014). Workplace mental health: Developing an integrated intervention approach. *BMC Psychiatry*, *14*(1), 131. DOI: 10.1186/1471-244X-14-131 PMID: 24884425

LaMontagne, A. D., Martin, A., Page, K. M., Reavley, N., Noblet, A., Milner, A., Keegel, T., Allisey, A., Papas, A., & Witt, K.. (2019). Developing an integrated approach to workplace mental health. In Hudson, H. L., & Nigam, J. A. (Eds.), *Total worker health* (pp. 211–227). American Psychological Association. DOI: 10.1037/0000149-013

Laplaud, N., Perrochon, A., & Gallou-Guyot, M. (2023). Management of post-traumatic stress disorder symptoms by yoga: An overview. *BMC Complementary Medicine and Therapies*, *23*, 258. DOI: 10.1186/s12906-023-04074-w

Lashari, S. A., Awang-Hashim, R., Lashari, T. A., & Kaur, A. (2023). Acculturation stress and social support for international students' adjustment in Malaysia: Does language proficiency matter? *Journal of Applied Research in Higher Education*, *15*(2), 496–508. DOI: 10.1108/JARHE-07-2021-0285

Lau, E. N. S. (2024). Implementing Contemplative Education for Enhancing Spirituality in Hong Kong Schools. *The Routledge International Handbook of Life and Values Education in Asia*, 441-452.

Leary, M. R., & Baumeister, R. F. (2000). The nature and function of self-esteem: Sociometer theory. In Vol. 32, pp. 1–62). Advances in Experimental Social Psychology. Elsevier., DOI: 10.1016/S0065-2601(00)80003-9

Leary, M. R., & Kowalski, R. M. (1990). Impression management: A literature review and two-component model. *Psychological Bulletin, 107*(1), 34–47. DOI: 10.1037/0033-2909.107.1.34

Lee, J., Lee, K., Lee, J., Hwang, J., & Park, D. (2024). Analysis of job stress, depression, and mindfulness among Korean physical therapists during the COVID-19 pandemic. *Work (Reading, Mass.), 80*(2), 741–749. DOI: 10.1177/10519815241289659 PMID: 40172849

Lee, M. Y., Zaharlick, A., & Akers, D. (2015). Impact of Meditation on Mental Health Outcomes of Female Trauma Survivors of Interpersonal Violence With Co-Occurring Disorders: A Randomized Controlled Trial. *Journal of Interpersonal Violence, 32*(14), 2139–2165. DOI: 10.1177/0886260515591277

Legare, C., Burger, O., Johnson, T., Mor, N., & Saldanha, N. (2022). Leverage the power of ritual to improve community health worker efficacy and public health outcomes: Lessons from Bihar, India. *The Lancet Regional Health. Southeast Asia, 1*, 100006. DOI: 10.1016/j.lansea.2022.04.002

Lehrer, P., Kaur, K., Sharma, A., Shah, K., Huseby, R., Bhavsar, J., Sgobba, P., & Zhang, Y. (2020, September). Heart Rate Variability Biofeedback Improves Emotional and Physical Health and Performance: A Systematic Review and Meta Analysis. [Erratum in: Appl Psychophysiol Biofeedback. 2021 Dec;46] [4] [:389. doi: 10.1007/s10484-021-09526-y. PMID: 32385728]. *Applied Psychophysiology and Biofeedback, 45*(3), 109–129. DOI: 10.1007/s10484-020-09466-z PMID: 32385728

Leiter, M. P., & Maslach, C. (2005). *Banishing burnout: Six strategies for improving your relationship with work.* Jossey-Bass.

Lemay, V., Hoolahan, J., & Buchanan, A. (2019). Impact of a yoga and meditation intervention on students' stress and anxiety levels. *American Journal of Pharmaceutical Education, 83*(5), 7001. DOI: 10.5688/ajpe7001 PMID: 31333265

Leow, S., Leow, K., & Ean, C. L. C. (2023). Satisfaction of basic psychological needs and eudaimonic well-being among first-year university students. *Cogent Social Sciences*, *9*(2), 2275441. DOI: 10.1080/23311886.2023.2275441

Levine, G. N., Lange, R. A., Bairey-Merz, C. N., Davidson, R. J., Jamerson, K., & Mehta, S. C.Jr, & American Heart Association Council on Clinical Cardiology; P. K., Michos, E. D., Norris, K., Ray, I. B., Saban, K. L., Shah, T., Stein, R., Smith, Cardiovascular and Stroke Nursing; and Council on Hypertension. (2017). Meditation and Cardiovascular Risk Reduction: A Scientific Statement From the American Heart Association. *Journal of the American Heart Association*, *6*(10), e002218. DOI: 10.1161/JAHA.117.002218

Leyland, A., Rowse, G., & Emerson, L. M. (2019). Experimental effects of mindfulness inductions on self-regulation: Systematic review and meta-analysis. *Emotion (Washington, D.C.)*, *19*(1), 108–122. DOI: 10.1037/emo0000425 PMID: 29578742

Liao, K. Y. H., & Wei, M. (2014). Academic stress and positive affect: Asian value and self-worth contingency as moderators among Chinese international students. *Cultural Diversity & Ethnic Minority Psychology*, *20*(1), 107–115. DOI: 10.1037/a0034071 PMID: 24491130

Lieberman, A. F., & Van Horn, P. (2011). *Psychotherapy with infants and young children: Repairing the effects of stress and trauma on early attachment*. Guilford Press.

Lincoln, Y. S., & Denzin, N. K. (Eds.). (2003). *Turning points in qualitative research: Tying knots in a handkerchief* (Vol. 2). Rowman Altamira.

Lindahl, J. R., Fisher, N. E., Cooper, D. J., Rosen, R. K., & Britton, W. B. (2017). The varieties of contemplative experience: A mixed-methods study of meditation-related challenges in Western Buddhists. *PLoS One*, *12*(5), e0176239. DOI: 10.1371/journal.pone.0176239 PMID: 28542181

Linton, M., Dieppe, P., & Medina-Lara, A. (2016). Review of 99 self-report measures for assessing well-being in adults: Exploring dimensions of well-being and developments over time. *BMJ Open*, *6*(7), e010641. DOI: 10.1136/bmjopen-2015-010641 PMID: 27388349

Livheim, F., Hayes, L., Ghaderi, A., Magnusdottir, T., Högfeldt, A., Rowse, J., Turner, S., Hayes, S. C., & Tengström, A. (2015). The effectiveness of acceptance and commitment therapy for adolescent mental health: Swedish and Australian pilot outcomes. *Journal of Child and Family Studies*, *24*(4), 1016–1030. DOI: 10.1007/s10826-014-9912-9

Lorenzini, J. A., Wong-Parodi, G., & Garfin, D. R. (2023). Associations between mindfulness and mental health after collective trauma: Results from a longitudinal, representative, probability-based survey. *Anxiety, Stress, and Coping*, *37*(3), 361–378. DOI: 10.1080/10615806.2023.2267454

Luu, K., & Hall, P. A. (2016). Hatha yoga and executive function: A systematic review. *Journal of Alternative and Complementary Medicine (New York, N.Y.)*, *22*(2), 125–133. DOI: 10.1089/acm.2014.0091 PMID: 26398441

Mackenzie, M. J., Wurz, A. J., Yamauchi, Y., Pires, L. A., & Culos-Reed, S. N. (2016). Yoga Helps Put the Pieces Back Together: A Qualitative Exploration of a Community-Based Yoga Program for Cancer Survivors. *Evidence-Based Complementary and Alternative Medicine : eCAM, 1832515*. Advance online publication. DOI: 10.1155/2016/1832515

Mahalik, J. R., Locke, B., Ludlow, L., Diemer, M., Scott, R. P. J., Gottfried, M., & Freitas, G. (2003). Development of the Conformity to Masculine Norms Inventory. *Psychology of Men & Masculinity*, *4*(1), 3–25. DOI: 10.1037/1524-9220.4.1.3

Maharishi Mahesh Yogi. (1977b). Foreword: The scientific age is rising to be the age of enlightenment. In Orme-Johnson, D. W., & Farrow, J. T. (Eds.), *Scientific Research on the Transcendental Meditation Program. 1*. Maharishi European Research University Press.

Maharishi Mahesh Yogi. (1986b). *Life supported by natural law: Lectures by Maharishi Mahesh Yogi*. Age of Enlightenment Press.

Mahfouz, J. (2018). Mindfulness training for school administrators: Effects on well-being and leadership. *Journal of Educational Administration, 56*(6), 602–619. DOI: 10.1108/JEA-12-2017-0171

Main, C. J., George, S. Z., & Foster, N. E. (2010). Psychosocial interventions and pain: Implications for physiotherapy. *Manual Therapy*, *15*(6), 486–490. DOI: 10.1016/j.math.2010.07.002

Mak, A. S., Bodycott, P., & Ramburuth, P. (2015). Beyond host language proficiency: Coping resources predicting international students' satisfaction. *Journal of Studies in International Education, 19*(5), 460–475. DOI: 10.1177/1028315315587109

Malhotra, A. K. (2017). *An Introduction to Yoga Philosophy: an annotated translation of the Yoga Sutras*. Routledge. DOI: 10.4324/9781315262635

Malhotra, S., & Patra, B. N. (2014). Prevalence of child and adolescent psychiatric disorders in India: A systematic review and meta-analysis. *Child and Adolescent Psychiatry and Mental Health*, *8*(1), 22. DOI: 10.1186/1753-2000-8-22 PMID: 25071865

Malik, S., Qin, H., & Oteir, I. (2021). Perceived Psychological, Linguistic and Socio-Cultural Obstacles: An Investigation of English Communication Apprehension in EFL Learners. *International Journal of Instruction, 14*(4), 733–752. DOI: 10.29333/iji.2021.14442a

Mamede, A., Merkelbach, I., Noordzij, G., & Denktas, S. (2022). Mindfulness as a protective factor against depression, anxiety and psychological distress during the COVID-19 pandemic: Emotion regulation and insomnia symptoms as mediators. *Frontiers in Psychology*, *13*, 820959. Advance online publication. DOI: 10.3389/fpsyg.2022.820959 PMID: 35432084

Manocha, R., Black, D., Sarris, J., & Stough, C. (2011). A randomized, controlled trial of meditation for work stress, anxiety and depressed mood in full-time workers. *Evidence-Based Complementary and Alternative Medicine : eCAM*, *2011*(1), 960583. DOI: 10.1155/2011/960583 PMID: 21716708

Markus, H. R., & Kitayama, S. (1991). Cultural variation in the self-concept. In *The self: Interdisciplinary approaches* (pp. 18–48). Springer New York. DOI: 10.1007/978-1-4684-8264-5_2

Marschke, E., Preziosi, R., & Harrington, W. (2011). Professionals and executives support a relationship between organizational commitment and spirituality in the workplace. *Journal of Business & Economics Research, 7*(8). Advance online publication. DOI: 10.19030/jber.v7i8.2320

Marshal, M. P., Dietz, L. J., Friedman, M. S., Stall, R., Smith, H. A., McGinley, J., Thoma, B. C., Murray, P. J., D'Augelli, A. R., & Brent, D. A. (2011). Suicidality and depression disparities between sexual minority and heterosexual youth: A meta-analytic review. *The Journal of Adolescent Health, 49*(2), 115–123. DOI: 10.1016/j.jadohealth.2011.02.005 PMID: 21783042

Maslach, C., & Leiter, M. P. (2016). Understanding the burnout experience: Recent research and its implications for psychiatry. *World Psychiatry; Official Journal of the World Psychiatric Association (WPA), 15*(2), 103–111. DOI: 10.1002/wps.20311 PMID: 27265691

Maslow, A. H. (1954). Motivation and personality. *Harper's.*

Matsumoto, D., Yoo, S. H., & Nakagawa, S. (2008). Culture, emotion regulation, and adjustment. *Journal of Personality and Social Psychology, 94*(6), 925–937. DOI: 10.1037/0022-3514.94.6.925 PMID: 18505309

Matsuzaka, S., Romanelli, M., & Hudson, K. D. (2021). "Render a service worthy of me": A qualitative study of factors influencing access to LGBTQ-specific health services. *SSM. Qualitative Research in Health, 1*, 100019. DOI: 10.1016/j.ssmqr.2021.100019

Matthews, A. K., Hughes, T. L., Johnson, T., Razzano, L. A., & Cassidy, R. (2002). Prediction of Depressive Distress in a Community Sample of Women: The Role of Sexual Orientation. *American Journal of Public Health, 92*(7), 1131–1139. DOI: 10.2105/AJPH.92.7.1131 PMID: 12084697

Mavroveli, S., Petrides, K. V., Rieffe, C., & Bakker, F. (2007). Trait emotional intelligence, psychological well-being and peer-rated social competence in adolescence. *British Journal of Developmental Psychology, 25*(2), 263–275. DOI: 10.1348/026151006X118577

McConnell, E. A., Janulis, P., Phillips, G.II, Truong, R., & Birkett, M. (2018). Multiple Minority Stress and LGBT Community Resilience among Sexual Minority Men. *Psychology of Sexual Orientation and Gender Diversity, 5*(1), 1–12. DOI: 10.1037/sgd0000265 PMID: 29546228

McElligott, D. (2010). Healing. *Journal of Holistic Nursing, 28*(4), 251–259. DOI: 10.1177/0898010110376321

McEwen, B. S. (1998). Protective and damaging effects of stress mediators. *The New England Journal of Medicine, 338*(3), 171–179. DOI: 10.1056/NEJM199801153380307 PMID: 9428819

McLaughlin, K. A., Koenen, K. C., Hill, E. D., Petukhova, M., Sampson, N. A., Zaslavsky, A. M., & Kessler, R. C. (2017). Trauma exposure and posttraumatic stress disorder in a national sample of adolescents. *Journal of the American Academy of Child and Adolescent Psychiatry, 52*(8), 815–830. DOI: 10.1016/j.jaac.2013.05.011 PMID: 23880492

Mehling, W. E., Gopisetty, V., Daubenmier, J., Price, C. J., Hecht, F. M., & Stewart, A. (2009). Body awareness: Construct and self-report measures. *PLoS One, 4*(5), e5614. DOI: 10.1371/journal.pone.0005614 PMID: 19440300

Mereish, E. H., & Bradford, J. B. (2014). Intersecting identities and substance use problems: Sexual orientation, gender, race, and lifetime substance use problems. *Journal of Studies on Alcohol and Drugs, 75*(1), 179–188. DOI: 10.15288/jsad.2014.75.179 PMID: 24411810

Mesquita, B. (2001). Emotions in collectivist and individualist contexts. *Journal of Personality and Social Psychology, 80*(1), 68–74. DOI: 10.1037/0022-3514.80.1.68 PMID: 11195892

Messenger, J. C., Ghosheh, N., & Bourne, M. (2017). *Working anytime, anywhere: The effects on the world of work.* International Labour Office.

Mestre, J. M., Guil, R., Lopes, P. N., Salovey, P., & Gil-Olarte, P. (2006). Emotional intelligence and social and academic adaptation to school. *Psicothema, 18*(suppl), 112–117. PMID: 17295967

Meyer, I. H. (2013). Prejudice, social stress, and mental health in lesbian, gay, and bisexual populations: Conceptual issues and research evidence. *Psychology of Sexual Orientation and Gender Diversity, 1*(S), 3–26. DOI: 10.1037/2329-0382.1.S.3

Meyer, I. H. (2003). Prejudice, social stress, and mental health in lesbian, gay, and bisexual populations: Conceptual issues and research evidence. *Psychological Bulletin, 129*(5), 674–697. DOI: 10.1037/0033-2909.129.5.674 PMID: 12956539

Meyer, I. H. (2015). Resilience in the study of minority stress and health of sexual and gender minorities. *Psychology of Sexual Orientation and Gender Diversity*, *2*(3), 209–213. DOI: 10.1037/sgd0000132

Michalski, C. A., Diemert, L. M., Helliwell, J. F., Goel, V., & Rosella, L. C. (2020). Relationship between sense of community belonging and self-rated health across life stages. *SSM - Population Health*, *12*, 100676. DOI: 10.1016/j.ssmph.2020.100676

Mishra, S. (2022). A Psychological Exploration Research on LGBT Community. *International Journal of Indian Psychology*, *10*(2). Advance online publication. DOI: 10.25215/1002.068

Monteiro, L. M., Musten, R. F., & Compson, J. (2015). Traditional and contemporary mindfulness: Finding the middle path in the tangle of concerns. *Mindfulness*, *6*(1), 1–13. DOI: 10.1007/s12671-014-0301-7

Moodley, R., & West, W. (2005). *Integrating traditional healing practices into counseling and psychotherapy*. SAGE Publications.

Morris, B. J. (2023). A brief history of lesbian, gay, bisexual, and transgender social movements. *American psychological association, Psychology topics, Sexual orientation and gender diversity. Preuzeto s:* https://www.apa.org/topics/lgbtq/history

Mueller, D., Bacalso, E., Ortega-Williams, A., Pate, D. J.Jr, & Topitzes, J. (2021). A mutual process of healing self and healing the community: A qualitative study of coping with and healing from stress, adversity, and trauma among diverse residents of a midwestern city. *Journal of Community Psychology, 49*(5), 1169–1194. DOI: 10.1002/jcop.22530

Mumtazah, L. (2024). The Role of Emotion Regulation in Increasing Resilience to Stress and Life Pressure. *Asian Journal of Multidisciplinary Research, 1*(2), 88–96. DOI: 10.59613/bs2n5f66

Murthy, R. S. (2017). National Mental Health Survey of India 2015–2016. *Indian Journal of Psychiatry, 59*(1), 21–26. DOI: 10.4103/psychiatry.IndianJPsychiatry_102_17 PMID: 28529357

Mustanski, B., Andrews, R., & Puckett, J. A. (2016). The effects of cumulative victimization on mental health among lesbian, gay, bisexual, and transgender adolescents and young adults. *American Journal of Public Health, 106*(3), 527–533. DOI: 10.2105/AJPH.2015.302976 PMID: 26794175

Narvaez, D. (2010). Building a sustaining classroom climate for purposeful ethical citizenship. In *International research handbook on values education and student wellbeing* (pp. 659–673). Springer Netherlands. DOI: 10.1007/978-90-481-8675-4_38

National centre of complementary and integrative health. (2022). Meditation and mindfulness: Effectiveness and safety. *NCCIH*. Retrieved August 3, 2025, from https://www.nccih.nih.gov/health/meditation-and-mindfulness-effectiveness-and-safety

Neff, K. (2003). Self-compassion: An alternative conceptualization of a healthy attitude toward oneself. *Self and Identity, 2*(2), 85–101. DOI: 10.1080/15298860309032

Neff, K. D., & Germer, C. K. (2013). A pilot study and randomized controlled trial of the mindful self-compassion program. *Journal of Clinical Psychology, 69*(1), 28–44. DOI: 10.1002/jclp.21923 PMID: 23070875

Nejadghaderi, S. A., Mousavi, S. E., Fazlollahi, A., Motlagh Asghari, K., & Garfin, D. R. (2024). Efficacy of yoga for posttraumatic stress disorder: A systematic review and meta-analysis of randomized controlled trials. *Psychiatry Research, 340*, 116098. DOI: 10.1016/j.psychres.2024.116098

Nidich, S., Mills, P. J., Rainforth, M., Heppner, P., Schneider, R. H., Rosenthal, N. E., Salerno, J., Gaylord-King, C., & Rutledge, T. (2018). Non-trauma-focused meditation versus exposure therapy in veterans with post-traumatic stress disorder: A randomised controlled trial. *The Lancet. Psychiatry, 5*(12), 975–986. DOI: 10.1016/S2215-0366(18)30384-5

Nishina, A., Juvonen, J., & Witkow, M. R. (2005). Sticks and Stones May Break My Bones, but Names Will Make Me Feel Sick: The Psychosocial, Somatic, and Scholastic Consequences of Peer Harassment. *Journal of Clinical Child and Adolescent Psychology, 34*(1), 37–48. DOI: 10.1207/s15374424jccp3401_4 PMID: 15677279

Noddings, N. (2005). Identifying and responding to needs in education. *Cambridge Journal of Education, 35*(2), 147–159. DOI: 10.1080/03057640500146757

Noggle, J. J., Steiner, N. J., Minami, T., & Khalsa, S. B. S. (2012). Benefits of yoga for psychosocial well-being in a US high school curriculum: A preliminary randomized controlled trial. *Journal of Developmental and Behavioral Pediatrics, 33*(3), 193–201. DOI: 10.1097/DBP.0b013e31824afdc4 PMID: 22343481

Nolen-Hoeksema, S., & Girgus, J. S. (1994). The emergence of gender differences in depression during adolescence. *Psychological Bulletin, 115*(3), 424–443. DOI: 10.1037/0033-2909.115.3.424 PMID: 8016286

Noorollahi, A., Shahabizadeh, F., & Nasri, M. (2024). Comparing The Effectiveness of Mindfulness-Based Therapy and Paradoxical Treatment on Distress Tolerance in Adolescents with Social Anxiety Symptoms. *International Journal of Education and Cognitive Sciences, 5*(3), 157–168. DOI: 10.61838/kman.ijecs.5.3.18

Number analytics. (2025). Rituals in modern society. Retrieved August 3, 2025, from https://www.numberanalytics.com/blog/rituals-in-modern-society

OECD. (2015). *Fit mind, fit job: From evidence to practice in mental health and work (Mental Health and Work).* OECD Publishing., DOI: 10.1787/9789264228283-

Ohrt, J., Webster, L., & De La Garza, M. (2014). The effects of a success skills group on adolescents' self-regulation, self-esteem, and perceived learning competence. *Professional School Counseling, 18*(1), 2156759X0001800113. https://doi.org/DOI: 10.1177/2156759X000180011

Orme-Johnson, D. W., Cavanaugh, K. L., Dillbeck, M. C., & Goodman, R. S. (2022). Field-effects of consciousness: A seventeen-year study of the effects of group practice of the transcendental meditation and tm-sidhi programs on reducing national stress in the united states. *World Journal of Social Science, 9*(2), 1. DOI: 10.5430/wjss.v9n2p1

Orme-Johnson, D., Alexander, C., Davies, J., Chander, H., & Larimore, W. (1988). International peace project: The effects of the maharishi Technology of the Unified Field. *The Journal of Conflict Resolution, 32*, 776–12. DOI: 10.1177/0022002788032004009

Ortiz, R., & Sibinga, E. (2017). The role of mindfulness in reducing the adverse effects of childhood stress and trauma. *Children (Basel, Switzerland), 4*(3), 16. DOI: 10.3390/children4030016

Oteir, I. N., & Al-Otaibi, A. N. (2019). Foreign language anxiety: A systematic review. *Arab World English Journal, 10*(3), 309–317. DOI: 10.24093/awej/vol10no3.21

Pachankis, J. E. (2007). The psychological implications of concealing a stigma: A cognitive-affective-behavioral model. *Psychological Bulletin, 133*(2), 328–345. DOI: 10.1037/0033-2909.133.2.328 PMID: 17338603

Pachankis, J. E., Rendina, H. J., Restar, A., Ventuneac, A., Grov, C., & Parsons, J. T. (2015). A minority stress—Emotion regulation model of sexual compulsivity among highly sexually active gay and bisexual men. *Health Psychology*, *34*(8), 829–840. DOI: 10.1037/hea0000180 PMID: 25528179

Pagis, M., & Tal, O. (2022). Collective mindfulness: Somatic attention to group and self in meditation practice in Israel. *Anthropology Today*, *38*, 13–16. DOI: 10.1111/1467-8322.12708

Paluska, S. A., & Schwenk, T. L. (2000). Physical activity and mental health: Current concepts. *Sports Medicine (Auckland, N.Z.)*, *29*(3), 167–180. DOI: 10.2165/00007256-200029030-00003 PMID: 10739267

Para, E. A. (2008). The Role of Social Support in Identity Formation: A Literature Review. *Graduate Journal of Counseling Psychology, 1*(1). http://epublications.marquette.edu/gjcp/vol1/iss1/9

Park, E. Y., Oliver, T. R., Peppard, P. E., & Malecki, K. C. (2023). Sense of community and mental health: A cross-sectional analysis from a household survey in Wisconsin. *Family Medicine and Community Health*, *11*(2). Advance online publication. DOI: 10.1136/fmch-2022-001971

Park, S., Ueno, S., & Sugita, M. (2025). The Impact of Resilience and Self-Regulation on L2 Proficiency among ESL Learners. *International Journal of TESOL Studies*, *7*(1). Advance online publication. DOI: 10.58304/ijts.20250107

Paulhus, D. L., & Reid, D. B. (1991). Enhancement and denial in socially desirable responding. *Journal of Personality and Social Psychology*, *60*(2), 307–317. DOI: 10.1037/0022-3514.60.2.307

Peng, A., & Patterson, M. M. (2022). Relations among cultural identity, motivation for language learning, and perceived English language proficiency for international students in the United States. *Language, Culture and Curriculum, 35*(1), 67–82. DOI: 10.1080/07908318.2021.1938106

Petrides, K. V., Mikolajczak, M., Mavroveli, S., Sanchez-Ruiz, M. J., Furnham, A., & Pérez-González, J. C. (2016). Developments in trait emotional intelligence research. *Emotion Review*, *8*(4), 335–341. DOI: 10.1177/1754073916650493

Philippine Department of Education. (2023). Good Manners and Right Conduct and Values Education Curriculum. https:// www. deped. gov. ph/ wp - content/ uploads/ MATATAG - GMRC - and - VE - Grades - 1 - 4 - and - 7. pdf

Pidgeon, A. M., & Keye, M. (2014). Relationship between resilience, mindfulness, and pyschological well-being in university students. *International Journal of Liberal Arts and Social Science*, *2*(5), 27–32. http://www.ijlass.org/data/frontImages/gallery/Vol._2_No._5/3.pdf

Pinderhughes, H., Davis, R. A., & Williams, M. (2015). *Adverse community experiences and resilience: A framework for addressing and preventing community trauma*. Prevention Institute.

Plöderl, M., & Tremblay, P. (2015). Mental health of sexual minorities. A systematic review. *International Review of Psychiatry (Abingdon, England)*, *27*(5), 367–385. DOI: 10.3109/09540261.2015.1083949 PMID: 26552495

Polanczyk, G. V., Salum, G. A., Sugaya, L. S., Caye, A., & Rohde, L. A. (2015). Annual research review: A meta-analysis of the worldwide prevalence of mental disorders in children and adolescents. *Journal of Child Psychology and Psychiatry, and Allied Disciplines*, *56*(3), 345–365. DOI: 10.1111/jcpp.12381 PMID: 25649325

Pollack, W. S. (1998). *Real boys: Rescuing our sons from the myths of boyhood*. Henry Holt and Company.

Porges, S. W. (2007). The polyvagal perspective. *Biological Psychology*, *74*(2), 116–143. DOI: 10.1016/j.biopsycho.2006.06.009 PMID: 17049418

Pretty, G. M. H. (2002). Young People's Development of the Community-Minded Self. *The Plenum Series in Social. Clinical Psychology*, •••, 183–203. DOI: 10.1007/978-1-4615-0719-2_10

Prezza, M., Amici, M., Roberti, T., & Tedeschi, G. (2001). Sense of community referred to the whole town: Its relations with neighboring, loneliness, life satisfaction, and area of residence. *Journal of Community Psychology*, *29*(1), 29–52. DOI: 10.1002/1520-6629(200101)29:1<29:aid-jcop3>3.0.co;2-c

Price, C. J., & Hooven, C. (2018). Interoceptive awareness skills for emotion regulation: Theory and approach of mindful awareness in body-oriented therapy (MABT). *Frontiers in Psychology*, *9*, 798. DOI: 10.3389/fpsyg.2018.00798 PMID: 29892247

Priya, K. R. (2012). Trauma Reactions, Suffering, and Healing among Riot-Affected Internally Displaced Children of Gujarat, India: A Qualitative Inquiry. *Qualitative Research in Psychology*, *9*(3), 189–209. DOI: 10.1080/14780887.2010.500353

Pruessner, L., Timm, C., Kalmar, J., Bents, H., Barnow, S., & Mander, J. (2024). Sven Barnow, & Mander, J. (2024). Emotion Regulation as a Mechanism of Mindfulness in Individual Cognitive-Behavioral Therapy for Depression and Anxiety Disorders. *Depression and Anxiety*, *2024*(1), 1–16. DOI: 10.1155/2024/9081139 PMID: 40226724

Pullen Sansfaçon, A., Medico, D., Suerich-Gulick, F., & Temple Newhook, J. (2020). "I knew that I wasn't cis, I knew that, but I didn't know exactly": Gender identity development, expression and affirmation in youth who access gender affirming medical care. *International Journal of Transgender Health*, *21*(3), 307–320. DOI: 10.1080/26895269.2020.1756551 PMID: 34993511

Purser, R. (2019). *McMindfulness: How mindfulness became the new capitalist spirituality*. Repeater.

Puyat, J. H., Gastardo-Conaco, M. C., Natividad, J., & Banal, M. A. (2021). Depressive symptoms among young adults in the Philippines: Results from a nationwide cross-sectional survey. *Journal of Affective Disorders Reports*, *3*, 100073. DOI: 10.1016/j.jadr.2020.100073

Qiu, Y. (2024). Social comparison on social media platforms: a media and communication perspective. In *SHS Web of Conferences* (Vol. 185, p. 03008). EDP Sciences. DOI: 10.1051/shsconf/202418503008

Qi, X., Tong, J., Chen, S., He, Z., & Zhu, X. (2020). Comparing the psychological effects of meditation-and breathing-focused yoga practice in undergraduate students. *Frontiers in Psychology*, *11*, 560152. DOI: 10.3389/fpsyg.2020.560152 PMID: 33281662

Qureshi, F., Misra, S., & Poshni, A. (2023). The partition of India through the lens of historical trauma: Intergenerational effects on immigrant health in the South Asian diaspora. *SSM. Mental Health*, *4*, 100246. DOI: 10.1016/j.ssmmh.2023.100246

Raguram, R., Venkateswaran, A., Ramakrishna, J., & Weiss, M. G. (2002). Traditional community resources for mental health: A report of temple healing from India. *BMJ (Clinical Research Ed.)*, *325*(7354), 38–40. DOI: 10.1136/bmj.325.7354.38

Rajan, G., & Sandhu, M. (2025). Investigating the Efficacy of an Integrative Positive Psychology Intervention (PPI) in Indian College Students: An Eclectic Approach Combining Mindfulness meditation, Guided Imagery, and Gratitude Journaling. *Journal of College Student Mental Health*, 1–25. DOI: 10.1080/28367138.2025.2513954

Rajgopal, T. (2020). Mental well-being at the workplace. *Indian Journal of Occupational and Environmental Medicine*, *24*(1), 1–5. DOI: 10.4103/0973-2284.276207 PMID: 32435108

Raj, P., & Dubey, A. (2024). Comprehending Health of the Transgender Population in India Through Bibliometric Analysis. *International Journal of Public Health*, *69*, 1606598. DOI: 10.3389/ijph.2024.1606598 PMID: 38665638

Ramaila, S. M. (2025). Fostering Holistic Development: The Integral Role of Educators in Nurturing Student Growth and Learning. In *Former Educators' Roles in Supporting Student Growth and Learning* (pp. 117-146). IGI Global Scientific Publishing.

Ranade, K., Shankarappa, M. R., Kumar, N., & Somaiya, A. (2025). In quest of an authentic identity - an exploratory study of mental health assessment of gender incongruence in urban India. *BMC Psychiatry*, *25*(1), 387. DOI: 10.1186/s12888-025-06740-4 PMID: 40240909

Raza, S. A., Ahmed, S., Asif, A., & Rani, A. (2023). The Impact of Burnout on the Psychological Well-being of ESL Students in Higher Education Environment. *Siazga Research Journal*, *2*(3), 147–156. DOI: 10.58341/srj.v2i3.21

Razi, N. I. M., & Rahmat, N. H. (2020). Barriers and motivation for learning English: A case study. *European Journal of English Language Teaching*, *6*(1). Advance online publication. DOI: 10.46827/ejel.v6i1.3301

Razza, R. A., Bergen-Cico, D., & Raymond, K. (2015). Enhancing preschoolers' self-regulation via mindful yoga. *Journal of Child and Family Studies*, *24*(2), 372–385. DOI: 10.1007/s10826-013-9847-6

Reb, J., Narayanan, J., & Chaturvedi, S. (2014). Leading mindfully: Two studies on the influence of supervisor trait mindfulness on employee well-being and performance. *Mindfulness*, *5*(1), 36–45. DOI: 10.1007/s12671-012-0144-z

Rechsteiner, K., Tol, V., & Maercker, A. (2019). "It should not have happened": Metaphorical expressions, idioms, and narrative descriptions related to trauma in an indigenous community in India. *International Journal of Qualitative Studies on Health and Well-being*, *14*(1). Advance online publication. DOI: 10.1080/17482631.2019.1667134

Remes, O., Brayne, C., van der Linde, R., & Lafortune, L. (2016). A systematic review of reviews on the prevalence of anxiety disorders in adult populations. *Brain and Behavior*, *6*(7), e00497. Advance online publication. DOI: 10.1002/brb3.497 PMID: 27458547

Rich, T., Chrisinger, B. W., Kaimal, R., Winter, S. J., Hedlin, H., Min, Y., Zhao, X., Zhu, S., You, S. L., Sun, C. A., Lin, J. T., Hsing, A. W., & Heaney, C. (2022). Contemplative Practices Behavior Is Positively Associated with Well-Being in Three Global Multi-Regional Stanford WELL for Life Cohorts. *International Journal of Environmental Research and Public Health*, *19*(20), 13485. DOI: 10.3390/ijerph192013485

Roberts, L., & Montgomery, S. (2016). Mindfulness-based Intervention for Perinatal Grief Education and Reduction among Poor Women in Chhattisgarh, India: A Pilot Study. *Interdisciplinary Journal of Best Practices in Global Development*, *2*(1), 1.

Robertson, M. M., Huang, Y. H., & Lee, J. (2009). Improving computer workstation setup to reduce musculoskeletal disorders. *Journal of Safety Research*, *40*(1), 53–59. DOI: 10.1016/j.jsr.2008.12.005 PMID: 19285587

Robinson, K. H., & Ferfolja, T. (2008). Playing it up, playing it down, playing it safe: Queering teacher education. *Teaching and Teacher Education*, *24*(4), 846–858. DOI: 10.1016/j.tate.2007.11.004

Roeser, R. W. (2014). The emergence of mindfulness-based interventions in educational settings. In *Motivational interventions* (Vol. 18, pp. 379–419). Emerald Group Publishing Limited. DOI: 10.1108/S0749-742320140000018010

Roeser, R. W., & Eccles, J. S. (2015). Mindfulness and compassion in human development: Introduction to the special section. *Developmental Psychology*, *51*(1), 1–6. DOI: 10.1037/a0038453 PMID: 25546594

Roeser, R. W., Skinner, E., Beers, J., & Jennings, P. A. (2012). Mindfulness training and teachers' professional development: An emerging area of research and practice. *Child Development Perspectives*, *6*(2), 167–173. DOI: 10.1111/j.1750-8606.2012.00238.x

Roeser, S. (2006). The role of emotions in judging the moral acceptability of risks. *Safety Science*, *44*(8), 689–700. DOI: 10.1016/j.ssci.2006.02.001

Rogers, J. M., Ferrari, M., Mosely, K., Lang, C. P., & Brennan, L. (2017). Mindfulness-based interventions for adults who are overweight or obese: A meta-analysis of physical and psychological health outcomes. *Obesity Reviews*, *18*(1), 51–67. DOI: 10.1111/obr.12461

Rosales-Ricardo, Y., Rizzo-Chunga, F., Mocha-Bonilla, J., & Ferreira, J. P. (2021). Prevalence of burnout syndrome in university students: A systematic review. *Salud Mental*, *44*(2), 91–102. DOI: 10.17711/SM.0185-3325.2021.013

Roselli, C. E. (2018). Neurobiology of gender identity and sexual orientation. *Journal of Neuroendocrinology*, *30*(7), e12562. DOI: 10.1111/jne.12562 PMID: 29211317

Ross, C. B., & Rocha Beardall, T. (2022). Promoting empathy and reducing hopelessness using contemplative practices. *Teaching Sociology*, *50*(3), 256–268. DOI: 10.1177/0092055X221092014

Rowkith, S., & Bhagwan, R. (2020). Honoring Tribal Spirituality in India: An Exploratory Study of Their Beliefs, Rituals and Healing Practices. *Religions*, *11*(11), 549. DOI: 10.3390/rel11110549

Ruecker, T. (2021, March). Retention and persistence in writing programs: A survey of students repeating first-year writing. In *Composition Forum* (Vol. 46). Association of Teachers of Advanced Composition.

Rugulies, R., Aust, B., Greiner, B. A., Arensman, E., Kawakami, N., LaMontagne, A. D., & Madsen, I. E. H. (2023). Work-related causes of mental health conditions and interventions for their improvement in workplaces. *Lancet*, *402*(10410), 1368–1381. DOI: 10.1016/S0140-6736(23)00869-3 PMID: 37838442

Russell, S. T., & Fish, J. N. (2016). Mental health in lesbian, gay, bisexual, and transgender (LGBT) youth. *Annual Review of Clinical Psychology*, *12*(1), 465–487. DOI: 10.1146/annurev-clinpsy-021815-093153 PMID: 26772206

Russell, V. (2020). Language anxiety and the online learner. *Foreign Language Annals*, *53*(2), 338–352. DOI: 10.1111/flan.12461

Ryan, C., Russell, S. T., Huebner, D., Diaz, R., & Sanchez, J. (2010). Family acceptance in adolescence and the health of LGBT young adults. *Journal of Child and Adolescent Psychiatric Nursing*, *23*(4), 205–213. DOI: 10.1111/j.1744-6171.2010.00246.x PMID: 21073595

Ryan, R. M., & Deci, E. L. (2001). On happiness and human potentials: A review of research on hedonic and eudaimonic well-being. *Annual Review of Psychology*, *52*(1), 141–166. DOI: 10.1146/annurev.psych.52.1.141 PMID: 11148302

S M Sehgal Foundation. (2021, December 29). Community participation in sustainable rural development in india. https://www.smsfoundation.org/role-of-community-participation-and-its-impact-on-sustainability-in-rural/

Saewyc E. M. (2011). RESEARCH ON ADOLESCENT SEXUAL ORIENTATION: DEVELOPMENT, HEALTH DISPARITIES, STIGMA AND RESILIENCE. *Journal of research on adolescence: the official journal of the Society for Research on Adolescence, 21*(1), 256–272. DOI: 10.1111/j.1532-7795.2010.00727.x

Saha, S., Lim, C. C. W., Cannon, D. L., Burton, L., Bremner, M., Cosgrove, P., Huo, Y., & McGrath, J. (2020). Co-morbidity between mood and anxiety disorders: A systematic review and meta-analysis. *Depression and Anxiety*, *38*(3), 286–306. DOI: 10.1002/da.23113 PMID: 33225514

Saldaña, J. (2021). Coding techniques for quantitative and mixed data. *The Routledge reviewer's guide to mixed methods analysis*, 151-160.

Salovey, P., & Mayer, J. D. (1990). Emotional intelligence. *Imagination, Cognition and Personality*, *9*(3), 185–211. DOI: 10.2190/DUGG-P24E-52WK-6CDG

Sanchez, B., & Kazen, H. (2021). Qualitative study on at-risk Hispanic adolescents engaged in social emotional learning and mindfulness practices. *International Journal of Educational Methodology*, *7*(4), 615–622. DOI: 10.12973/ijem.7.4.615

Sandberg, B., Hurmerinta, L., & Menzfeld, M. (2024). Volunteerism and community healing. *Community Development (Columbus, Ohio)*, *55*(6), 795–809. DOI: 10.1080/15575330.2023.2301695

Sanderson, K., & Andrews, G. (2006). Common mental disorders in the workforce: Recent findings from descriptive and social epidemiology. *Canadian Journal of Psychiatry*, *51*(2), 63–75. DOI: 10.1177/070674370605100202 PMID: 16989105

Sandfort, T. G. M., de Graaf, R., ten Have, M., Ransome, Y., & Schnabel, P. (2014). Same-Sex Sexuality and Psychiatric Disorders in the Second Netherlands Mental Health Survey and Incidence Study (NEMESIS-2). *LGBT Health*, *1*(4), 292–301. DOI: 10.1089/lgbt.2014.0031 PMID: 26609539

Sarason, S. B. (1974). *The psychological sense of community: Prospects for community psychology*. Brookline Books.

Sarubin, N., Nothdurfter, C., Schüle, C., Lieb, M., Uhr, M., Born, C., Zimmermannc, R., Bühner, M., Konopka, K., Rupprecht, R., & Baghai, T. C. (2014). The influence of Hatha yoga as an add-on treatment in major depression on hypothalamic–pituitary–adrenal-axis activity: A randomized trial. *Journal of Psychiatric Research*, *53*, 76–83. DOI: 10.1016/j.jpsychires.2014.02.022 PMID: 24655586

Savafi, S., Bazzazian, S., & Sirtori, C. R. (2024). The effectiveness of mindfulness training on social adjustment, self-esteem, and hope among transgender individuals in Tehran. *Journal of Neurology & Neuroscience Disorders*, *10*(1), 1–8. DOI: 10.17352/jnnsd.000057

Scherer, S., Talley, C., & Hill, O. (2021). Mindfulness and Silent Sitting in the Classroom. In *A Human Values Pathway for Teachers: Developing Silent Sitting and Mindful Practices in Education* (pp. 55–78). Springer Singapore. DOI: 10.1007/978-981-16-0200-9_6

Schmidt, S. (2004). Mindfulness and healing intention: Concepts, practice, and research evaluation. *Journal of Alternative and Complementary Medicine (New York, N.Y.)*, *10*(Suppl 1), S7–S14. DOI: 10.1089/ACM.2004.10.S-7

Schnabel, L. (2018). Sexual Orientation and Social Attitudes. *Socius: Sociological Research for a Dynamic World, 4*, 2378023118769550. Advance online publication. DOI: 10.1177/2378023118769550

Schneider, R. H., Dillbeck, M. C., Yeola, G., & Nader, T. (2024). Peace through health: Traditional medicine meditation in the prevention of collective stress, violence, and war. *Frontiers in Public Health, 12*. Advance online publication. DOI: 10.3389/fpubh.2024.1380626

Schonert-Reichl, K. A., & Lawlor, M. S. (2010). The effects of a mindfulness-based education program on pre-and early adolescents' well-being and social and emotional competence. *Mindfulness, 1*(3), 137–151. DOI: 10.1007/s12671-010-0011-8

Schonert-Reichl, K. A., Oberle, E., Lawlor, M. S., Abbott, D., Thomson, K., Oberlander, T. F., & Diamond, A. (2015). Enhancing cognitive and social–emotional development through a simple-to-administer mindfulness-based school program for elementary school children: A randomized controlled trial. *Developmental Psychology, 51*(1), 52–66. DOI: 10.1037/a0038454 PMID: 25546595

Schultz, P. P., & Ryan, R. M. (2015). The "why,""what," and "how" of healthy self-regulation: Mindfulness and well-being from a self-determination theory perspective. In *Handbook of mindfulness and self-regulation* (pp. 81–94). Springer New York. DOI: 10.1007/978-1-4939-2263-5_7

Segal, Z., Williams, M., & Teasdale, J. (2012). *Mindfulness-based cognitive therapy for depression*. Guilford press.

Sekhon, S., & Gupta, V. (2023). *Mood Disorder*. PubMed; StatPearls Publishing. https://www.ncbi.nlm.nih.gov/books/NBK558911/

Selye, H. (1956). Stress and psychiatry. *The American Journal of Psychiatry, 113*(5), 423–427. DOI: 10.1176/ajp.113.5.423 PMID: 13362640

Semlyen, J., King, M., Varney, J., & Hagger-Johnson, G. (2016). Sexual orientation and symptoms of common mental disorder or low wellbeing: Combined meta-analysis of 12 UK population health surveys. *BMC Psychiatry, 16*(1), 67. Advance online publication. DOI: 10.1186/s12888-016-0767-z PMID: 27009565

Serquina, E. A., & Batang, B. L. (2018). Demographic, Psychological Factors and English Proficiency of ESL Students. *TESOL International Journal, 13*(4), 182–191.

Serrano, I. M. A., Cuyugan, A. M. N., Cruz, K., Mahusay, J. M. A., & Alibudbud, R. (2023). Sociodemographic characteristics, social support, and family history as factors of depression, anxiety, and stress among young adult senior high school students in metro Manila, Philippines, during the COVID-19 pandemic. *Frontiers in Psychiatry, 14*, 1225035. DOI: 10.3389/fpsyt.2023.1225035 PMID: 37772068

Shah, R., Gao, Z., & Mittal, H. (2015). Culture. In *Innovation, Entrepreneurship, and the Economy in the US, China, and India* (pp. 55–65). Elsevier. https://doi.org/DOI: 10.1016/B978-0-12-801890-3.00004-6

Shaikh, A., Kamble, P., Daulatabad, V., Singhal, A., Madhusudhan, U., & John, N. A. (2024). Mental health challenges within the LGBTQ community: A societal imperative. *Journal of Family Medicine and Primary Care, 13*(9), 3529–3535. DOI: 10.4103/jfmpc.jfmpc_321_24 PMID: 39464965

Shami, S., Venu, C. D. V. P., Shanampoodi, G. B., & Rajeswari, T. S. (2025). Impact Of English Language Learning On Mental Health: Exploring The Relationships Between Language Anxiety, Self-Esteem, And Depression. *Journal of Neonatal Surgery, 14*(9S, 9s), 328–333. DOI: 10.52783/jns.v14.2668

Shapiro, S. L., Brown, K. W., & Astin, J. A. (2012). Toward the integration of meditation into higher education: A review of research. *Teachers College Record, 113*(3), 493–528. DOI: 10.1177/016146811111300306

Shapiro, S. L., & Carlson, L. E. (2009). *The Art and Science of Mindfulness: Integrating Mindfulness into Psychology and the Helping Professions*. American Psychological Association. DOI: 10.1037/11885-000

Sharma, R. (2021). Rights of LGBTQ in India and the Struggle for Societal Acceptance. *Issue 3 Int'l JL Mgmt. & Human., 4*, 18, http://doi.one/10.1732/IJLMH.26695

Sharma, D., & Sharma, B. R. (2024). The impact of yoga and meditation on mental and physical well-being. *Journal of Ayurveda and Integrated Medical Sciences*, *9*(5), 144–153. DOI: 10.21760/jaims.9.5.23

Sharma, M., & Haider, T. (2013). Yoga as an alternative and complementary treatment for patients with low back pain: A systematic review. *Journal of Evidence-Based Complementary & Alternative Medicine*, *18*(1), 23–28. DOI: 10.1177/2156587212458693

Shelov, D. V., Suchday, S., & Friedberg, J. P. (2009). A pilot study measuring the impact of yoga on the trait of mindfulness. *Behavioural and Cognitive Psychotherapy*, *37*(5), 595–598. DOI: 10.1017/S1352465809990361 PMID: 19751539

Sherab, K., & Schuelka, M. J. (2023). Happy students in Bhutan. In *Routledge eBooks* (pp. 56–75). https://doi.org/DOI: 10.4324/9781003037262-4

Shirom, A. (2005). Reflections on the study of burnout. *Work and Stress*, *19*(3), 263–270. DOI: 10.1080/02678370500376649

Sibinga, E., Webb, L., Ghazarian, S. R., & Ellen, J. M. (2016). School-based mindfulness instruction: An RCT. *Pediatrics*, *137*(1), e20152532. DOI: 10.1542/peds.2015-2532 PMID: 26684478

Silva, A. (2024). Socio-cognitive mindfulness is a well-being booster: A serial mediation model to test the mindfulness reappraisal hypothesis with managers. *Evidence-Based HRM: A Global Forum for Empirical Scholarship, 13*(1), 1–16. https://doi.org/DOI: 10.1108/EBHRM-09-2023-0240

Simonsson, O., Stenfors, C., Goldberg, S., Hendricks, P., & Osika, W. (2023). Altered states of leadership: Mindfulness meditation, psychedelic use, and leadership development. *Frontiers in Psychology*, *14*, 1151626. Advance online publication. DOI: 10.3389/fpsyg.2023.1151626 PMID: 37476092

Singh, A. A., Meng, S. E., & Hansen, A. W. (2014). "I am my own gender": Resilience strategies of trans youth. *Journal of Counseling and Development, 92*(2), 208–218. DOI: 10.1002/j.1556-6676.2014.00150.x

Slemp, G. R., Jach, H. K., Chia, A., Loton, D. J., & Kern, M. L. (2019). Contemplative interventions and employee distress: A meta-analysis. *Stress and Health, 35*(3), 227–255. DOI: 10.1002/smi.2857

Slimmen, S., Timmermans, O., Mikolajczak-Degrauwe, K., & Oenema, A. (2022). How stress-related factors affect mental wellbeing of university students A cross-sectional study to explore the associations between stressors, perceived stress, and mental wellbeing. *PLoS One, 17*(11), e0275925. DOI: 10.1371/journal.pone.0275925 PMID: 36342914

Smith, B., Metzker, K., Waite, R., & Gerrity, P. (2015). Short-Form Mindfulness-Based Stress Reduction Reduces Anxiety and Improves Health-Related Quality of Life in an Inner-City Population. *Holistic Nursing Practice, 29*(2), 70–77. DOI: 10.1097/HNP.0000000000000075 PMID: 25658929

Snapp, S. D., Watson, R. J., Russell, S. T., Diaz, R. M., & Ryan, C. (2015). Social support networks for LGBT young adults: Low cost strategies for positive adjustment. *Family Relations, 64*(3), 420–430. DOI: 10.1111/fare.12124

Snyder, B. (2020). *Yoga and mindfulness as a vehicle for language acquisition and social-emotional health for fifth grade ELL language arts students* (Master's thesis, William Paterson University of New Jersey). ProQuest Dissertations & Theses Global.

Sofianopoulou, K., Bacopoulou, F., Vlachakis, D., Kokka, I., Alexopoulos, E., Varvogli, L., Chrousos, G. P., & Darviri, C. (2021). Stress Management in Elementary School Students: A Pilot Randomised Controlled Trial. *EMBnet.Journal, 26*(1), e976. DOI: 10.14806/ej.26.1.976 PMID: 34621631

Sonnentag, S., Binnewies, C., & Mojza, E. J. (2010). Staying well and engaged when demands are high: The role of psychological detachment. *The Journal of Applied Psychology, 95*(5), 965–976. DOI: 10.1037/a0020032 PMID: 20718528

Sood, S. (2018). Cultivating a yogic theology of collective healing: A yogini's journey disrupting white supremacy, hindu fundamentalism, and casteism. *Race and Yoga*, *3*(1). Advance online publication. DOI: 10.5070/R331034279

Soomro, M. A., Rajper, M. A., Koondhar, M. A., & Khan, I. K. (2023). The Relationship between Perceived Psychological Barriers, Anxiety, and Rural Affiliation of Pakistani College Students to Communicate in English. *VFAST Transactions on Education and Social Sciences*, *11*(1), 29–37. DOI: 10.21015/vtess.v11i1.1380

Southwick, S. M., Bonanno, G. A., Masten, A. S., Panter-Brick, C., & Yehuda, R. (2014). Resilience definitions, theory, and challenges: Interdisciplinary perspectives. *European Journal of Psychotraumatology*, *5*(1), 25338. DOI: 10.3402/ejpt.v5.25338 PMID: 25317257

Sowmya, D. S. (2025). Embracing Self-Compassion: A Cornerstone of Student Well-Being. In *Nurturing Student Well-Being in the Modern World* (pp. 103-140). IGI Global.

Sparks, K., Faragher, B., & Cooper, C. L. (2001). Well-being and occupational health in the 21st-century workplace. *Journal of Occupational and Organizational Psychology*, *74*(4), 489–509. DOI: 10.1348/096317901167497

Spijker, J., & Claes, S. (2014). [Mood disorders in the DSM-5]. *Tijdschrift voor Psychiatrie*, *56*(3), 173–176. https://pubmed.ncbi.nlm.nih.gov/24643826/ PMID: 24643826

Srinivasan, S. P., & Chandrasekaran, S. (2020). Care of transgender individuals in India: A clinical perspective. *Indian Journal of Social Psychiatry*, *36*(4), 284–288. DOI: 10.4103/ijsp.ijsp_88_20

Srinivasan, S. P., & Chandrasekaran, S. (2025). Mental Health Status and Its Psychosocial Correlates Among Help-Seeking Transgender Individuals: Experiences from a Clinic in South India. *Transgender Health*, *10*(2), 201–209. DOI: 10.1089/trgh.2022.0150 PMID: 40309069

Srivastava, S. (2023). The evolution of education: Navigating 21st-century challenges. *International Journal for Multidisciplinary Research*, *5*(5), 1–9.

Srivastava, S., Khan, M., Kumari, A., & Jain, A. (2024). Does workplace ostracism lead to workplace withdrawal? Testing the moderating–mediating effects of rumination and mindfulness in Indian hospitality industry. *Journal of Organizational Effectiveness: People and Performance*, *11*(4), 873–891. DOI: 10.1108/JOEPP-08-2023-0328

Stedham, Y., & Skaar, T. (2019). Mindfulness, trust, and leader effectiveness: A conceptual framework. *Frontiers in Psychology*, *10*, 1588. Advance online publication. DOI: 10.3389/fpsyg.2019.01588 PMID: 31354589

Steele, L. S., Ross, L. E., Dobinson, C., Veldhuizen, S., & Tinmouth, J. M. (2009). Women's Sexual Orientation and Health: Results from a Canadian Population-Based Survey. *Women & Health*, *49*(5), 353–367. DOI: 10.1080/03630240903238685 PMID: 19851942

Steinberg, L. (2005). Cognitive and affective development in adolescence. *Trends in Cognitive Sciences*, *9*(2), 69–74. DOI: 10.1016/j.tics.2004.12.005 PMID: 15668099

Subhash, M., Jithesh, M., Rahmath, P. K., & Anjali, A. (2024). Integrated management with Ayurveda, yoga and counselling in gender dysphoria with conduct disorder. *Ayushdhara*, *10*(6), 158–164. DOI: 10.47070/ayushdhara.v10i6.1448

Sulastri, S., Andriani, C., & Fitria, Y. (2017). The factors forming formal and non-formal leadership based on Minangkabau culture in Padang. *Asia Pacific Management and Business Application*, *6*(1), 15–30. DOI: 10.21776/ub.apmba.2017.006.01.2

Sultan, S. (2012). Students' perceived competence affecting level of anxiety in learning English as a foreign language. *Pakistan Journal of Psychological Research*, *27*(2), 225–239.

Sun, Y., Lamoreau, R., O'Connell, S., Horlick, R., & Bazzano, A. N. (2021). Yoga and mindfulness interventions for preschool-aged children in educational settings: A systematic review. *International Journal of Environmental Research and Public Health*, *18*(11), 6091. DOI: 10.3390/ijerph18116091 PMID: 34198737

Swain, J., Hancock, K., Hainsworth, C., & Bowman, J. (2015). Mechanisms of change: Exploratory outcomes from a randomised controlled trial of acceptance and commitment therapy for anxious adolescents. *Journal of Contextual Behavioral Science*, *4*(1), 56–67. DOI: 10.1016/j.jcbs.2014.09.001

Tajik, M. A., Manan, S. A., Schamiloglu, U., & Namyssova, G. (2024). Gaps between policy aspirations and enactment: Graduate students' struggles with academic English amidst a turbulent transition to the EMI environment in Kazakhstani universities. *Current Issues in Language Planning*, *25*(2), 212–235. DOI: 10.1080/14664208.2023.2283651

Tang, Y. Y., Hölzel, B. K., & Posner, M. I. (2015). The neuroscience of mindfulness meditation. *Nature Reviews. Neuroscience*, *16*(4), 213–225. DOI: 10.1038/nrn3916 PMID: 25783612

Tasan, M., Mede, E., & Sadeghi, K. (2021). The effect of pranayamic breathing as a positive psychology exercise on foreign language learning anxiety and test anxiety among language learners at tertiary level. *Frontiers in Psychology*, *12*, 742060. DOI: 10.3389/fpsyg.2021.742060 PMID: 34659061

Telles, S., Singh, N., & Joshi, M. (2010). Post traumatic stress symptoms and heart rate variability in Bihar flood survivors following yoga: A randomized controlled study. *BMC Psychiatry*. Advance online publication. DOI: 10.1186/1471-244X-10-18

Tempone-Wiltshire, J. (2024). The Role of Mindfulness and Embodiment in Group-Based Trauma Treatment. *Psychotherapy and Counselling Journal of Australia*, *12*(1). Advance online publication. DOI: 10.59158/001c.94979

Tessler, R. C., & Schwartz, S. H. (1972). Help seeking, self-esteem, and achievement motivation: An attributional analysis. *Journal of Personality and Social Psychology*, *21*(3), 318–326. DOI: 10.1037/h0032321 PMID: 5060750

Thayer, J. F., & Lane, R. D. (2000). A model of neurovisceral integration in emotion regulation and dysregulation. *Journal of Affective Disorders*, *61*(3), 201–216. DOI: 10.1016/S0165-0327(00)00338-4 PMID: 11163422

Theisen-Womersley, G. (2021). *Trauma and resilience among displaced populations*. Springer., DOI: 10.1007/978-3-030-67712-1_13

Thomson, C. J., Lesser, I. A., & Hatfield, G. L. (2024). Psychological and physiological effects of an acute bout of yoga before a simulated academic exam in university students. *Journal of American College Health*, •••, 1–11. DOI: 10.1080/07448481.2024.2308267 PMID: 38330344

Thomson, G. (2021). Collective Healing: Towards a Conceptual Framework, Genocide Studies and Prevention. *International Journal (Toronto, Ont.)*, *15*(3), 33–48. DOI: 10.5038/1911-9933.15.3.1843

Toghiani, M., Ghasemi, F., & Sharifi, T. (2019). The effectiveness of acceptance and commitment group therapy on social anxiety in female dormitory residents in Isfahan University of Medical Sciences. *Journal of Education and Health Promotion*, *8*(1), 41. DOI: 10.4103/jehp.jehp_111_18 PMID: 30993134

Toomey, R. B., & Russell, S. T. (2013). The Role of Sexual Orientation in School-Based Victimization: A Meta-Analysis. *Youth & Society*, *48*(2), 176–201. DOI: 10.1177/0044118X13483778 PMID: 26997680

Toukan, E., & Tawil, S. (2024). A new social contract for education: Rebuilding trust in education as a common good. *Prospects*, *54*(2), 259–275. DOI: 10.1007/s11125-024-09702-y

Treleaven, D. A. (2018). *Trauma-sensitive mindfulness: Practices for safe and transformative healing*. WW Norton & Company.

Trojan, S. (2020). *Integrating mindfulness strategies and English as a second language instruction* (Capstone project No. 485). Hamline University, School of Education and Leadership. https://digitalcommons.hamline.edu/hse_cp/485

Van Dam, N. T., Van Vugt, M. K., Vago, D. R., Schmalzl, L., Saron, C. D., Olendzki, A., Meissner, T., Lazar, S. W., Kerr, C. E., Gorchov, J., Fox, K. C. R., Field, B. A., Britton, W. B., Brefczynski-Lewis, J. A., & Meyer, D. E. (2018). Mind the hype: A critical evaluation and prescriptive agenda for research on mindfulness and meditation. *Perspectives on Psychological Science*, *13*(1), 36–61. DOI: 10.1177/1745691617709589 PMID: 29016274

Van Gordon, W., Sapthiang, S., & Shonin, E. (2022). Contemplative psychology: History, key assumptions, and future directions. *Perspectives on Psychological Science*, *17*(1), 99–107. DOI: 10.1177/1745691620984479 PMID: 34185604

Van Gordon, W., Shonin, E., Dunn, T., Garcia-Campayo, J., & Griffiths, M. (2017). Van Gordon, W., Shonin, E., Dunn, T., Garcia-Campayo, J., & Griffiths, MD (2017). Meditation Awareness Training for the treatment of fibromyalgia: A randomised controlled trial. *British Journal of Health Psychology*, *22*, 186–206. DOI: 10.1111/bjhp.12224 PMID: 27885763

Varghese, F., Nolan, J., Bihm, E., Salagame, K., Khanna, R., & Ali, S. (2017). Transformational leadership and Asian Indian values: Duty, selfless service, and nonviolence. *The Counseling Psychologist*, *45*(6), 810–829. DOI: 10.1177/0011000017723080

Veerman, A. L., & Ganzevoort, R. R. (2001). Communities Coping with Collective Trauma. *Psychiatry*, *101*, 141–148.

Veisiy, N., Arjmandnia, A. A., Vakili, S., & Gholamali Lavasani, M. (2022). The effect of training emotional self-regulation strategies on social competence, academic performance and behavioral problems of students with learning disabilities with comorbidity of attention deficit/hyperactivity disorder. *Journal of Psychological Science*, *21*(116), 1613–1629. DOI: 10.52547/JPS.21.116.1613

Vilvens, H. L., Frame, D. L., & Owen, P. C. (2021). Promoting the inclusion of mindfulness and contemplative practices in the college classroom. *Pedagogy in Health Promotion*, *7*(2), 148–158. DOI: 10.1177/2373379920925849

Wandrekar, J. R., & Nigudkar, A. S. (2020). What do we know about LGBTQIA+ mental health in India? A review of research from 2009 to 2019. *Journal of Psychosexual Health, 2*(1), 26–36. DOI: 10.1177/2631831820918129

Wang, C., & Sun, T. (2020). Relationship between self-efficacy and language proficiency: A meta-analysis. *System, 95*, 102366. DOI: 10.1016/j.system.2020.102366

Wang, F., & Szabo, A. (2020). Effects of yoga on stress among healthy adults: A systematic review. *Alternative Therapies in Health and Medicine, 26*(4), 58–64. PMID: 32088671

Wang, H., & Guan, B. (2018). The positive effect of authoritarian leadership on employee performance: The moderating role of power distance. *Frontiers in Psychology, 9*, 357. Advance online publication. DOI: 10.3389/fpsyg.2018.00357 PMID: 29628902

Wang, S., Shih, S., & Kuo, L. (2024). Exploring mindfulness interventions for stress resilience in newly graduated nurses: A qualitative study. *Tzu-Chi Medical Journal, 36*(4), 452–459. DOI: 10.4103/tcmj.tcmj_250_23 PMID: 39421497

Webb, J., Padro, M., Thomas, E., Davies, A., Etzel, L., Rogers, C., & Heredia, N. (2022). Yoga at every size: A preliminary evaluation of a brief online size-inclusive yoga and body gratitude journaling intervention to enhance positive embodiment in higher-weight college women. *Frontiers in Global Women's Health, 3*, 852854. Advance online publication. DOI: 10.3389/fgwh.2022.852854 PMID: 35720811

Webster, E. M. (2022). The impact of adverse childhood experiences on health and development in young children. *Global pediatric health, 9*, 2333794X221078708.

Wei, D., Wang, X., You, X., Luo, X., Hao, C., Gu, J., Peng, S., Yang, X., Hao, Y., Silenzio, V. M. B., Li, J., & Hou, F. (2020). Prevalence of depression, anxiety and suicide among men who have sex with men in China: A systematic review and meta-analysis. *Epidemiology and Psychiatric Sciences*, *29*, e136. Advance online publication. DOI: 10.1017/S2045796020000487 PMID: 32536353

Wei, F. Y. F., Wang, Y. K., & Klausner, M. (2012). Rethinking college students' self-regulation and sustained attention: Does text messaging during class influence cognitive learning? *Communication Education*, *61*(3), 185–204. DOI: 10.1080/03634523.2012.672755

Weisner, L. (2020). Individual and community trauma: Individual experiences in collective environment. Illinois criminal justice information authority center for violence prevention and intervention research. https://researchhub.icjia-api.cloud/uploads/Individual%20and%20Community%20Trauma-%20Individual%20Experiences%20in%20Collective%20Environments-200715T15003405.pdf

Weisz, J. R., Kuppens, S., Ng, M. Y., Eckshtain, D., Ugueto, A. M., Vaughn-Coaxum, R., Jensen-Doss, A., Hawley, K. M., Krumholz Marchette, L. S., Chu, B. C., Weersing, V. R., & Fordwood, S. R. (2017). What five decades of research tells us about the effects of youth psychological therapy: A multilevel meta-analysis and implications for science and practice. *The American Psychologist*, *72*(2), 79–117. DOI: 10.1037/a0040360 PMID: 28221063

West, J., Liang, B., & Spinazzola, J. (2017). Trauma Sensitive Yoga as a complementary treatment for posttraumatic stress disorder: A Qualitative Descriptive analysis. *International Journal of Stress Management*, *24*(2), 173–195. DOI: 10.1037/str0000040

Wilson, G., & Gillies, R. M. (2005). Stress associated with the transition from high school to university: The effect of social support and self-efficacy. *Australian Journal of Guidance & Counselling*, *15*(1), 77–92. DOI: 10.1375/ajgc.15.1.77

Wimmer, L., Bellingrath, S., & Von Stockhausen, L. (2020). Mindfulness training for improving attention regulation in university students: Is it effective? And do yoga and homework matter? *Frontiers in Psychology*, *11*, 719. DOI: 10.3389/fpsyg.2020.00719 PMID: 32411045

Wisconsin department of health services. (2020). *In This Together: Understanding the Effects of Collective Trauma*. https://www.dhs.wisconsin.gov/publications/p02779.pdf

Wittgens, C., Fischer, M. M., Buspavanich, P., Theobald, S., Schweizer, K., & Trautmann, S. (2022). Mental health in people with minority sexual orientations: A meta-analysis of population-based studies. *Acta Psychiatrica Scandinavica*, *145*(4), 357–372. DOI: 10.1111/acps.13405 PMID: 35090051

Wong, S. Y., Mak, W. W., Cheung, E. Y., Ling, C. Y., Lui, W. W., Tang, W., Wong, R. L., Lo, H. H., Mercer, S., & Ma, H. S. (2011). A randomized, controlled clinical trial: the effect of mindfulness-based cognitive therapy on generalized anxiety disorder among Chinese community patients: protocol for a randomized trial. *BMC Psychiatry*, *11*(1), 187. Advance online publication. DOI: 10.1186/1471-244X-11-187 PMID: 22126115

Woodyard, C. (2011). Exploring the therapeutic effects of yoga and its ability to increase quality of life. *International Journal of Yoga*, *4*(2), 49–54. DOI: 10.4103/0973-6131.85485

World Health Organization. (2022). *WHO guidelines on mental health at work*. World Health Organization.

Xuan Mai, L., Ngoc, L. K., & Thao, L. T. (2024). Factors hindering Student participation in English-speaking classes: Student and Lecturer perceptions. *SAGE Open*, *14*(3), 21582440241266297. DOI: 10.1177/21582440241266297

Yarns, B. C., Abrams, J. M., Meeks, T. W., & Sewell, D. D. (2016). The Mental Health of Older LGBT Adults. *Current Psychiatry Reports*, *18*(6), 60. Advance online publication. DOI: 10.1007/s11920-016-0697-y PMID: 27142205

Zaccaro, A., Piarulli, A., Laurino, M., Garbella, E., Menicucci, D., Neri, B., & Gemignani, A. (2018). How breath-control can change your life: A systematic review on psycho-physiological correlates of slow breathing. *Frontiers in Human Neuroscience, 12*, 409421. DOI: 10.3389/fnhum.2018.00353 PMID: 30245619

Zahn-Waxler, C., Shirtcliff, E. A., & Marceau, K. (2008). Disorders of childhood and adolescence: Gender and psychopathology. *Annual Review of Clinical Psychology, 4*(1), 275–303. DOI: 10.1146/annurev.clinpsy.3.022806.091358 PMID: 18370618

Zasiekina, L., & Zhuravlova, O. (2019). Acculturating stress, language anxiety and procrastination of international students in the academic settings. *Psycholinguistics, 26*(1), 126–140. DOI: 10.31470/2309-1797-2019-26-1-126-140

Zeidner, M., Matthews, G., & Roberts, R. D. (2009). *What we know about emotional intelligence: How it affects learning, work, relationships, and our mental health*. Boston Review., DOI: 10.7551/mitpress/7404.001.0001

Zhao, Y., Llorente, A. M. P., & Gómez, M. C. S. (2021). Digital competence in higher education research: A systematic literature review. *Computers & Education, 168*, 104212. DOI: 10.1016/j.compedu.2021.104212 PMID: 36568577

Zhou, L., & Xing, H. (2025). Individualization of Religious Rituals and Their Healing Functions in a Mobile Society—Empirical Evidence from China. *Religions, 16*(4), 521. DOI: 10.3390/rel16040521

Zinner, E. S., & Williams, M. B. (Eds.). (1999). *When a community weeps: Case studies in group survivorship*. Brunner/Mazel.

Zoogman, S., Goldberg, S. B., Hoyt, W. T., & Miller, L. (2015). Mindfulness interventions with youth: A meta-analysis. *Mindfulness, 6*(2), 290–302. DOI: 10.1007/s12671-013-0260-4

About the Contributors

Shubhangni Jain aspires to explore more aspects of psychology further in the field of education & hone their knowledge further. Also, it will allow them to interact with fresh minds with whom they would be able to share & demonstrate knowledge both theoretical and empirical. As an entry- level psychologist, they intend to contribute to the development and progress of the esteemed organization. They are confident that they possess excellent communication skills, attitude & mindset related to various aspects of the field with good interpersonal skills, which are required for the job. They are also confident that they have good knowledge of psychological research methods and practices, including clinical psychology work experience in solving psychological problems.

Akanksha Singh is a passionate psychologist, academician, and researcher who blends scientific rigor with a deep understanding of human experiences. Currently an Assistant Professor at Chitkara University, India, her work spans forensic and psycho-social domains, including victimology, minority stress, and LGBTQIA+ mental health, reflected in her SCOPUS and PubMed-indexed publications. With an interdisciplinary foundation in forensic science and psychology, she explores human behavior—from crime and victim experiences to identity, mental health, and behavioural outcomes. Beyond academics, Dr. Singh is a dedicated mentor and innovator, actively guiding students, leading neurocognitive lab initiatives, and fostering inclusive, impact-driven learning environments. Trained in queer-affirmative practices, statistical analysis, and scientific communication, she is a dynamic educator and social advocate committed to inclusive, evidence-based education and meaningful societal impact.

Shweta Sharma s an Assistant Professor of Psychology at Amity University, Gurugram. She is a dedicated psychologist, researcher, and academician with a strong commitment to advancing mental health awareness and psychological well-being. With extensive experience in academia and research, Dr. Sharma has worked as a psychology faculty member, research associate, and research assistant, actively contributing to various research projects. Her expertise spans teaching, psychological assessment and diagnosis, and the development and implementation of therapeutic interventions. Dr. Sharma is highly skilled in research writing, including the preparation of research papers, synopses, books, and academic projects. She possesses strong communication abilities and is proficient in both Hindi and English. Additionally, she is well-versed in the use of word processing, spreadsheet, and presentation tools, along with advanced data analysis software essential for teaching and research.

***

Ojeshavi Arya is currently pursuing M.Sc. in Clinical Psychology at the National Forensic Sciences University, Delhi. Her research interests lie in the areas of indigenous practices, artificial intelligence, mental health, well-being, therapeutic modalities, and the understanding of minority groups such as individuals with disabilities and refugees. She is particularly intrigued by the intersection of culture, identity, personality, upbringing, and parenting, and how these factors influence individual behavior. Through her work, she aims to bring these nuanced interactions and their implications to the forefront of psychological research.

Divya Dubey serves as Faculty at Jindal Institute of Behavioural Sciences (JIBS), O. P. Jindal Global University, Sonipat, Haryana. Dr. Dubey has completed her Ph.D. in Forensic Psychology from Amity University, Lucknow Campus. She has completed her Masters from Lucknow University with specialization in Clinical and Organizational Psychology. She completed her one-year Professional Post-Graduate

Diploma in Forensic Psychology from National Forensic Sciences University (NFSU), Gandhinagar, Gujarat, where she got trained in number of tools used in detection of deception as Polygraph, Layered Voice Analysis (LVA), Brain Electrical Oscillation Signature Profiling (BEOS) and Suspect Detection System (SDS). She studied Professional Diploma in Criminal Profiling and Crime Scene Analysis from The Forensic Criminology Institute, Alaska, United States and earned Diplomat Status in Criminal Profiling from International Association of Forensic Criminologist (IAFC). She also has a licence in operating Layered Voice Analysis (LVA 6.50), Professional Investigation Focus Tool from Nemesysco, Israel. She also worked as a Project Assistant in one of the DST Project in the Department of Cognitive and Brain Sciences at Indian Institute of Technology (IIT) Gandhinagar, Gujarat, India. She also worked as a counsellor in Sabarmati Jail, Ahmedabad, Gujarat and Tihar Jail, New Delhi, providing Psychological First Aid to offenders and also worked on their correctional programme. She has also worked as a Consultant in Risk and Threat department in Cyber security organization in Dubai, where she is responsible in imparting training and lectures on LVA 6.50 to Government and Private entities, including Dubai Police and Ministry of Defence, Abu Dhabi. She also worked as an Executive Director in one of the consultancy in Dubai, A to Z Consultancy, Dubai. She also worked as an Adjunct Faculty in Amity University, Dubai. She was invited as a subject expert on News channel, Zee Hindustan in the capacity of a Forensic Psychologist to discuss Psychological Autopsy in Sushant Singh case. Courses Taught: Divya Dubey taught various courses including Introduction to Forensic Psychology, Psychological Practices in Law, Introduction to Personality Theories and Foundations of Physiological Psychology to Masters students at Amity University, Dubai. Dr. Dubey is also teaching electives, Law Enforcement and Crime Prevention, Psychology of Peace and Conflict and Core paper in Forensic and Investigative Psychology at O. P Jindal Global University. She has also receives invitations from International and National forum as a subject expert and eminent speaker to train students and professionals from diverse background. She also presented papers in a various International and National Conferences and has also published papers in a Scopus Indexed Journal.

Marie Grace A. Gomez is Professor 4 at the Counselor Education Area, College of Education, University of the Philippines-Diliman. She teaches counseling and research courses at the undergraduate and graduate levels. She has a bachelor's degree in Political Science, a Master of Arts in Education (Guidance) degree, a Doctor of Philosophy degree in Guidance and another doctorate in Special Education. She is currently working on a graduate degree in Clinical Psychology. All degrees were earned from the University of the Philippines-Diliman. She has served as a classroom teacher, guidance counselor, and administrator in the basic and tertiary education settings. Her community extension projects involve counseling and assessment of children, persons with disability, children in conflict with the law, drug surrenderees, sexually abused children, medical personnel, women with mental health issues in institutional settings, and persons affected by COVID-19. Her researches are in education, persons with disability, program development, and development of assessment instruments. She has published and presented research both locally and internationally and is constantly invited to referee journal articles submitted for publication. She is a member of the Pi Gamma Mu Honor Society, the Pi Lambda Theta Honor Society for Teachers an the Phi Kappa Phi Honor Society. She was a recipient of the UP Presidential Scholarship Award, the UP International Publication Award, the One-UP Professorial Chair for Teaching and Research, and the One-UP Professorial Chair Award for Teaching and Public Service. She served as lead researcher for the Philippines on comprehensive sexuality education research by the United Nations Education Scientific and Cultural Organization (UNESCO) and the Leonard Cheshire UK. She has received the 2022 Most Outstanding Professional Teacher Award in the field of Academe and Research from the Philippine Federation for Professional Associations.

Nishtha Grover is an Assistant Professor at the School of Behavioral Forensics, National Forensic Sciences University (NFSU) and a doctoral scholar at Christ (Deemed to be University). She holds a double master's degree and specializes in the interdisciplinary application of psychology within forensic and academic contexts. Her research interests include positive psychology, child and adolescent psychology, trauma-focused therapy, and psychotherapy, with a focus on promoting psychological resilience, mental well-being, and evidence-based therapeutic interventions. She has served as a resource person and chaired numerous national and international conferences, reflecting her recognition within the academic and professional community. Her work emphasizes integrating scientific research with practical applications to support mental health, forensic assessment, and therapeutic outcomes.

Liza Legaspino is currently taking up Doctor of Philosophy in Curriculum and Instruction at Philippine Normal University– Manila, where she also earned her Master of Arts in Education with a specialization in Early Childhood Education. At the same university, she graduated cum laude with a bachelor's degree in Early Childhood Education. Before joining the Department of Education as a curriculum specialist, she was a part-time professor at Philippine Normal University and San Beda College Alabang, teaching early childhood education and professional education courses. Miss Liza was also a textbook author and previously worked as a preschool teacher and a grade school language teacher at Manresa School. She is a resource speaker on different topics related to Early Childhood Education, social and emotional learning, creativity, teacher education, curriculum, and motivation. At present, she is a Senior Education Program Specialist under the Bureau of Curriculum Development, DepEd Central Office. She is one of the crafters of the revised Kindergarten and Life and Career Skills Curriculum and is also involved in other national programs such as the National Reading Program, Strengthened Senior High School, Financial Education, Homeroom Guidance, Peace Education, and part of the technical working group of the Filipino SEL Framework in collaboration with ChildFund Philippines and SEAMEO INNOTECH.

Kenneth Leow, PhD, is an Assistant Professor and Program Director of PhD in Social and Behavioral Science in the Department of Psychology at Heriot-Watt University, Malaysia. His research examines human motivation, social support, and well-being in social contexts through the framework of Self-Determination Theory (SDT). Dr. Leow's contribution to this field lies in bridging theoretical insights from SDT with practical applications in educational settings. By identifying key social and motivational factors that enhance resilience, his research aims to foster supportive academic environments through meaningful community engagement. This work is particularly significant given the increasing mental health challenges faced by many schools and universities in the post-pandemic environment.

Yueh Yea Lo, PhD, is a Senior Lecturer in the Department of Language and Literacy Education, Faculty of Education, Universiti Malaya, and serves as the UM SDG 4 Champion, committed to advancing inclusive and quality education. Her research focuses on writing, technology-enhanced learning, cross-cultural communication, and resilience, reflecting her dedication to language education and learner well-being. Dr. Lo has published in reputable journals like SAGE Open, PLOS ONE and Humanities and Social Sciences Communications. She has also earned recognition through awards including Best Oral Presentation (2023), Gold Awards for Teaching Innovation (2023), and Best Paper Award (2025) at the International Scholar Conference. As Program Coordinator, she mentors students and leads transformative initiatives. Actively engaged in professional networks, she is also a frequent guest speaker for community outreach program, promoting educational sustainability and learner engagement.

Abinash Sahoo is a dedicated and enthusiastic Bachelor of Physiotherapy (BPT) student at Centurion University of Technology and Management (CUTM), Odisha, With a strong academic foundation in physical rehabilitation sciences, he is passionate about advancing knowledge in physiotherapy and community health. Beyond academics, he is actively engaged as a social worker, demonstrating a deep sense of responsibility and commitment towards improving community well-being. His areas of interest include physical rehabilitation, workplace wellness, preventive health, and community-based physiotherapy initiatives.

Jona Kristen M. Valdez is a Licensed Guidance Counselor who currently serves as the Supervising Education Program Specialist for the Good Manners and Right Conduct and Values Education (GMRC and VE) program, the Homeroom Guidance Program (HG), and the Career Guidance Program (CGP) of the Department of Education- Central Office. Her expertise encompasses curriculum and policy development, program management, research and training. She has conducted workshops and served as a resource person for various initiatives, including programs implemented by other government agencies and organizations. She earned her Bachelor's Degree in Psychology from Miriam College and completed her Master of Education with a major in Guidance and Counseling at Roosevelt College (now FEU Roosevelt). Currently, she is pursuing her PhD in Educational Philosophy and History at the University of the Philippines-Diliman.

Index

A

B

C

D

E

F

G

I

J

K

T

W

Y